Attention Deficit Disorder

Yale University Press Health & Wellness

A Yale University Press Health & Wellness book is an authoritative, accessible source of information on a health-related topic. It may provide guidance to help you lead a healthy life, examine your treatment options for a specific condition or disease, situate a healthcare issue in the context of your life as a whole, or address questions or concerns that linger after visits to your healthcare provider.

Thomas E. Brown, Ph.D., *Attention Deficit Disorder: The Unfocused Mind in Children and Adults*

Ruth Grobstein, M.D., Ph.D., *The Breast Cancer Book: What You Need to Know to Make Informed Decisions*

James Hicks, M.D., *Fifty Signs of Mental Illness: A Guide to Understanding Mental Health*

Mary Jane Minkin, M.D., and Carol V. Wright, Ph.D., *A Woman's Guide to Menopause and Perimenopause*

Mary Jane Minkin, M.D., and Carol V. Wright, Ph.D., *A Woman's Guide to Sexual Health*

Catherine M. Poole, with DuPont Guerry IV, M.D., *Melanoma: Prevention, Detection, and Treatment*, 2d ed.

Attention Deficit Disorder

The Unfocused Mind in Children and Adults

Thomas E. Brown, Ph.D.

Yale University Press New Haven & London

Designed by Rebecca Gibb. Set in Scala type by Integrated Publishing Solutions. Printed in the United States of America.

Library of Congress Cataloging-in-Publication Data
Brown, Thomas E., Ph. D.
Attention deficit disorder : the unfocused mind in children and adults / Thomas E. Brown
p.   cm. — (Yale University Press health & wellness)
Includes bibliographical references and index.
ISBN 0-300-10641-6 (alk. paper)
1. Attention-deficit hyperactivity disorder. 2. Attention-deficit disorder in adults.
I. Title. II. Series.
RJ506.H9B765 2005
616.85'89—dc22
2005040895

A catalogue record for this book is available from the British Library. The paper in this book meets the guidelines for permanence and durability of the Committee on Production Guidelines for Book Longevity of the Council on Library Resources.

10 9 8 7 6 5 4 3 2

To my wife, Bobbie, with continuing love and gratitude for all you are, all you give, and all we share together

As physicians strive to gather more data, to see more, to be more objective, to be more scientific, they are often experienced by their patients as not listening. . . . Listening is central to learning about and coming to understand a sufferer. . . . The healer learns about the sufferer in direct proportion to the quantity and quality of his listening.

—Stanley W. Jackson, M.D., "The Listening Healer in the History of Psychological Healing" (1992)

The untangling of the complexity has barely begun. . . . But even at its early stages, the whole business of the matter of the mind requires a global view if we are to get anywhere.

—Gerald M. Edelman, M.D., Ph.D., *Bright Air, Brilliant Fire: On the Matter of the Mind* (1992)

Contents

Preface

Over the past decade hundreds of thousands of children, adolescents, and adults have been diagnosed and treated for attention deficit disorder (ADD) or attention-deficit hyperactivity disorder (ADHD). Advocacy groups for individuals and families affected with ADD/ADHD are burgeoning not only in the United States and Canada, but also in the United Kingdom, Germany, Australia, Mexico, Norway, Spain, Japan, and many other diverse cultures around the world.

Despite this popular groundswell and a tremendous amount of scientific evidence supporting the validity of the ADHD diagnosis and the safety and effectiveness of available treatments, a large segment of those in the popular media and many individuals remain skeptical; they consider ADD a trivial problem that is often overdiagnosed and overtreated. Most of this skepticism is based on simple ignorance about the complex nature of the disorder, its often devastating effects on individuals and families, and the safe, effective benefits obtained by the vast majority of those who receive appropriate treatment.

Over the past twenty years I have assessed and helped to provide treatment for thousands of children, adolescents, and adults who suffer from attention deficit disorders. I have studied and participated in relevant scientific research. I have traveled throughout the United States and in twenty-five other countries to consult with professionals and laypersons about ADHD and to offer lectures and professional education workshops. These experiences have convinced me that there is a continuing and widespread need for a clear, scientifically based explanation of what ADD/ADHD is, what it isn't, and how it can effectively be recognized and treated.

Thirty-six years ago, when I began studying psychology at Yale, we did not have the powerful imaging tools that now make it possible to look within the living human brain and observe moment to moment changes in its neural networks. We were, however, taught another way to learn about problems of brain function: to listen carefully to the way patients describe their experiences.

I have written *Attention Deficit Disorder* to describe what I've learned from conversations with thousands of children, adolescents, and adults who have ADHD. I hope it will be of interest to a wide range of readers in the general public: those who encounter these problems in themselves, family, or friends, and those who simply want to gain a fresh perspective on the fascinating complexity of the human brain. I hope it will also be useful for psychologists, educators, psychiatrists, pediatricians, family practice physicians, internists, social workers, human resource managers, counselors, and other professionals who want to better provide understanding and appropriate support to individuals who suffer from the difficulties described here.

The path to writing this book began one day as I listened to a very bright high school student describe frustrations that interfered daily with his schoolwork. He complained that he could read fluently, but moments later could not recall what he had just read. He said that his mind repeatedly took long excursions in almost every class. Often he was unable to stay focused enough to catch more than snippets of the lecture or class discussion. He explained that despite good intentions to prepare homework and write papers, he ended up procrastinating on assignments and got the inevitable poor results. Something about his description of these persistent struggles made them sound more like problems of "can't" than problems of "won't."

The boy's descriptions led me to suspect he had an attention deficit disorder that had remained undiagnosed because he was bright and not hyperactive or disruptive. A trial of stimulant medication brought sudden and dramatic improvements in virtually all of his attentional impairments.

That experience ignited my curiosity. How could someone with so much ability, such an intense desire for success, be chronically impaired in so many ways and then overcome these difficulties almost overnight using just a few small daily doses of a short-acting medication?

The following pages are filled with many real-life examples obtained from children, adolescents, and adults suffering from ADHD. These are intertwined with explanations of current research in neuroscience, psychology, and psychiatry that I find helpful in understanding the complex problems of how this disorder can be recognized and effectively treated.

The first chapter poses the perplexing question of ADHD: How can apparently normal persons have chronic difficulty "maintaining focus" for tasks they see as important, while they are able to pay attention very well to less important tasks that interest them? Is this just a simple problem of "willpower?" I argue that, despite appearances, the core problem in ADHD is not lack of willpower, but chronic, often lifelong impairment of the "executive" or management functions of the brain.

In Chapter 2 I use everyday examples to describe six clusters of cognitive problems reported by most persons with ADD. Some of these symptoms are included in the diagnostic criteria for ADHD in *DSM-IV,* the psychiatric diagnostic manual; some are not. These include chronic difficulties with (1) organizing, prioritizing, and getting started, (2) focusing, sustaining, and shifting attention, (3) regulating alertness, sustaining effort, and determining processing speed, (4) managing frustration and modulating emotions, (5) utilizing working memory and accessing recall, and (6) monitoring and self-regulating action. These cognitive functions interact to serve as the management system of the mind. Chronic impairments of these functions constitute what I call "ADD syndrome."

Understanding this syndrome requires at least a minimal grasp of how the brain operates. In Chapter 3 I offer basic explanations of how the brain works to manage daily life: how it uses short-term term memory to get things done; how it selects moment by moment what things are most important to pay attention to; and how it regulates itself to be alert and "open for business" when needed. The chapter includes information about how two specific chemicals manufactured in the brain regulate these functions, and what happens when those chemicals do not work adequately.

Problems of ADD syndrome are different at different ages. In Chapter 4 I describe how parents and teachers build a supportive environment, or "scaffolding," to help young children gradually develop self-management skills to behave carefully, to cooperate with others, to communicate, and to work to learn to read and write. I also explain how, despite scaffolding, these tasks are much more difficult for children with ADD syndrome.

Chapter 5 explains how that scaffolding is gradually withdrawn as teenagers are required to take more responsibility for managing their time and homework, dealing with their emerging sexuality and developing relationships, working for money and driving a car, and, eventually, leaving home to function more independently. I describe impairments of adolescents with ADD syndrome as they encounter these tasks.

Some adults have less difficulty with ADD syndrome once they get out of school. Others experience increasing difficulty as they struggle to find and hold a job, advance careers, develop relationships, manage households and finances, and negotiate partnerships and childcare. I describe the effects of ADD syndrome on these tasks in Chapter 6.

All the problems of ADD syndrome are experienced by everybody sometimes. Chapter 7 raises the question of how clinicians can differentiate the impairments of ADD syndrome from normal problems of inattention. Here, too, I challenge the validity of popular but overly simplistic efforts to evaluate the impairments of ADD.

Research has established that persons diagnosed with ADHD are as much as six times more likely than others to suffer from one or more other psychiatric or learning disorders at some time during their life. In Chapter 8 I describe a variety of disorders of learning, emotion, or behavior that often overlap with ADD syndrome. I propose that executive function impairments of ADD syndrome are an integral part of many different psychiatric and learning disorders, and I suggest some possible helpful changes to current diagnostic models.

In Chapter 9, I explain options to alleviate ADD syndrome impairments with treatment. The first step in any treatment program is to provide accurate information to the patient and family about the nature and course of ADD impairments. Since ADD syndrome is biochemically based, the most effective treatment is usually medication. Recently, new medications and new delivery systems for older medications have been developed. I outline what is now known about safety, effectiveness, side effects, and practical aspects of these medication treatments. The usefulness and limitations of behavioral treatments, accommodations, and other supports for ADD syndrome are also described. I emphasize that it is important to design for each patient a personalized treatment plan.

In Chapter 10, I provide examples of how untreated ADD syndrome tends to erode hope, and how it can cause severe suffering to individuals and families. This chapter also describes fears, prejudices, and other factors that are barriers to seeking, obtaining, and sustaining adequate treatment. I contrast strategies that offer "unrealistic hope" with interventions that nurture "realistic hope" in the daily lives of individuals and families suffering from ADD syndrome.

Many children, adolescents, and adults whom I have treated over the past twenty years have contributed to what is written here. Their names and identifying data have been removed, but I remain very grateful for their comments and stories, which have infused my understanding and these pages with essential details of real life. I also appreciate deeply the encouragement of patients, parents, and professional colleagues as I worked to write and publish these materials; their enthusiasm has sustained me during the long process of turning ideas and images into sentences and paragraphs.

For helpful comments on earlier versions of the manuscript I am indebted to Dr. Jay Giedd, Dr. Anthony Rostain, Dr. Rosemary Tannock, and Dr. Margaret Weiss. Wendy Hill is the medical illustrator who provided the excellent drawings that illustrate the text. Our son, Dave Brown, helpfully challenged my hesitations about trying to write for a wider audience and our daughter, Liza Somilleda, contributed perceptive comments on the entire manuscript. I am especially indebted to Jean Thomson Black, my editor at Yale University Press; she has played a pivotal role in helping me to target and shape this manuscript. My sincere thanks also go to Julie Carlson, manuscript editor, who kindly provided skilled guidance to improve the clarity and flow of each chapter. Most of all, I am grateful to my beloved wife, Bobbie, who has skillfully helped me to rework my excessively professorial prose into a much more readable text. To her I am grateful not only for helping me to nurture this book to completion, but also for the countless ways in which her sensitivity, wisdom, wit, and love sustain my work and my life.

Introduction

Often people think of "focus" as holding a camera still and adjusting the lens for a clear picture of an unmoving object. That is not the meaning of focus in the title of this book. Rather, focus refers here to a complex, dynamic process of selecting and engaging what is important to notice, to do, to remember, moment to moment. Much as a careful driver focuses on the task of driving a car in heavy traffic by actively looking ahead while also checking mirrors, observing road signs, braking, and so on (all while monitoring dashboard gauges, keeping in mind the speed limit and destination, and ignoring the temptation to look too long at interesting sights), a person employs this very active, rapidly shifting, repeatedly readjusted deployment of attention and memory as the "focus" needed to plan and control ongoing activity. Such focus is extremely difficult for the 7 to 10 percent of the world's population who suffer from a syndrome of cognitive impairments currently known as attention deficit disorder (ADD) or attention-deficit hyperactivity disorder (ADHD).

"Syndrome" is a term that describes a cluster of symptoms that tend to appear together. For example, nasal congestion, sore throat, headache, fatigue, and fever often appear together as a syndrome commonly referred to as a "cold." One single cause or a variety of different causes might lead to one common syndrome.

In this book, the term "ADD syndrome" is used to refer to a cluster of impairments in the management system of the mind. The *DSM-IV,* the diagnostic manual of the American Psychiatric Association, describes currently accepted diagnostic criteria for attention-deficit hyperactivity disorder (ADHD). The concept of ADD syndrome introduced in this book is not intended to be a new diagnosis, replacing existing diagnostic categories. I am simply proposing a new way of looking at these impairments, of which many, but not all, are encompassed in current diagnostic criteria for ADHD. Other labels have been proposed for this cluster of impairments: "Attention Deficit Disorder," "Executive Dysfunction," "Minimal Brain Dysfunction," "Regulatory Control Disorder," and "Dysexecutive Syndrome," to name a few. The concept of ADD syndrome described here includes many impairments described by these various labels, impairments that often appear together and tend to respond to similar treatments.

Compared to others of the same age and developmental level, persons with ADD syndrome tend often to have an "unfocused mind" not only for driving, but also for many other important tasks of daily life. This does not mean that persons with ADD syndrome are never able to focus adequately. Nor does it mean that those without ADD syndrome are always well focused. ADD syndrome is not like pregnancy, an all-or-nothing status with no in-between. It is more like depression. Every person feels sad sometimes, but a person is not diagnosed and treated for depression simply because he feels unhappy for a few days or even a few weeks. It is only when depressive symptoms are persistent and significantly impairing that the diagnosis of depression is appropriately made. Similarly, persons with ADD syndrome are not constantly unfocused, but they are much more persistently and pervasively impaired in these cognitive functions than most other people.

My purpose in writing this book is to describe more adequately the complex ADD syndrome as it occurs in children, adolescents, and adults. My understanding of ADD syndrome is not universally accepted. Some researchers prefer less cognitive, more behavioral models to describe this disorder. In these pages the reader will find a new, somewhat controversial understanding of ADD syndrome, including how it can be recognized and how it can be treated effectively.

Sometimes an effective treatment for a disorder is discovered by accident, before there is a full understanding of what is being treated or why the treatment works. An effective treatment for ADD syndrome was accidentally discovered in 1937 by Charles Bradley, a Rhode Island physician who was seeking a medication to alleviate severe post-spinal-tap headaches in behavior-disordered children he was studying. The amphetamine compound he tried was not helpful for the headaches, but teachers reported dramatic, though short-lived, improvement in the children's learning, motivation, and behavior while they were on this medication. Gradually this treatment gained wider use for hyperactive children with disruptive behavior problems.

Our understanding of what would later be called ADD syndrome expanded significantly during the 1970s when researchers noticed that hyperactive children tend also to have chronic problems with inattention that, like problems with hyperactivity, improve in response to stimulant treatment. In 1980 the American Psychiatric Association first used the term "attention deficit disorder" as an official diagnosis. At that time they recognized chronic impairment of attention, with or without hyperactive behavior problems, as a psychiatric disorder. The 1980 version of the diagnostic manual also noted that although this disorder usually originates during childhood, impairments to attention sometimes persist into adulthood. A 1987 revision of the manual changed the name of this condition to Attention-Deficit/Hyperactivity Disorder; since that time the official name has continued to bind inattention to hyperactive behavior problems, largely neglecting the independent importance of the syndrome's cognitive impairments.

Over the past decade, specific medicines have proven safe and very useful to many children, adolescents, and adults throughout the world who suffer from ADD syndrome. Yet very little has been published to explain in understandable terms the complex nature of attention and the wide variety of these chronic cognitive problems associated with ADHD.

In this book, I emphasize the crippling effects of chronic inattention problems on development and functioning throughout the lifespan. I also suggest that the current diagnosis of ADHD encompasses only part of a much wider range of cognitive impairments that are often responsive to medication treatment. And I propose that a cluster of cognitive impairments associated with ADHD, here called ADD syndrome, affects not only those diagnosed with ADHD, but also many people with a wide variety of other conditions, some of whom might benefit from treatments used for ADHD.

Like most clinicians of my generation and, unfortunately, many of the current generation, I learned very little about impairments to attention during my professional training. We were taught to recognize little children, mostly boys, who were extremely hyperactive and often responded to treatment with stimulant medications. And we were told that these hyperactive children often had difficulty paying attention to their teachers and parents. But our education about attention problems generally stopped there.

In the ensuing thirty years of clinical work, I have learned much more about the complex nature of attention. The impetus for most of this learning came from my patients: children, adolescents, and adults struggling with learning, working, social relationships, and family life. As they described to me the wide variety of their chronic problems with inattention, I began to appreciate the complexity of attention and its crucial importance in everyday life. Indeed, by describing the wide range of cognitive functions that improve when treatment is effective, these patients have helped me see the interconnectedness of the attentional networks of the mind.

Although this book is built on a clinical understanding of patients with problems of inattention, it also incorporates information from current research in psychology, psychiatry, and neuroscience. By integrating recent findings in these rapidly changing fields with the clinical study of how inattention affects patients day by day, we can better understand previously mysterious processes within the brain—and better support patients with symptoms of ADHD.

Many people of all ages continue to suffer needlessly from chronic impairments of attentional functions. I hope through this book to share my understanding, acquired over years of clinical experience and research, that many of these complex impairments are treatable. I want to challenge common misunderstandings of ADD syndrome and to advocate for those who suffer from the disorder. In addressing ADD syndrome, we have an important opportunity both to relieve widespread suffering and to learn more about the vast, fascinating complexities of the human brain's attention and management systems.

Chapter 1   Misconceptions about Focus and Willpower

MYTH: ADD is just a lack of willpower. Persons with ADD focus well on things that interest them; they could focus on any other tasks if they really wanted to.

FACT: ADD looks very much like a willpower problem, but it isn't. It's essentially a chemical problem in the management systems of the brain.

Most individuals who suffer chronically from an impaired ability to pay attention are able to focus their attention very well on activities that interest them. So why can't they pay attention during other activities that they recognize as important? To answer this riddle, we have to look more carefully at the many aspects of attention, recognizing that processes of attention in the human brain are more complex and subtle than we might have imagined. One way to understand the complexity of attention is to listen carefully to patients with ADHD as they describe their struggles with inattention. Meet a patient of mine, a teenaged hockey player whom I'll call Larry:

> Larry, a sturdy, sandy-haired high school junior, was sitting in my office with his parents as we began our first session together. While introducing the family, the parents mentioned that Larry's hockey team had just won the state championship. Proudly they told of how well he had played. As goalie he had successfully blocked thirty-four shots in the championship game and led his team to victory. Larry smiled modestly, but with obvious and well-deserved pleasure.

Then Larry's father stated their dilemma. "When he is playing hockey, Larry is amazing in how he pays attention to all the action. He knows where that puck is every second. He protects the goal and at the same time he watches what the other guys are doing and helps keep his team organized and motivated. He is always totally involved and on top of his game."

"But at school," his father continued, "it's an entirely different story. We know that Larry is very bright. His IQ test scores show he's in the superior range, in the top 3 percent. Usually he scores high on semester exams and he did very well on the PSAT, but his day-to-day work and his report card grades are always up and down, from A+ to almost failing."

"We know Larry wants to get good grades. He's always talking about how he wants to become a doctor and how he needs to get his grades up so he'll get into a good college and then medical school. But for years he has been totally inconsistent in his schoolwork. Once in a while we see him burning the midnight oil to do some reading or write a paper, but most of the time he procrastinates and avoids his schoolwork. We're constantly getting complaints from his teachers, the same frustrations every year."

"They say that once in a while Larry will make some comment in class that shows how smart he is, how well he understands whatever they are working on. Once in a while he'll write an excellent paper or do an amazing job on an assignment. But most of the time, the teachers are complaining that Larry is uninvolved and out to lunch. He's not a behavior problem, but he is gazing out the window or staring at the ceiling. They say that in class discussions he often doesn't even know what page they are on. And we're always getting reports that his homework is late or just not done."

"How can Larry be so amazingly good at paying attention to his hockey, and yet be so amazingly poor at paying attention to his schoolwork?"

Larry had been staring at the carpet as his father spoke, but then he raised his head. His eyes were moist as he quietly said to his parents, "I don't know why it keeps happening. I'm just as frustrated and even more worried about this than you are. When I saw my last report card, I went to my room and cried."

"I know what I have to do and I really want to do it because I know how important it is for all the rest of my life. I try to get into it like I'm into hockey. Sometimes I can get into it for a while, for this assignment or that class. But mostly I just can't make it happen."

"I really want to, and I know I should be able to do it; I just can't. I just can't make myself pay steady attention to my work for school anywhere near the way I pay attention when I'm playing hockey."

A very similar dilemma was experienced by Monica, a shy girl in fifth grade who hung her head as her mother angrily described to me her problems in school.

Her teachers say she can't pay attention for more than three minutes at a time. I know that's not true! I've watched her play Nintendo. She can play those video games for three hours at a time without moving. And the teacher says she's "easily distracted." That's nonsense! When she's playing those video games she's locked onto that screen like a laser. When she's into those games the only way you can get her attention is to jump in her face or just turn off the TV.

I've done everything I can think of to get her to shape up in school. I've gotten daily reports from school and praised her when she did well. I've tried to bribe her with rewards for good work. I've tried punishing her, taking away her Nintendo or making her do long time-outs in her room. None of it works. I know she can pay attention when she really wants to. I don't know what else I can do. She's not a dumb kid and she's not a bad kid, but if she doesn't start paying attention to her schoolwork pretty soon, she's never going to do any better in school than I did. I never finished high school and I really regret it. I want something better for her. If only I could get her to pay attention to her schoolwork the way she pays attention to those video games.

Everyone I've ever evaluated for chronic problems with inattention has some domains of activity where they can pay attention without any difficulty. Some are artistic; they intently sketch and draw. Others are childhood engineers constructing marvels with Lego blocks and, in later years, repairing car engines or designing computer networks. Some others are musicians who push themselves for hours to learn chords for a new song or to compose a new piece of music.

Attention and "Willpower"

The examples of Larry and Monica bring us back to the central riddle of chronic inattention: How can someone who is very good at paying attention for some activities be unable to pay enough attention to other tasks that they know are important and really want to accomplish? When I have asked this question of patients with ADHD, most answer with something like: "It's easy! If it's something I'm really interested in, I can pay attention. If it's not interesting to me, I can't pay attention, regardless of how much I might want to."

Most people respond to this answer with skepticism. "That's true for anyone," they say. "Anybody's going to pay attention better for something they're interested in than for something they're not."

But for some individuals there is an important difference. When faced with something boring that they know they have to do, that's important to them, most people can make themselves focus on the task at hand. Yet some lack this ability unless the consequences of not paying attention are very immediate and severe. One middle-aged businessman, Henry, whom I had diagnosed with attention deficit disorder, once reported:

> I've got a sexual example for what it is like to have ADD. It's like having impotence of the mind. If the task you are trying to do is something that turns you on, you're "up" for it and you can per-

form. But if the task you are trying to do is not intrinsically interesting, if it doesn't turn you on, then you can't "get it up." You can't make it happen. It's just not a willpower kind of thing.

Facets of Attention

What do we mean by "paying attention"? Over one hundred years ago, William James wrote:

> Everyone knows what attention is. It is the taking of possession by the mind, in clear and vivid form, of one out of what seem several possible objects or trains of thought. Focalization, concentration of consciousness [is] its essence. It implies withdrawal from some things in order to deal effectively with others, and it is a condition which has a real opposite in the confused, dazed, scatter-brained state which . . . is called distraction. (1890, vol. 1, pp. 403–404)

James held what I call "the spotlight theory" of attention: the notion that attention is a solitary, powerful beam focused by the mind on some "objects or trains of thought" (in James's words) selected from the many other perceptions and ideas that might otherwise be attended to in that same moment.

This "spotlight theory" is too simple. It describes only certain types of attention—visual attention, for example, in which one looks steadily at one point rather than flitting around aimlessly to see many different points, or simple auditory attention, in which one listens to one sound, or a series of sounds, while ignoring others. But when we look carefully at the descriptions of Larry and Monica, for example, we notice that they do many things at once. They are not only watching and listening to what is happening on the screen or on the ice, but also engaging in complex actions that may occur simultaneously or in rapid-fire sequence. As Monica plays her video games, she is not simply staring at the TV, but also actively monitoring rapid movements of many objects on the screen, deciding which ones might enrich or destroy her icon. She responds quickly by pressing control buttons and guiding her icon with adept movements of the controls. Monica keeps track of her score and her levels in the game, all while recalling and engaging strategies useful in earlier games. She also contains her alternating feelings of frustration and triumph so that she can attend to the game without overreacting to its ever-changing ups and downs.

Likewise, Larry's success on the hockey rink depends on multifaceted and simultaneously implemented aspects of attention. He not only tracks the puck in its quick movements around the ice, but also monitors his teammates and opposing players, trying to anticipate moves and to alert his defensemen to dangers and opportunities. Simultaneously, he keeps track of the passage of time—how many minutes or seconds are left in the period, or how soon a player will be released from the penalty box.

Larry also notices subtle cues of flagging effort in his teammates and calls out to encourage and challenge them. He stops himself from thinking too much about a goal he just blocked or one that just got by him into the net. He keeps in mind and tries to follow tips given by his coach in practice last week or during the momentary time out. And he tries to ignore provocative actions and comments from opposing players or spectators. All this and much more is included in Larry's paying attention while he is playing hockey.

Larry's father suggested even broader meanings of attention when he spoke of how Larry exercised year round in the gym to stay in shape for hockey and how he pushed himself hard to build strength, endurance, and skills during team practices. He elaborated on how Larry planned his daily schedule to be on time to every practice. And he told of how carefully Larry managed his equipment, keeping his skates sharp and his pads and uniform in good repair. He related how this boy attended special training clinics and studied plays of college and professional goalies so he could use their strategies to improve his moves on the ice. From this description it was clear that Larry gave intense and continuing attention to hockey in a wide variety of complex ways.

The Many Components of Inattention

If "attention" is more than just a simple "beam of focus," we can reason that "inattention" is multifaceted as well. When teachers and parents complained about Larry and Monica's poor attention to their schoolwork, they were not using a simple "focus the spotlight" concept of attention— that is, they were not complaining simply about these students not listening to the class discussion or not watching what was being written on the blackboard. They were talking about a much broader, more complex range of attentional functions.

Larry's problems with lack of attention to schoolwork included a chronic failure to engage himself with the various tasks of school. He reported not only excessive distractibility, but also chronic difficulty in getting started on assigned work; he would intend to do it, but procrastinate until it was too late. He told of poor planning, losing track of what readings were assigned or what math problems were to be done. This boy who was so careful with his skates and hockey equipment often lost his textbooks and couldn't find the notes he needed to do his homework. He told of how he often would start an assignment and then lose interest in it, setting aside the task to do something else and frequently not returning to it.

Larry also complained about his memory for schoolwork. Although he had become a virtual encyclopedia of statistics and other detailed information about many hockey players, he reported chronic forgetfulness about directions given by the teacher or the content of readings he had done for class. Often he was unable to recall for an exam information he had studied carefully and seemed to have mastered just the day before.

Larry said he often felt drowsy in class and while he was trying to read texts assigned for homework. He described how he had to struggle to stay awake in those situations, even when he had slept well the night before and was not overtired. This sluggishness was in sharp contrast to the heightened alertness he felt anytime he was thinking about or engaged in tasks related to hockey.

Inattention as a Disorder

When we look carefully at the details of Larry's chronic academic difficulties, it is clear that this boy's inattention is broad-based and complex. It includes problems of excessive distractibility, procrastination, difficulties in organizing his work, avoidance of tasks requiring sustained mental effort, insufficient attention to details, losing track of belongings, failure to finish assigned tasks, and excessive forgetfulness in daily activities.

What do all of these problems have in common? They are all impairments in facets of "attention"—impairments that are elements of what I describe in Chapter 2 as "ADD syndrome." And all of these chronic difficulties are listed among the inattention symptoms of the disorder ADHD in *DSM-IV,* the fourth edition of the diagnostic manual published by the American Psychiatric Association (2001). "Inattention" as it is described in *DSM-IV* is a broad term. Under its umbrella are a wide variety of cognitive impairments recognized as chronic, but not necessarily constant. The diagnostic manual notes: "Signs of the disorder may be minimal or absent when the person is under very strict control, is in a novel setting, is engaged in especially interesting activities, is in a one-to-one situation . . . or while the person experiences frequent rewards for appropriate behavior" (p. 79).

Everyone experiences difficulty in exercising these various aspects of attention from time to time. But those who legitimately are diagnosed as having ADHD by *DSM-IV* criteria are persons who manifest ADHD symptoms "to a degree that is maladaptive and inconsistent with developmental level" (p. 83). In other words, they must have these symptoms to a degree that makes consistent trouble for them in ways that most persons of the same age and developmental level do not often experience. Moreover, the ADHD symptoms must produce "clear evidence of clinically significant impairment in social, academic or occupational functioning" (p. 84). That is, the ADHD must disrupt significantly the individual's schoolwork, employment, and/or relationships with other people.

ADHD is not like pregnancy, where one either does or does not have the characteristics, where there is no "almost" or "a little bit." ADHD is more like depression, which occurs along a continuum of severity. Everyone occasionally has symptoms of a depressed mood. But being unhappy for a few days does not qualify one for the diagnosis of depression. It is only when symptoms of depression significantly interfere with an individual's activities over a longer time that he or she is eligible for such a diagnosis.

Moreover, for inattention impairments to be considered a disorder, they not only have to be chronic and impairing, but also have to be present in a cluster. These multiple aspects of inattention constitute a *syndrome,* a grouping of symptoms that often occur together and characterize a specific disorder. Put another way, the impairments described in the examples of Larry and Monica are like a string of Christmas tree lights, each of which may appear separate when viewed from a distance, but are actually linked. And as with Christmas tree lights—certainly the older, less reliable versions—when one flickers or fails, the others usually do the same.

This example of Christmas tree lights is not perfect. Cognitive functions of attention are not wired in series like the old light strings. And they are not simple or discrete as are the separate bulbs. Each attentional function I've described is, in fact, itself a cluster of complex functions. Yet despite the limitations of this metaphor, chronic symptoms of inattention do appear as a syndrome and patients can be successfully diagnosed on the basis of these symptoms. In fact, individuals diagnosed with ADHD, by definition, have chronic impairments in not just a few, but in at least six of the nine inattention symptoms listed in *DSM-IV* and often some of the hyperactive-impulsive symptoms as well. I discuss components of the ADD syndrome in more detail in Chapter 2.

ADD Syndrome and Impaired Executive Functions

For decades the syndrome now known as ADHD was seen simply as a childhood behavior disorder characterized by chronic restlessness, excessive impulsivity, and an inability to sit still. Late in the 1970s it was recognized that these hyperactive children also had significant and chronic problems paying attention to tasks or listening to their teachers. This discovery paved the way for changing the name of the disorder in 1980 from "hyperkinetic disorder" to "attention deficit disorder" and to recognizing that some children suffer from chronic problems of inattention without any significant hyperactivity. That change from an exclusive focus on hyperactivity and impulsive behavior to a primary focus on inattention as the principal problem of the disorder was the first major paradigm shift in understanding this syndrome.

In recent years another major shift in understanding ADHD has been developing. Increasingly researchers are recognizing that the syndrome of ADHD symptoms overlaps with impairments in what neuropsychologists call "executive functions." F. Xavier Castellanos (1999) pointed this out:

> ADHD is not merely a deficit of attention, an excess of locomo-
> tor activity or their simple conjunction. . . . The unifying abstrac-
> tion that best encompasses the faculties principally affected in
> ADHD has been termed executive function (EF), which is an
> evolving concept . . . there is now impressive empirical support
> for its importance in ADHD. (p. 179)

The concept of executive functions refers not to corporate activities of business executives, but to facets of the cognitive management functions of the brain. Although there is not yet an established consensus definition of executive functions, most researchers agree that the term should be used to refer to brain circuits that prioritize, integrate, and regulate other cognitive functions. Executive functions, then, manage the brain's cognitive functions; they provide the mechanism for "self-regulation" (Vohs and Baumeister 2004).

A Metaphor for Executive Functions

Imagine a symphony orchestra in which each musician plays his or her instrument very well. If there is no conductor to organize the orchestra and start the players together, to signal the introduction of the woodwinds or the fading out of the strings, or to convey an overall interpretation of the music to all players, the orchestra will not produce good music.

Symptoms of ADD can be compared to impairments not in the individual musicians, but in the orchestra's conductor. As is clear in the cases of Larry and Monica, persons diagnosed with ADD usually are able to pay attention, to start and stop their actions, to keep up their alertness and effort, and to utilize their short-term memory effectively when engaged in certain favorite activities. This successful functioning of persons with ADD in preferred activities indicates that these people are not totally unable to exercise attention, alertness, or effort. They can play their instruments very well—sometimes. The problem of persons with ADD lies in their chronic inability to activate and manage these functions in the right way at the right time. Impairment lies not at the level of the individual musicians (those functions work perfectly well under certain circumstances), but at the level of the conductor, who has to start and guide all of the individual players.

This notion that the core attentional problems in ADD are impairments of executive functions is quite different from William James's "spotlight" concept of attention. The new paradigm describes the complex and rapidly shifting integration of multiple aspects of attention to achieve multiple tasks. Yet this notion does resonate with James's description of attention as "withdrawal from some things in order to deal effectively with others." The concept of executive functions is a way of describing how the brain's various cognitive functions are managed—by being continually shifted and reconfigured—to "deal effectively" with the moment-by-moment demands of life.

One way to consider this broader view of attention as executive functions is to observe situations where tasks are not dealt with effectively. Martha Bridge Denckla (1996) has written about patients with high intelligence and no specific learning disabilities who have chronic difficulties in dealing effectively with tasks. She compares these persons to a disorganized cook trying to get a meal on the table.

> Imagine a cook who sets out to cook a certain dish, who has a well-equipped kitchen, including shelves stocked with all the necessary ingredients, and who can even read the recipe in the cookbook. Now imagine, however, that this individual does not take from the shelves all the ingredients relevant to the recipe, does not turn on the oven in a timely fashion so as to have it at the proper heat when called for in the recipe, and has not defrosted the central ingredient. This individual can be observed dashing to the shelves, searching for the spice next mentioned in the recipe, hurrying to defrost the meat and heat the oven out of sequence. Despite possession of all equipment, ingredients

and recipe, this motivated but disheveled cook is unlikely to get dinner on the table at the appointed hour. (p. 264)

The "motivated but disheveled cook" sounds very much like a person with severe ADD who tries to accomplish a task, but is unable to "get it together." Individuals with ADD often describe themselves as intensely wanting to accomplish various duties for which they are unable to activate, deploy, and sustain the needed executive functions.

Executive Functions and Intelligence

Denckla introduced her tale of the disorganized cook as an example of impairment seen in some patients who have "excellent intelligence" (p. 264). This comment is important because it indicates that such disorganization can be independent of general intelligence. It is quite possible for an individual to be extremely bright on standard measures of intelligence and still have severe impairments of executive functions such as those often seen in ADD.

I have evaluated persons with a wide range of intellectual abilities. Some of my patients diagnosed with ADD are extremely bright, employed as university professors, research scientists, physicians, attorneys, and senior executives in business. The intellectual abilities of others are distributed across the high-average, average, and low-average ranges of IQ. An individual's overall level of "smarts" as measured by standard IQ tests appears to have very little to do with whether they meet the diagnostic criteria for ADD.

Executive Functions and Awareness

A forty-three-year-old man came to my office with his wife to be evaluated for attentional problems. Both of the couple's children had recently been diagnosed with ADD and had benefited from treatment. When I explained that most children diagnosed with ADD have a parent or other close relative with ADD, both parents laughingly announced, "Those apples haven't fallen far from the tree." All agreed that the father had more ADD symptoms than either of the children. Here's how the wife described her husband:

Most of the time he's totally spaced out. Last Saturday he set out to fix a screen upstairs. He went to the basement to get some nails. Downstairs he saw that the workbench was a mess so he started organizing the workbench. Then he decided he needed some pegboard to hang up the tools. So he jumped into the car and went to buy the pegboard. At the lumberyard he saw a sale on spray paint, so he bought a can to paint the porch railing and came home totally unaware that he hadn't gotten the pegboard, that he had never finished sorting out the workbench, and that he had started out to fix the broken screen that we really needed fixed. What he needs is a lot more awareness of what he is doing. Maybe that medicine our kids are taking can give him that.

From this wife's description one might conclude that the central problem of ADD is essentially a lack of sufficient self-awareness. She seems to believe that if only her husband were more steadily aware of what he is doing, he would not be so disorganized, jumping from one task to another without completing any single one. But most people do not require constant self-awareness to complete routine tasks. For most people, most of the time, operations of executive functions occur automatically, outside the realm of conscious awareness. For example, while driving a car to the local supermarket, experienced drivers do not usually talk themselves through each step of the process. They do not have to say to themselves: "Now I put the key in the ignition, now I put my foot on the brake, now I turn on the engine, now I check my mirrors and prepare to back out of my driveway," and so on. Most experienced drivers move effortlessly through the steps involved in starting the car, negotiating traffic, navigating the route, observing traffic regulations, finding a parking place, and parking the car. In fact, while they do these complex tasks they may be tuning their radio, listening to the news, thinking about what they intend to fix for supper, and carrying on a conversation with a passenger. Effective execution of multiple and concurrent tasks involved in driving to the supermarket requires extensive use of executive functions, most of which operate without any conscious effort. Many other routine tasks of daily life—for example, preparing a meal, shopping for groceries, doing homework, or participating in a meeting—involve similar self-management in order to plan, sequence, monitor, and execute the complex sequences of behavior required. Yet for most actions, most of the time, this self-management operates without full awareness or deliberate choice. The problem of the "unaware" husband is not that he fails to think enough about what he is doing. The problem is that the cognitive mechanisms that should help him stay on task, without constantly and consciously weighing alternatives, are not working effectively.

Gerald Edelman and Giulio Tononi (2000) have described how much of our cognitive life

> is the product of highly automated routines. When it comes to talking, listening, reading, writing or remembering, we are all like accomplished pianists. When we read, all kinds of neural processes are going on that allow us to recognize letters irrespective of the font and size, to parse them into words, to enable lexical access and to take care of syntactic structure. There was certainly a time in which we had consciously to learn about letters and words in a laborious way, but afterward these processes become effortless and automatic. . . .
>
> This pervasive automatization in our adult lives suggests that conscious control is exerted only at critical junctures, when a definite choice or a plan has to be made. In between, unconscious routines are continuously triggered and executed so that consciousness can float free of all these details and proceed to plan and make sense of the grand scheme of things . . . only the last levels of control or of analysis are available to consciousness, while everything else proceeds automatically. (pp. 57–58)

Even the simpler example of keyboarding on a computer illustrates the point. If one can type fluently without stopping to consciously select and press each individual key, one's mind is left free to formulate ideas and to convert these into words, sentences, and paragraphs that can convey ideas to a reader. Interrupting one's writing to focus on and press keys one at a time costs too much time and effort; it cannot be done very often if one is to write productively. Grainne Fitzsimons and John Bargh (Fitzsimmons and Bargh 2004, Bargh 2005) have summarized research showing that progress on many complex tasks rests on one's ability to carry out most of the task using such "automatic self-regulation."

Executive Functions and the Brain's Signaling System

Recognition of the amazing fact that executive functions generally operate without conscious awareness offers an important caveat to my use of the orchestra conductor as a metaphor for executive functions. Some might take my metaphor literally and assume that there is a special consciousness in the brain that coordinates other cognitive functions. One might picture a little man, a homunculus, a central executive somewhere behind one's forehead, exercising conscious control over cognition like a miniature Wizard of Oz. Thus, if there is a problem with the orchestra's playing, one might attempt to speak to the conductor, requesting or demanding needed improvements in performance.

Indeed, this presumed "conductor" or controlling consciousness is often the target of encouragement, pleas, and demands by parents, teachers, and others as they attempt to help those who suffer from ADD. "You just need to make yourself focus and pay attention to your schoolwork the way you focus on those video games you love to play!" they say. "You've got to wake up and put the same effort and energy into your studies that you put into playing hockey!"

Those who care about persons with ADD and witness their poor performance in important tasks routinely prod them to deal with their "impotence" in the face of those tasks by insisting: "Just make yourself do it! We can all see that you have the ability. It's just a matter of realizing what is really important and exercising willpower!" Alternatively, they may impose punishments on the person with ADD or shame them for their failure to "make themselves" do consistently what they ought to do. These critics seem to assume that the person with ADD needs only to speak emphatically to the "conductor" of their own mental operations to get the desired results.

But in reality there is no conscious conductor within the human brain. Further, each individual can only use what is made available by his or her own neural networks. If the person's neural networks for executive functions are impaired, as they are in ADD, then that individual is likely to be proportionally impaired in the management of a wide range of cognitive functions regardless of how much he or she may wish otherwise.

There is now considerable evidence that persons appropriately diagnosed with ADD suffer from significant impairments in executive functions of the brain. These functions are not all localized in a single area of the brain; they are decentralized, with many supported by complex networks within the prefrontal cortex. Some essential components of executive functions are supported by the amygdala and other subcortical structures, while other executive functions depend on the reticular formation and portions of the cerebellum located in the posterior of the brain. Figure 3 in Chapter 3 shows these and other critical regions and structures of the brain.

Complex neuronal networks link the various structures in the brain that sustain executive functions. Rapid-fire messages of input and output travel these networks via low-voltage electrical impulses that can traverse the entire system in much less than a millisecond. The efficient movement of these electrical impulses along the network depends on the rapid release and reuptake of neurotransmitter chemicals, which carry each message across synapses, or the connections between neurons, much as a spark jumps the gap of a sparkplug.

To do this work, each of the 100 billion neurons in the brain depends on one of the fifty or so neurotransmitter chemicals manufactured within the brain. Without the effective release and reuptake of the needed neurotransmitter chemical, that portion of the neural network cannot effectively carry its messages. There is now considerable evidence that executive functions of the brain impaired in ADD depend primarily, though not exclusively, on two particular neurotransmitter chemicals: dopamine and norepinephrine.

The most persuasive evidence for the importance of these two transmitter chemicals in ADD impairments comes from medication treatment studies. Over two hundred well-controlled studies have demonstrated effectiveness of stimulant medications in alleviating symptoms of ADHD. Although these medications are not effective for all persons with ADHD, they work effectively to alleviate ADHD symptoms for 70 to 80 percent of those diagnosed with this disorder. And the medications used to treat ADHD symptoms tend to alleviate many symptoms of ADHD simultaneously.

The primary action of medications used for ADD is to facilitate release and to inhibit reuptake of dopamine and norepinephrine at neural synapses of crucially important executive functions. As Antonio Damasio (1994) emphasized,

> Without basic attention and working memory there is no prospect of coherent mental activity. . . . They are necessary for the process of reasoning, during which possible outcomes are compared, ranking of results are established, and inferences are made. (p. 197)

ADD medications help to release dopamine or norepinephrine across the synaptic gap between neurons and to hold it there long enough to pass the message along. Medications that do not act powerfully to facilitate release and to block reuptake of dopamine and norepinephrine tend not to be effective in alleviating ADD symptoms.

Improvement produced by stimulants generally can be seen within thirty to sixty minutes after an effective dose is administered. When the medication has worn off, ADD symptoms generally reappear at their former level. Stimulants thus do not cure ADD symptoms; they only alleviate them while each dose of medication is active. In this sense, taking stimulants is not like taking doses of an antibiotic to wipe out an infection; it is more like wearing eyeglasses that correct one's vision while the glasses are being worn, but do nothing to fix one's impaired eyes. This effect has been demonstrated repeatedly in over two hundred medication treatment studies that were double-blind: that is, neither the doctors nor the patients knew during the study who was being given real stimulant medication and who was being treated with placebos.

Given the often dramatic alleviation of ADD symptoms experienced by 70 to 80 percent of persons diagnosed with ADHD when they take stimulant medications, it is very difficult to sustain the notion that ADHD impairments are a matter of a lack of willpower. Prior to beginning medication treatment most ADHD patients have made heroic, though often erratic, efforts to improve their situation with willpower alone. Usually such efforts barely work, if at all, and cannot be sustained.

Some argue that improvement in ADD symptoms requires not only willpower, but also intensive behavioral treatments. Results of a major study sponsored by the National Institute of Mental Health (MTA, 1999) challenged this assumption. In the study, 576 children diagnosed with ADHD were randomly assigned to one of four groups, which received either:

Comprehensive behavioral treatment with no medication,

Carefully managed medication treatment with no other treatment,

A combination of comprehensive behavioral treatment with medication management, or

Community treatment with a pediatrician or another caregiver of the family's choice.

The results of this study were striking. Stimulant medication alone, carefully monitored for each child, was of significantly greater help than the best battery of behavioral supports that could be developed without medication. More surprising, children who received the combined treatment (medication and comprehensive behavioral treatment) showed no better improvement of their core ADHD symptoms than did children treated only with carefully managed medications. Combined treatments were more helpful with some related problems, but nonmedication treatments, even at their best, did not improve the core symptoms of ADHD anywhere near as much as did the carefully monitored medication treatment. This study, described with many others in Chapter 9, stands as powerful evidence that impairments of attention and memory associated with ADHD result primarily from malfunctions in parts of the brain's neural networks that depend on the chemicals dopamine and norepinephrine.

Much more remains to be learned about how the brain's complicated neural networks operate to sustain the broad range of functions encompassed in "attention." Yet it is clear that impairments of executive functions, those brain processes that organize and activate what we generally think of as attention, are not the result of insufficient willpower. So in fact there is an answer to the mystery of inattention illustrated by the experiences of Larry and Monica. Neural chemical impairments of the brain's executive functions cause some individuals who are good at paying attention to specific activities that interest them to have chronic impairment in focusing for many other tasks, despite their wish and intention to do otherwise.

Chapter 2   Six Aspects of a Complex Syndrome

MYTH: ADD is a simple problem of being hyperactive or not listening when someone is talking to you.

FACT: ADD is a complex disorder that involves impairments in focus, organization, motivation, emotional modulation, memory, and other functions of the brain's management system.

Imagine a large carton filled with photographs taken throughout your life. The carton is filled with snapshots of you and various family members roller skating or riding bikes, fishing off a pier or swimming in a lake, dressing up for Halloween or setting off for the first day of school. Some are posed with you in your Scout or Little League uniform or in costume for a dance recital. Others are candid shots taken around a birthday cake, in the midst of holiday celebrations, or at other memorable moments.

Given a box of such photos all mixed together, you might want to sort them to take a more systematic look. There are many ways you could do the sorting. You might put together all photos of a certain kind of activity, regardless of time or place: all of the holidays, vacation shots, or birthday parties. Or you might sort according to age periods, for example, all elementary school snapshots together, then all high school photos, then those taken in college, and so on. Yet whatever sorting scheme is used to organize your photographs, and regardless of how many snapshots are in each group, those photos can capture only fragmentary, fleeting glimpses of actual life experiences. Descriptions of the process of attention are like those snapshots.

Attention is an incredibly complex, multifaceted function of the mind. It plays a crucial role in what we perceive, remember, think, feel, and do. And it is not just one isolated activity of the brain. The continuous process of attention involves organizing and setting priorities, focusing and shifting focus, regulating alertness, sustaining effort, and regulating the mind's processing speed and output. It also involves managing frustration and other emotions, recalling facts, using short-term memory, and monitoring and self-regulating action.

This understanding of the wide-ranging facets of attention has emerged from my study of children, adolescents, and adults diagnosed with attention deficit disorder. Observing the problems that result when attention fails has allowed me to notice the effects of attentional processes on multiple aspects of daily life. Documenting the interconnected improvements that occur when attentional impairments are effectively treated has shown me the subtle but powerful linkages between attention and multiple aspects of the brain's management system. All of these observations have led me to conclude that attention is essentially a name for the integrated operation of the executive functions of the brain.

In this chapter I have gathered vignettes from many patients who have described problems resulting from failures of attention. These snapshots are organized under six clusters shown in Figure 1. Each cluster encompasses one important aspect of the brain's executive functions. Although each has a one-word label (for example, activation, focus, effort, and so on), these clusters are not single qualities like height, weight, or temperature. Each cluster is more like a basket encompassing related cognitive functions that depend on and interact continuously with the others, in ever-shifting ways. Together these clusters describe executive functions, the management system of the brain.

The arrangement used in this chapter is just one of many possible ways to describe executive functions and to clump symptoms of inattention reported by most persons with ADD. Until we know much more about underlying neural processes, any descriptive model is likely to be a bit arbitrary. But regardless of how the clusters are arranged, these executive functions tend to operate in an integrated way. Most persons diag-

Executive Functions Impaired in ADD Syndrome

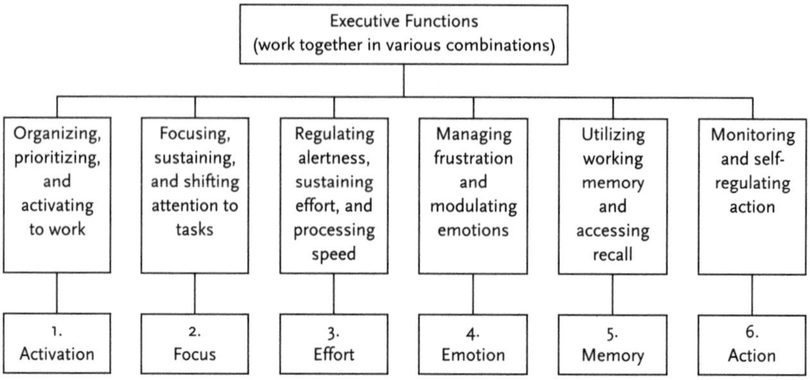

Figure 1 Executive functions impaired in ADD syndrome. *Source:* Brown 2001c.

nosed with ADHD report significant chronic difficulties in at least some aspects of each of these six clusters. Impairments in these clusters of cognitive functions tend to show up together; they appear clinically to be related.

In addition, these clusters of cognitive functions tend to improve together. When an individual with ADD is treated with appropriate medication and shows significant improvement in one of these six clusters, some significant improvement is usually seen in aspects of the other five clusters as well.

Since these clusters of symptoms often appear together in persons diagnosed with ADD and often respond together to treatment, it seems reasonable to think of these symptoms of impairment as a "syndrome." Because this syndrome consists primarily, though not exclusively, of symptoms associated with the disorder currently classified as attention-deficit hyperactivity disorder, I refer to it as "ADD syndrome." Taken together, the six clusters in this model describe my understanding of the executive functions of the brain.

Although this description of the brain's executive functions is derived primarily from studying persons with ADHD, it should be noted that these executive functions can become impaired in other ways as well. In Chapter 8 I describe how impairments of executive functions similar to ADD syndrome can result from other causes, other psychiatric disorders, and even from later stages of normal aging. In this chapter I use examples from individuals with ADHD to describe how each of the six clusters works and, for some, doesn't work.

Cluster 1: Organizing, Prioritizing, and Activating for Tasks

Although many people associate ADD with impulsive and hyperactive behavior where affected individuals are too quick to speak or act, difficulties in getting started on tasks are a primary complaint of many individuals with ADD syndrome. Though they may be impulsive in some domains of activity, those with this syndrome often complain that procrastination is a major problem, particularly when they are faced with tasks that are not intrinsically interesting. Often these individuals lament that they keep putting off important tasks until the task has become an emergency. Only when faced with dire consequences in the very immediate future are they able to get themselves motivated enough to begin. This persistent problem in getting started was described by a patient of mine, an attorney, who was quite successful in many aspects of his work, but who nevertheless sought evaluation and treatment. His chronic procrastination, together with other ADD symptoms, had put him at serious risk of getting fired.

> All my life I've had trouble getting started on my work when I have to work by myself. I don't have any trouble when I'm talking with clients or working with other lawyers or working with the secretaries. But when I'm in my office and I've got paperwork to do, I just can't get myself started. A couple of times a week I set aside several hours for paperwork that I want to get done. I need to get it done because I don't get paid until it's done. I block out several hours to do it and I'm in my office with all the materials I need in front of me. But I just can't get myself to start it. Usually I end up turning on my computer and sitting in the office doing email, checking some news sites, and playing video games. I have to shut it off every time the secretary comes in so she doesn't see what I'm doing.
>
> The end of the day comes and my work isn't even started. I go home and have a bite to eat and watch some TV. Then about

10 p.m. I suddenly remember: "Oh, my God. I've got that report to do! I have to get it in by 8 a.m. tomorrow or I'm going to be in very serious trouble at work." At that point I don't have any problem getting started. I get on my home computer and work very efficiently from 10 p.m. to 2 a.m. and produce an excellent report. But it's a hell of way to have to live.

Like this attorney, many individuals with ADD syndrome chronically delay starting tasks until they are face-to-face with the immediate pressure of a final deadline. They know the task needs to be done, but they ignore it until the last possible moment. They have a significant, chronic problem with cognitive activation.

The Neurochemistry of Motivation

This chronic problem in getting started on necessary tasks raises important questions about motivation. Many persons with ADD report that they often are aware of specific tasks they need, want, and intend to do, but are unable to get themselves to begin the necessary actions. Often these are routine tasks such as completing homework assignments, laundering clothes, or submitting invoices or expense account reports to obtain reimbursement. Or they may be important, less common tasks like completing a thesis for a degree, asking for a raise or promotion, or filing income tax returns on time.

Sometimes the potential reward or penalty is clear and immediate; sometimes the ultimate consequence is more uncertain and further down the road. In either situation many persons with ADD syndrome often feel unable to *make* themselves initiate the actions needed until they are in a "Mayday" situation.

This difficulty in activation for work tasks is often improved when the person with ADD syndrome is successfully treated with medication. One college student, for example, reported that his initial trial of stimulant medication helped him to get going on his work in ways that before treatment he had often intended to try, but only rarely attempted.

In my classes this week I took incredibly good notes, much better organized and with a lot more of the important details. It came so naturally to write it all down. Usually I say I'm going to get all that stuff down, but I never get to it. You can see the difference here in my notebook. I've got lots of pages of really good notes for every class this week. Usually I just have the date and one or two phrases with a bunch of doodles.

That medication made me feel more like doing my homework too. I just pulled out my books and started to do it. I can't say I enjoyed it, but I did feel kind of satisfied just having it done. So many times I have walked into class unprepared, without having done the assigned reading, just hoping that I wouldn't be called on.

The striking phrase in this student's comments is "made me *feel more like doing* my work." By contrast, many unmedicated patients with ADD syndrome report that they often are aware of a need to do a particular task, but "just *don't feel like doing* it." The student's report indicates that the stimulant medication changed his immediate readiness to engage in the task at hand by modifying the neural chemistry of his brain.

A further clue to the chemistry of motivation can be found in the reactions of persons with ADD syndrome who have taken an excessively high dose of stimulant medication. Under too high a dose, some patients report as one of my patients did: "It wasn't pleasant. I had this feeling that I needed to be doing something, even though there wasn't anything I needed to do. It was a kind of restless feeling. I felt like a workaholic on a forced vacation. Just couldn't relax and enjoy. I was all 'psyched up' for work even when there wasn't any work that needed to be done." Excessive doses of stimulants can transiently produce a compulsion to work. Thus disinterest and procrastination can often be alleviated with appropriate doses of stimulants, whereas excessively high doses of stimulants can produce an excessive drive to work, even when there is no work to do.

Setting and Maintaining Priorities

Persons with ADD syndrome often complain that they have much more difficulty than most others in sorting out and assigning priorities to various tasks. One woman described it this way:

My husband said I couldn't organize a two-car funeral. It made me mad, but I guess he's right. When I have a bunch of things to do, they all seem equally important. Like when I'm cleaning the house. I try to straighten up the living room a little and I pick up yesterday's newspaper and then I start reading it. Then I go upstairs to get the vacuum cleaner and when I'm up there I see an envelope of photos I got developed last week. I sit down to put them in the album and then I get involved in looking at the other pictures in the album.

It happens even with paying the bills. Often I just dump all the day's mail in a big basket and don't even sort it out. Last month our mortgage bank and our electric company both phoned us because I hadn't paid them. We had the money, but for two months in a row I had left our mortgage statement and our electric bill in a pile of junk mail. I just don't seem to be able to say to myself, "OK, I've got all these things to take care of, this should be first and then this and then this. I'm not good at figuring out how to use whatever time or energy I have to take care of what I've got to do.

Her description highlights several components in what might otherwise be assumed to be a single function. She describes a problem in scanning a range of tasks and discriminating among them; in assigning different weights of priority to various tasks confronting her. What needs to be done first, second, and third? This person has problems relating parts to a whole. She seems to see "cleaning the house" as a collection of discrete tasks, almost like separate trees, without much awareness of how these trees are all aspects of one forest.

Many routines of our daily life involve organizing, prioritizing, and sequencing jobs according to their importance, their urgency, and the availability of resources. Usually, but not always, critical variables include time or money, which cause very practical constraints to quickly come into play. Most people cannot afford to buy everything they want, and all of us have fewer than twenty-four waking hours in a day to spend doing what we want or need to do. Estimates have to be made, priorities have to be assigned, and expenditures have to be sequenced and allocated. If not, or if these decisions are not realistic, one is likely to be "a day late" and/or "a dollar short," with potentially escalating consequences.

Of course we all differ in how reflective we are about organizing and sequencing our priorities. Some of us work with scrupulous attention to budgets that guide every purchase and use Palm Pilot schedules to control virtually every minute of our day. Others of us are more casual about how we spend our time and money. Persons with ADD syndrome, regardless of how much they "try" on such matters, report chronic difficulties in organizing themselves from moment to moment and from day to day. They complain that they often have trouble completing tasks for deadlines, getting to appointments on time, or keeping their checking account balanced.

When they describe specifics of their difficulties with organizing themselves, persons with ADD syndrome often indicate a recurrent failure to notice critical details. A salesman with ADD syndrome whom I evaluated realized one day as we were talking that his chronic tardiness for appointments resulted from his never factoring realistic travel time into his schedule. He would set up an appointment on the East Side of Manhattan to begin thirty minutes after concluding another appointment on the West Side. This allowed no time for stopping in the bathroom, taking the elevator down to ground level, getting a taxi, and getting stuck in traffic. When I questioned him about his lateness, the salesman showed that he had all of the relevant information he needed to make a realistic estimate, but he repeatedly failed to use the information in his day-to-day planning.

Others with ADD syndrome report similar problems with their finances. Often these difficulties involve failures to estimate time properly or to calculate the relationship between expenditures and income. The "disorganized homemaker," for example, reported that she simply let her bills pile up with junk mail over a period of a couple of months, forgetting to pay mortgage and electric bills until receiving reminder calls. She knew that those bills were important and needed to be paid promptly, but when they arrived it seemed to her a long time before the payment would be overdue. With little sense of how soon the future would become the present, she made no effort to store the bills where she would easily remember to pay them at the appropriate time.

Many people with ADD syndrome have problems regarding money. They tend to make purchases—sometimes relatively small ones like a new shirt, book, or CD; other times larger ones like expensive clothing, computers, and so on—on the basis of how much money they anticipate taking in. Frequently they do not take into account how much of their incoming money is already committed to standing expenses like monthly rent or car payments. This difficulty is especially acute with "plastic money." Many are shocked to discover how much they have run up in high-interest credit card debt. They tend to think of each purchase as a discrete event without realizing how these purchases and the associated interest fees are accumulating.

A similar tendency to ignore realistic limitations is often seen in the "to do" lists kept by some persons with ADD syndrome. Though they may be very intelligent about other things, many seem clueless about how many tasks they can actually accomplish within a single day or week. Many create lists with thirty or more items for a single day, some of which are time-consuming projects that no one could actually accomplish in a month. They seem to have great difficulty figuring out how long a task will take and then prioritizing by putting some items ahead of others, deferring some to another day, or simply recognizing some as currently not possible.

Cluster 2: Focusing, Sustaining, and Shifting Attention to Tasks
One of the most common complaints of persons with ADD syndrome is that they cannot focus their attention on a task and keep focusing as long as necessary. Sometimes their problem is one of selection. They find it very hard to focus on the particular stimulus that requires attention: the voice on the telephone or the words printed on the page.

One high school student compared his problem to the difficulty of keeping the radio signal when driving too far away from the radio station.

In my classes I always get part of what's being talked about. But no matter how hard I try, I keep losing track of what's happening. Like in Geometry I'll be listening while the teacher explains how to do this problem, and then I just drift off for a little bit. I come back and try to figure out where he is on this thing now, and then pretty soon I lose it again. And then I'll get another piece of it, but usually I don't know how he got to that because I had drifted off. Same thing happens in English and in History and in everything else. I just can't keep my mind on what's happening in class for more than a few minutes. I'm always drifting in and out.

It's sort of like what happens when you're listening to your car radio and you drive too far away from the station you're listening to. You know how the voice or the music starts going in and out on you? That's the way it is for me when I'm trying to listen to somebody talk. And lots of times it happens when I'm reading or trying to work on a paper. Most of the time I just can't keep myself tuned to what I'm trying to do.

Everyone experiences from time to time this difficulty in selecting and holding focus. Over a century ago, William James (1890) described inability to focus as a state of distraction into which most people fall several times a day:

> The eyes are fixed on vacancy, the sounds of the world melt in to confused unity, the attention is dispersed . . . and the foreground of consciousness is filled, if by anything, by . . . surrender to the empty passing of time. In the dim background of our mind we know meanwhile what we ought to be doing, dressing ourselves, answering the person who has spoken to us, trying to make the next step in our reasoning. But somehow we cannot *start*. (p. 404)

James observed that this inability to focus, to pay attention to what one intends to do, is experienced by most people several times daily. But persons with ADD syndrome report that they struggle much more often than the rest of us throughout the day, and often minute by minute, to hold their focus on the task at hand.

Many persons with ADD syndrome have chronic trouble focusing their attention on reading, especially if the material is assigned rather than self-selected. A college student described his difficulty this way:

> Reading assignments always take me a long time. It's because I can never get the meaning from reading a paragraph just once. My eyes can go over every word and I feel like I understand what I have read at the moment of the reading, but then it just doesn't stick inside my head. If I have to answer any questions about what I've just read, or if I have to talk with someone about it, I always have to go back and read it again a couple of times more in order to really understand what I've read.
>
> One of my tutors said that I am a "passive reader," that I just don't get active enough in paying attention to what I am reading. It's strange, though—I don't usually have this problem when I'm reading science fiction or other things I've picked for myself. But no matter how hard I try, I just can't get hooked into what I'm reading when I have to read something that I haven't chosen.

This difference between reading something self-selected and reading assigned materials is reminiscent of the distinctions described in Chapter 1 where Larry could attend very well to playing hockey and Monica could attend intently to video games, but neither was able to mobilize similar engagement for schoolwork. People with ADD syndrome often describe themselves as unable to focus and sustain their attention unless the task is intrinsically interesting to them.

When this problem arises in reading it illustrates what the repeating reader's tutor probably meant by "passive reading." One's eyes may go over each sentence and one may have a feeling of understanding the words, but the meaning of the sentence or passage is not actually grasped. Recognition of the words is not accompanied by enough actively focused attention to capture the meaning and encode it in working memory.

People who don't suffer from ADD syndrome may experience this "passive reading" if they try to read while they are very tired. Their eyes may go over each word of the passage, but after a few pages they realize that they haven't the foggiest notion of what they have just tried to read. Although the sounds of each word may have been adequately decoded, the message of the words has not. Comprehension of the meanings of sentences and paragraphs is an active process that requires the sustained, active engagement of the reader's focused attention.

Another facet of the problem of not being able to focus on an intended task is excessive distractibility. Even when they have focused on a task, whether reading, listening, or trying to do some other work, persons with ADD syndrome often feel themselves drawn away by distractions. Like anyone else they see and hear things going on around them and they have many thoughts continually going through their head. But unlike most others, who readily block out distractions in order to do what needs to be done, persons with ADD syndrome have chronic and severe difficulty screening out those distracting stimuli. They cannot ignore the myriad thoughts, background noises, and perceptions in the surrounding environment.

> I really try to keep my mind on what my teacher is saying, but I just can't stay with it for long. All this other stuff keeps popping into my head. I'll be listening to what she says and then somebody drops a pencil and I have to stretch my neck and look over and see where it fell. Then I'll be listening to the teacher again for a couple of minutes and pretty soon I'm thinking about some TV show I saw the night before. I still hear her, but I'm not getting what she's saying.
>
> And then I'll stop myself and start listening to try to figure out what's been going on. Then in a couple of seconds I'll start wondering about what I am going to do after school today and who I could call to go out tonight. And then I'm looking at the clock and wondering how soon this class is going to be over. All this stuff is going on in my head at one time. It's like you're watching TV and you've got four different stations coming in on one channel. It's kind of hard to keep following the one you're trying to listen to.

This junior high school student quoted is typical of many individuals with ADD syndrome in his persisting difficulty with filtering out distractions. This is not simply a problem of immaturity. Children and adolescents have no monopoly on excessive distractibility, and the problem is not limited to students sitting in boring classrooms. Many adults with ADD syndrome report persistence of this problem, which can cause trouble in their jobs, driving, and social relationships.

> I don't miss much of anything, except what I'm supposed to be paying attention to. When I'm working in my cubicle, I'm always listening in on what everybody else is doing. I just can't help myself. If one of the secretaries is talking on the phone two cubicles over, I'm listening in and trying to figure out what they're talking about. Meanwhile, I'm checking out what's going on across the hall at the coffee machine and who just went into the bathroom. It's not easy when I'm trying to follow a couple of different phone conversations at the same time.
>
> Then too, I'm often "out to lunch" at meetings. If we're all sitting in the conference room reviewing some project, I'll be looking out the window watching some squirrel climb up a tree or checking out the clouds going by or the guy mowing the lawn. Or I just drift off thinking of "whatever" and then, all of a sudden, I catch myself and realize that I've spaced out and have totally lost track of the group's conversation.
>
> The scariest times with this are when I'm driving along the expressway and suddenly catch myself looking too long at a billboard while I'm coming up way too fast on a car that is slowing down in front of me because of a traffic jam that I hadn't seen coming. More than a few times I've had to hit my brakes fast and hard to prevent a collision. This "getting distracted" can get pretty dangerous.

Shifting Focus

This driver's comment about staring too long at a billboard illustrates another problem often reported by persons with ADD syndrome: difficulty in shifting focus. The same individuals who have chronic difficulty with getting distracted and drifting off task report that they sometimes have the opposite problem: they are unable to stop focusing on one thing and redirect their focus to another when they need to. Some call this "hyperfocus." They describe it as "locking on" to some task, sight, or sound they are interested in while totally ignoring or losing track of everything else, including some things they ought to attend to, like looking ahead while driving the car or answering someone who has directly spoken to them. This is what Monica's mother described in Chapter 1 as her daughter locking onto video games "like a laser" so that one can get her attention only by "getting in her face" or turning off the television. Many persons with ADD syndrome report that they get stuck in this way while using their computer.

> When I log on to the Internet, I come under a hypnotic spell. Usually it starts out with just checking my e-mail. Then I get caught up for a while reading various Listservs I subscribe to and writing responses to notes from my friends. After that I usually switch over to check on the various news sites to see what has been happening. And then I think of some other site I like that I haven't visited for a long time, so I head for that. It always seems like just a few minutes, but then I'll look over at the clock and see that I've been online for three or four hours.
>
> My wife tells me that she tries to talk to me while I'm online, but I don't even hear her. I guess I just shut the whole world out and totally immerse myself in whatever I'm doing on the computer. Even when I know I should get off to help put our kids to bed or to do some work I need for the office the next morning, I just can't pull myself away from it.
>
> Sometimes this same thing happens at work. Last week I got so involved in researching online for a project I had been assigned that I totally lost track of time and was twenty-five minutes late for a meeting with my boss. I knew I had the meeting and I had planned to be right on time because he's a stickler for promptness. He wasn't too happy when he had to send his secretary to get me for the meeting.

The problem of becoming engrossed doesn't happen only with computers. Sometimes it occurs in conversation. Friends and relatives often report that persons with ADD syndrome frequently persevere in talking about something in which they're interested when the conversation has already moved on to other topics. This problem may be especially common during arguments, when the individual with ADD syndrome is presenting a particular point of view with such intensity that he is unable to take into account other perspectives.

Some persons with ADD syndrome report similar problems in writing. While trying to compose a letter, responses to an essay exam, a report, or some other written project, they find themselves stuck on one phrase or one particular sentence, working and reworking it in an effort to make it perfect. Meanwhile, their time to complete the exam has elapsed, their interest in completing their letter has dissipated, or their deadline for completion of the project has passed.

Maintaining effective attention requires the ability to select the most important of countless external and internal stimuli—and screen out those that intrude on awareness. Yet it also requires the ability to shift one's focus of attention as needed, to attend to other words, images, sounds, feelings, topics, and matters. People with ADD syndrome often report chronic difficulty in focusing their attention, in sustaining their focus of attention, and in shifting their focus of attention as needed to meet the demands of learning, work, social interactions, and the countless tasks of daily life. As in the other clusters of symptoms described here, these difficulties occur occasionally for everyone. But for persons with ADD syndrome they seem to be more persistent, pervasive, and problematic.

Cluster 3: Regulating Alertness, Sustaining Effort, and Processing Speed

Many with ADD syndrome report that they frequently become very drowsy—to the point where they can hardly keep their eyes open—when they have to sit still and be quiet. Some describe themselves as "borderline narcoleptic." Usually this is not a problem when they are physically active or actively engaged in conversation. But it can pose serious difficulties when they are trying to listen to a lecture or proceedings of a meeting. Getting drowsy is especially problematic when they try to read, particularly if what they are reading is not especially interesting to them. Similar difficulties occur for many when they sit down to write an essay or report. Some report the same drowsiness when they are driving long distances on a highway, without the stimulation of having to negotiate heavy traffic or the possibility of observing many people. As one college student described it:

> I'm OK if I'm on my feet and moving around, or if I'm talking a lot. But if I have to sit still and be quiet, I start getting drowsy. The worst is if I have to sit through a long lecture or in a double period seminar or meeting where you can't talk or I just don't have much to say. My eyelids get so heavy. I have to struggle to keep them open. It's really embarrassing to be sitting there obviously nodding off, especially if you happen to be sitting up front where the professor is looking right at you. Now you may think this is just because I'm up partying too late the night before, but that's not it. A lot of other guys in my dorm stay up late, but I always go to bed early.
>
> Last spring at the end of the semester, I had gone to bed really early the night before so I could be alert. It was the last class of the term and the professor was going to be telling us what to study for the final exam. So I got there early and had my notebook ready and as soon as he came in and started talking I was taking really good notes. The next thing I knew the class was over and I was just waking up as everybody was picking up their stuff and walking out. I had great notes on the first eight or ten minutes of class, and then I just nodded off and fell sound asleep.

This problem of drowsiness in ADD syndrome is not simply a matter of being overtired; it can occur when the person is well rested. Often individuals with this difficulty report that they become suddenly reinvigorated when they join in conversation at the meeting or if something especially interesting arises in what they are reading. Likewise, the drowsiness disappears when the lecture or meeting ends and they get up to begin some other activity.

From these clinical descriptions, it appears that this problem of drowsiness when sitting still and being quiet is related not to being overtired, but rather to chronic difficulties in sustaining alertness. It is as though individuals with ADD syndrome cannot stay alert unless they are engaged actively in a behavior that provides steady motoric, social, or cognitive feedback. They seem to need to feel themselves in motion, hear their own voices, or be very actively engaged in internal conversation with what they are trying to read.

Though the problem of daytime drowsiness afflicts many with ADD syndrome even when they are not tired, heavy eyelids sometimes appear for a different reason. Many with ADD syndrome report that they are often tired during the day because they have chronic and severe difficulties in settling into sleep, even when they are very tired and want to fall asleep. This is the opposite pole of the same problem: difficulty in regulating alertness.

Parents often report that their children with ADHD have chronic difficulty falling asleep, even when the hour is late and the kids are obviously exhausted. Some adults with ADHD have similar problems. Here is one example:

> My mother tells me that from my first few months she always had a hard time getting me to settle down for sleep. I was never much of a nap-taker and always a night owl. She always said I didn't want to close my eyes because I was afraid I would miss out on some interesting action. I don't know what the reason is, but I do know that even today I still have a lot of trouble getting myself to fall asleep. I can be dead tired, my eyes blurry and almost ready to collapse, but then I lie down on my bed and I just can't get my head to shut off so I can get to sleep. It just keeps going over whatever I've been thinking about. Usually I have to listen to music or watch TV so I can block that other stuff out and get to sleep.
>
> Once I get to sleep, I usually sleep like a dead person. They could drop a bomb in my bedroom and I wouldn't even notice.

That was a big problem when I was in high school. I was always missing my bus and late for school. It took my parents about ten tries to get me up every day. They would make noise and pull the covers off of me and I'd just mumble or swear at them and roll over and go back to sleep. This is even when I had especially asked them to get me up on time so I wouldn't lose credit for my early classes.

It was even worse when I got to college because I couldn't wake up from any alarm clock and my roommates never wanted to take on the job of getting me out of bed. The only thing that worked was when I lived in the fraternity house and could make the pledges do it. Later, when I got married, my wife took it over.

This vignette illustrates dual aspects of the problem in regulating alertness commonly reported by persons with ADD syndrome. It is as though they get stuck in whatever level of activation they are in, unable to release themselves from full consciousness to enter sleep, or sleeping so soundly that efforts to awaken them resemble efforts to raise the dead.

In addition to chronic problems in regulating alertness and vigilance, many persons with ADD syndrome also report great difficulty in sustaining effort for work tasks. Though they may have a virtually inexhaustible reservoir of energy for tasks intrinsically interesting to them, they tend quickly to run out of steam when engaged in jobs that require sustained effort with little immediate reward. Here is one example:

If I'm doing something that I can get done quickly in one chunk, I'm usually OK. I love it when people in the office call me to troubleshoot some problem in dealing with a client or even to help them fix some glitch in their computer. If I could do that kind of quick fix stuff all the time I would be a great worker.

It's the long-term projects I have trouble with, the kind of thing where you can't get it done in one chunk in a few minutes or even in a few hours or a whole day—those projects where you have to keep chipping away at it because it just can't be done even in one day. I fade out fast on those things. I start out saying to myself, "OK, I'm really going to apply myself to this job and keep working steadily on it, one chunk a day until it's finished." But pretty soon I'm getting bored and losing interest. So I usually end up just saying to myself, "Hurry up, slap-dash. Let's just get this damn thing done without worrying about how good it is." Or sometimes I don't even get that far. I just put it off until it becomes more of an emergency. My mind is much more of a sprinter. I've never been much as a long-distance runner.

The example of this "sprinter" highlights an important question: how does a person keep going to complete a task that doesn't offer an immediate reward? Another clue to the dilemma comes from a college student:

In our psychology course we just finished studying about laboratory rats and how they keep pressing this little bar in their cage longer if they get a reward like a food pellet only once in a while. On the results chart you could see how a rat that got a food pellet for every press of the bar would quickly quit pressing the bar if you stopped giving the pellets. But those rats that got the pellets only once in a while, they kept up pressing for a long time after the pellets stopped coming. I guess they figured that if they kept up pressing a little longer, sooner or later another one of those pellets would be coming to them.

I think I'm a lot like the rat that has to be getting a pellet for every press of the bar, otherwise I just lose interest and give it up. I know I'd be a lot better off if I could keep myself going longer. I always stop reading a book if it doesn't seem interesting in the first chapter. I just can't keep myself at it for long if those pellets don't come quick and often.

Even when they do expend significant effort, many persons with ADD syndrome report that they require an extraordinarily long time to complete certain types of tasks because of a tediously slow processing speed. They often complain that it takes them a particularly long time to read and write. Sometimes slow processing time in reading results from the need to reread repeatedly. In writing, the problem of excessive slowness may be due to the getting-stuck problem (also known as "sticky perseveration"). But for many with ADD syndrome, there is a chronic problem with slow processing speed that is different from these earlier described difficulties. One high school student described it with an analogy about a computer modem.

> It takes me so long to get things written down. When I am taking notes on what the teacher is saying, I'm always trying to write down something from sentence two while everybody else in class is taking notes on sentence nine. I just can't keep up and write things down as fast as others in the class. Even if I'm just copying sentences off the chalkboard, it always takes me longer to get it copied than it does everybody else.
>
> And it's not just when I'm taking notes. When I am writing an essay or sentences to answer on a test, I never can get it out fast enough, regardless of how hard I try. My mind is fast in thinking about things and in getting ideas, but I'm so slow in getting things written down. I feel like I'm a Pentium IV computer with a really slow modem. It takes half of forever to upload or download the information I need.

Like many with ADD syndrome, this high-school student suffers from a tediously slow processing speed that restricts how much he can write at once. Mel Levine (2003) has described this output problem in written expression; he laments that many with such difficulties are seen as lazy, when they actually are impaired in their ability to coordinate and integrate the multiple skills required for writing.

Although individuals with ADHD often have a slow processing speed for certain tasks, in other situations many have trouble slowing themselves down enough to minimize errors. Boys with ADHD studied by Virginia Douglas (1999) were both too slow and too fast. Their reaction times for some cognitive tasks were too slow, but on other, more demanding tasks they had difficulty slowing themselves down enough to perform carefully. They were unable to regulate their processing speed appropriately for changing task demands.

Cluster 4: Managing Frustration and Modulating Emotions

The diagnostic criteria for attention-deficit hyperactivity disorder in the *DSM-IV* do not include any items referring to emotions. Yet many clinicians report that patients with ADHD struggle with managing their emotions. Paul Wender (1987, 1995) described how individuals with ADHD have "affective lability" and frequently demonstrate a bored or demoralized mood, irritable complaining, angry outbursts, or insufficiently controlled excitability. Wender also noted that individuals with ADHD appear to have a low tolerance for frustration and often find it difficult to persevere through the many stresses of daily life; they readily experience feeling "overwhelmed" or "stressed out."

My own clinical research with children, adolescents, and adults has led to similar conclusions. ADD symptom rating scales I have developed from studying each of these age groups include a cluster of symptoms related to managing frustration and modulating emotions (Brown 1996a, 1996b, 1996c, 2001a, 2001b, 2001c). In analyzing reports from patients with ADHD, I have found that their problems with emotions seem to fall into two closely related types: a very low threshold for frustration, and chronic difficulty in regulating subjective emotional experience and expression.

All persons vary over time and situation in their threshold for frustration. If one is overtired, in a hurry, or very tense, even small frustrations such as dropping a pencil or having to stop briefly at a red light may bring a quick surge of frustration and irritation. Yet most individuals, most of the time, tend to react proportionally to frustration. Minor frustrations usually elicit low-level annoyance, moderate frustrations cause somewhat stronger irritation, and major frustrations may produce proportionate anger.

In contrast, many with ADD syndrome report disproportionate emotional reactions to frustration: a short fuse, a low threshold for irritability. A middle-aged salesman with ADD syndrome described it this way:

> I went to the diner for a late lunch. It was mid-afternoon and the place was fairly quiet. Most everybody else had already eaten. I was eating my sandwich and was in a pretty good mood. Then this guy sitting behind me got his sandwich and he was chewing

too loud. "Chomp, chomp, chomp" with every bite. The sound of his noisy chewing quickly got on my nerves. It was driving me nuts. It was like I had a computer virus in my head and it was taking up all the space. That's all I could think about—the obnoxious sound of his chomping on his sandwich.

Suddenly I realized my fists were clenched and I was seriously thinking about getting up and smacking this guy in the mouth! I didn't do it because I didn't want to get arrested. But if I had been at home I would have been yelling at somebody. After a few minutes, it was all over. He was still making the same noises, but then it didn't bother me anymore. I just went on with my lunch and started thinking about something else. That sort of thing happens to me a lot though. Some frustration that most people would consider a zero, one, or two on a ten-point scale of frustration hits me as though it were a seven, eight, or nine.

This man's analogy to a computer virus illustrates an aspect of emotional experience described by many with ADD syndrome: a feeling that an emotion, in this case irritation, floods one's mind, taking up all available space. This overwhelming intensity of feeling then can cause one to lose perspective and become, for a few moments or much longer, so preoccupied with that particular feeling that other relevant thoughts and feelings are displaced, ignored, or overlooked.

The immediacy of the emotion then can have too much influence on thought and action, causing one to speak or act in ways that don't adequately take account of other feelings, ideas, or information that may also be important. One high school student with ADD syndrome described this as the cause of his difficulties on the school debate team:

All my friends said I should join our school's debate team because they know how much I love to argue. I get really intense in any argument. Once I get started I have to prove my point. I get into it so much that I'm like a bulldozer, running right over everybody else's arguments, pushing their points down and pushing my points so much that they just have to give in. Lots of times I get to talking really loud and practically shouting them down. My approach didn't work very well on the debate team.

Last week I got kicked off the team. The coach said I have good potential, but I just don't know how to listen and tie my points to what the other team has been saying. He said I need to learn to debate more like somebody playing chess and not so much like somebody playing football. He's probably right, but even when I try to calm myself down, I have a really hard time hold-ing back from pushing my point. When I'm into my thing I just can't listen very much to what the other guys are saying. It's like there just isn't enough room in my head for what they are say-ing because I'm so much into what I feel and what I want to say.

Friends and family members often complain of this intense single-mindedness of persons with ADD syndrome, because it can be very an-noying and sometimes hurtful. They report that the individual with ADD syndrome often reacts to even minor frustrations with intense outbursts of anger. Sometimes the tirade includes very harsh words or actions. One wife of a man with ADD syndrome described her experience this way:

It doesn't take much for my husband to lose his temper. Usually he is in a pretty good mood, but then all of a sudden some little frustration will set him off. Maybe someone else has eaten the last of his favorite breakfast cereal or one of our kids forgets to bring the trash cans from the driveway into the garage. All of a sudden he'll be shouting at the top of his lungs and getting in your face about how nobody in the house cares about anything and how we are all inconsiderate and lazy and worthless, never doing anything right regardless of how many times he reminds us. So far he has never hit any of us, but in those moments it al-ways seems like he just might.

Usually this lasts for just a few minutes and then later he'll always apologize. But it's hard to forget those comments he makes. Seems like when he gets mad, all he can feel or think

about is how mad he is. He just can't remember that the people
he is yelling at are people he loves and cares about. He forgets
that we can get hurt by what his says, especially when he comes
on so strong with it. I've tried to talk with him about this and
he always feels bad afterwards, but it keeps on happening.
I know he loves me and loves our kids, but sometimes you
wonder.

This vignette illustrates a problem described by many with ADD syndrome. It resembles the "computer virus in the head" dilemma in the earlier example. A computer virus can suddenly gobble up all available space
in a computer's operating system, crowding out all of the workspace so
the system cannot function. In a similar way, the overly intense frustration
often experienced by many persons with ADD syndrome can flood their
mind so much that, for the moment, they forget the vulnerability of the
loved ones whom they attack. Usually, as in this case, the outburst is intense, but totally verbal. Some individuals with ADD syndrome are less re-
strained in their anger. They often react to frustration by lashing out—
throwing objects, banging doors, punching walls, driving recklessly, or
pushing or hitting people.

Everyone has had some experiences where, in a moment of intense
anger, they have said or done things hurtful to other people who did not
deserve such treatment. What is different for many with ADD syndrome
is that they tend to have a very low threshold for frustration and, as a result,
they experience these intense outbursts with greater frequency and intensity than most others. Unfortunately it is the people closest to them—
their parents, siblings, spouse, children, or other loved ones—who most
often bear the brunt of such unrestrained attacks.

Irritability and anger are not the only emotions that are problematic
for persons with ADD syndrome. Many individuals with ADD have equal
or greater difficulty modulating other emotions, such as hurt or sadness,
worry or anxiety. The salesman who had become so irritated by the loud
chewing also told a story about his problem with a different emotional
response:

Last week in the office I was walking down the hall when I saw this friend who works in another department. He was looking at some papers while he was walking. I said a friendly "Hi" and thought he would stop and visit for a couple of minutes because I hadn't seen him for a long time. But he just barely looked up and mumbled a quick "Hi" back to me and kept right on walking.

Most people would just blow that off right away, figuring he was just in a hurry to get someplace or preoccupied with whatever he was reading. Not me. I got to thinking about it over and over. I kept wondering, "Why wasn't he more friendly? Have I done something to piss him off? Did I do something that annoyed somebody else in his department and now they're all mad at me?"

All these thoughts kept going round and round in my head. It was like that computer virus thing again only this time it went on for most of the afternoon. I didn't get anything done for the rest of that day. That sort of getting too sensitive and too worried thing happens to me way too often.

While he recognized that there was probably a reason for the other man's behavior that had little to do with him, the salesman continued to ruminate for several hours, wondering about possible causes for the other man's actions. Once again, the emotional "virus" was taking up a disproportionate share of the workspace in his head. Many with ADD syndrome describe themselves as "overly sensitive" and reacting too intensely to even minor slights or criticism.

A different problem in regulating emotions was described by a forty-five-year-old man with ADD who noticed it only when he confronted that problem in his son and was reminded by his wife about his own similar tendencies:

I've never been a very patient person. When I get an idea in my head about something I want to do, or something I want to get, or something I want to buy, that wish takes on such intense urgency that I feel I've got to have this NOW! It almost doesn't matter how expensive it is, or how inconvenient it might be for me or somebody else, or whether I'll be using time or money today for this when I know I need that time or money tomorrow for something else that is more important. I feel this relentless drive to do everything I can to get whatever it is I want and to get it now, overcoming whatever obstacles might be put in my way.

And then if I am able to get it, after a few minutes it usually isn't all that satisfying. I just had to have it, and then I've got it, and then I'm off to my next thing. I've always been that way, but I didn't realize it until I got mad at my ten-year-old son for pulling the same kind of stuff. After I finished yelling at him for it, my wife said to me, "Can't you see that he's only doing the same things you do yourself?" She was right.

Some others with ADD syndrome report that they often have difficulty modulating feelings of sadness, discouragement, or depression. One high school student said that his friends called him "dark cloud."

Most of the time I walk around feeling like "Everything sucks. Everything always sucks. Everything always will suck. What's the use? Why bother?" I can get out of that feeling when something interesting happens: shooting hoops with my buddies, hanging with my girlfriend, going to a concert, or watching wrestling on TV. But then as soon as the interesting part is over, I go right back to feeling really bored and thinking about how everything sucks.

I'm not really depressed. I usually sleep OK and eat OK and I never feel like killing myself. I just feel really bored a lot of the time and don't very often feel much like talking with anybody else or getting myself started on doing something. Some of my friends who feel this same way smoke a lot of weed. I'm not one of those "stoners." This is just me. It's the way I've always been.

The mother of this fifteen-year-old corroborated his self-description. She said that since infancy he had always been rather shy and didn't seem to enjoy things very much. She told how it had always been difficult to get him to smile or laugh except when they saw slapstick comedy movies. According to her he did have a few friends and spent time with them, but the mother reported that even with his friends he had very little to say and didn't show much pleasure.

What was striking about this adolescent boy was the change that occurred after his ADHD was diagnosed and treated with stimulant medication. Not only did the medication help to alleviate his difficulties with sustaining attention, completing tasks, and so on; it also brought a marked improvement in his ability to initiate and sustain conversations with friends and family. The stimulant also seemed to facilitate more spontaneous smiling and laughter. His family described him "coming out of his shell." The boy himself reported, "I don't know why, but when I'm on this medicine I don't feel so bored. I feel a lot more relaxed and more like I want to say things and talk with other people. My friends say I'm more "with it" when I'm on it. But when it wears off or if I don't take it, I still have that "everything sucks" feeling.

Not every patient with ADD syndrome experiences such improvements in mood and social interaction when on stimulant medication, but many do. Whether their mood problems respond to stimulant medications or not, it appears that many with ADD syndrome suffer from chronic problems in managing frustration and modulating emotions. Some have much more difficulty with one class of emotions than another—for example, they are very consistently irritable or tend always to be overanxious, or they are chronically oversensitive or consistently unhappy and withdrawn. Others appear to have many more problems than their peers with modulating virtually every emotional response.

Some with ADD syndrome also meet full criteria for another disorder that more directly reflects problems with managing one or more emotions, for example, an anxiety, depressive, or bipolar mood disorder. I discuss this overlap, which occurs very frequently, in Chapter 8. At issue in these various examples is simply that persons with ADD syndrome, with or without any additional psychiatric disorder, tend to suffer from chronic problems in managing frustration and other emotions. These chronic problems appear to be an integral aspect of ADD syndrome and not just overlap with other disorders. In addition, like other symptoms of ADD syndrome, they often respond to treatment with stimulants.

Cluster 5: Utilizing Working Memory and Accessing Recall

When asked about memory, many persons with ADD syndrome describe a peculiar contradiction. Many report that they are quite good at accessing long-term memories, for example, they can recall details from experiences years earlier. Yet most complain of chronic difficulties in their ability to hold one thought or bit of information in mind while simultaneously doing something else. They often forget what they were just about to say or the purpose for which they have just walked into a room. They tend to forget where they have most recently placed their keys, what they have done with a needed document, or whom they have just dialed on the telephone.

Chronic difficulties with memory appear to be a core problem in ADD syndrome, but the impairments are not generally with long-term storage memory; instead they involve "working memory," a term that has been used in many different ways, most of which are unrelated to the older term "short-term memory." Working memory has several functions. An important one is to hold one bit of information active while working with another. One patient described his impairment of this essential function as lacking a "hold" button in his memory.

> I'm really good at remembering things from a long time ago. I can tell you the whole story line from movies I saw just once years ago and haven't seen since. But even though I'm the best in my family for remembering things from way back, I'm the worst at remembering what happened just a few minutes ago. If I call the Information operator to get a phone number, I can never remember it long enough to dial it. I always have to write it down or I'll mix up the numbers.
>
> I'll go into a room to get something and then I'm standing there scratching my head and wondering what I came in there for. Or I'll go to the store to get five things I need to fix dinner. If I don't write them down I'll only be able to pick up one of them;

I can't remember the other four to save my life. It's like my
mind is a multiline phone where the hold button doesn't work.
If I am trying to remember one thing and then I set it aside even
for just a minute to think about or do something else, I totally
lose what I was trying to hold onto.

Working memory, then, is not short-term memory. It does not function as the queue on a computer's printer, simply holding information
briefly while it awaits further processing. Working memory, instead, is
like a very active computational unit that not only holds information, but
also actively processes this current information in connection with the
vast files of longer-term memory. In other words, working memory might
be compared to the RAM of a computer combined with its file manager
and search engine.

Working memory is essential for participation in a group discussion or
in individual conversation where one has to try to understand what someone is saying while formulating a response. People with ADD syndrome
often have a great deal of difficulty with these concurrent functions.

It's so frustrating when we're having class discussions. The
teacher will ask a question and I'll have a good answer for it, so
I'll raise my hand. And then she calls on somebody else first
and I have to listen to this other kid say his answer. Then she
comes back and asks me to say my answer. When she does that
I just have to shrug and say, "I don't know." By then I've not
only forgotten what I was going to answer; I've even forgotten
the question.

When I'm just talking with friends, lots of times I just interrupt and say what I've got to say. I know that if I'm polite and
wait until the other person has stopped talking, I won't ever be
able to remember what I was going to say. The problem is that
while I'm trying to keep in mind what I want to say, often I am
not paying enough attention to what the other person is trying to
say to me. Usually both my thought and theirs gets washed away
from my mind.

This student clearly illustrates how impairments of working memory can interfere with both receptive and expressive aspects of communication between individuals and within groups. His complaint, common among persons with ADD syndrome, highlights the difficulty in maintaining reciprocal communication when working memory function is impaired.

Another aspect of working memory involves the retrieval of information from the files of longer-term memory. One student described how his impairments of working memory interfered with his taking tests.

> It's so frustrating when I study hard for tests and then can't remember what I learned. I'll study hard and learn everything we're supposed to know. My friends quiz me and I've got it all down. Then, the next day I go in to take the test, figuring that I'm going to get a good grade. And then when I'm actually taking the test, a big chunk of what I knew so well the night before just evaporates. It's like I have a file in my computer and can't remember the file name to pop it up. I know the stuff is in there, but I just can't get to it, so I can't put it down on the test. Then a few hours after the test, something will jog my memory and it's all back again. It's not that I didn't have it in there. It was in my mind, I just couldn't retrieve it when I needed it.

The student's complaints about being unable to recall lessons studied and seemingly mastered the night before illustrate a distinct type of memory problem: defective retrieval of learned information. His comparison to forgetting the name of a computer file is apt. Persons with ADD syndrome often complain that they have chronic difficulty pulling up from the files of longer-term memory the information needed to do a task at hand. Sometimes the problem is recalling the name of someone whose face has just been recognized as familiar. Sometimes the problem lies in retrieving information or procedures needed to answer a question or solve a problem.

Many aspects of academic work depend heavily on the effective functioning of working memory. When reading, one needs to hold in mind the sounds symbolized by the first part of a word while decoding the sound of later syllables to recognize the word as a whole. One then has to retrieve from memory the meanings associated with that word and hold those in mind while linking them to meanings of other words to get the full meaning and context of the entire sentence. This process happens automatically for fluent readers as they rapidly link up and absorb layers of meaning built on words, sentences, paragraphs, chapters, and so on. Persons whose working memory is significantly impaired, however, may experience great difficulty in understanding an entire text, even if they are quite competent in decoding each word. Reading comprehension is built on the effective functioning of working memory in conjunction with an active, sustained attention to the text.

Working memory is also essential for doing math, even simple arithmetic. If one cannot keep in mind what quantities have been borrowed or need to be carried from one column to another in calculations, one's answers are not likely to be correct. And if one cannot keep in mind the sequence of operations, then much of algebra, geometry, and higher math becomes incomprehensible.

Written expression also places strong demands on working memory. One college student described how working memory problems interfered with her writing:

> When I write sentences to answer exam questions or to write an essay or a term paper, I keep getting lost. I start out with one thing I am trying to say and then I get going on that one thing and forget about what I was supposed to hook it up with. Usually my answer doesn't really fit very well with the question.
>
> It's even worse in longer writing projects like an essay or a term paper. There I'll make a point and then forget to explain it enough. Or I'll just wander off the path. Teachers are always writing in the margins, "Elaborate this more" or "How did you get from what you just said to this?" One teacher said that I keep forgetting where I am supposed to be going. She's right. When I have to write longer things it's like I'm just wandering around in what I write. I can't stick to the topic and then explain the different parts to get to wherever I'm supposed to take it.

To write a paragraph, letter, or essay, one has to consider simultaneously many elements: Who is the audience? What is the major point? How can I connect subordinate points to the main idea? Especially with longer or more complex writing tasks, it is necessary to hold several viewpoints in mind while putting words and images together understandably. This process presents a major challenge to working memory.

There has not been much research on students who have problems with written expression, but preliminary studies indicate that persons with ADHD demonstrate a disproportionately high incidence of impairment in this respect. For reasons explained in Chapters 4 and 8, it is likely that working memory impairments of ADD syndrome play a significant role in creating difficulties with written expression among ADHD students.

Working memory is involved not only in academic tasks, but also in countless aspects of everyday life, as one holds briefly in mind the continuing flow of perceptions of current external events—sounds just heard, images just observed, impressions just formed. Akira Miyake and Priti Shah (1999) describe how working memory plays a crucial role in moment-by-moment integration of memories held "internally" in long-term memory stores and those transient memories currently coming in from "external" sources:

> During the performance of many (if not all) complex everyday cognitive tasks, the processing of external information and internal information needs to interact dynamically, going back and forth between information distributed across the internal mind and the external world. . . . Working memory . . . may serve as the important interface between external representations and internal representations. (p. 466)

Problems with integrating internal and external information can have a substantial influence on one's ability to link new information being acquired with other information already in mind. One illustration is a student who had great difficulty taking his SAT, a test required for college admission.

I took my SAT last week. I know I did really poorly because I wasn't able to finish a bunch of the reading comprehension questions. They give you this passage of three or four paragraphs to read and then you have to answer five multiple-choice questions about what you have just read. Most of them are really dense reading, with lots of details. And the questions are tricky, often hinging on very specific details in the text.

It took me so long on each question! I couldn't remember what I had just finished reading. I would read the passage and then for each question I needed to read it all over again to find the answer. I had to keep reading this same passage over and over again. I tried reading the questions first so I'd know what details to look for, but by the time I did that and then got back to the paragraphs, I had forgotten the questions. This kind of thing happens to me a lot.

Sometimes this need to reread is due to the "passive reading" problem described in the vignette earlier in this chapter. In other situations, it appears that the reader has actively engaged with the text, but is simply not able to hold its meaning in mind while reading subsequent parts or when addressing questions immediately following the reading.

The difference between problems of working memory and problems of insufficient attention has been a matter of debate among researchers. Neuroscientists studying memory functions have argued that what is currently referred to as working memory is not simply a memory unit of the mind, but a complex system that involves both "working attention" and "working memory" serving together to manage the continuous flow of information in the mind. Chronic impairments in this complex system are an important aspect of the ADD syndrome.

Cluster 6: Monitoring and Self-Regulating Action

Most descriptions of the disorder now known as ADHD emphasize problems with hyperactive and impulsive behavior. Many persons identified with this disorder tend to act without sufficient forethought, or are chronically restless and hyperactive, finding it very difficult to slow down and adequately control their actions. Children with ADHD have often been seen as wild, restless, and impulsive, unable sufficiently to control their words and bodies and so needing much more supervision from teachers and parents than others of the same age. One mother described her son's behavior:

> My son is six years old, but he usually acts like he is only three or four. When he wants something he just goes for it. He just can't wait. He almost got hit by a car last summer because he chased a ball out into the street and didn't even stop to look. In kindergarten last year he was always in trouble because he grabbed toys or crayons away from other kids. When they were supposed to sit on the circle and listen for show and tell, he was always interrupting with his own comments; he had to tell about something he was thinking about. He couldn't just listen to another kid or even to the teacher. When he was supposed to draw a picture or copy some shapes, he was always in a hurry. If he tried to do what they asked him to draw or write, he did it too fast and it was too messy.
>
> This year he is repeating kindergarten, but I'm afraid he won't be ready for first grade even next year. He just doesn't seem to be able to slow down enough to listen to the directions or to do anything carefully. He's way behind other kids his age in self-control.

This mother's description shows many different ways in which her six-year-old son is substantially behind his peers in his ability to monitor and control his actions. He acts impulsively and doesn't slow down enough to listen to others, to follow directions, or to do assigned tasks carefully. Chronic and extreme problems of this sort are typical of many young children with ADD syndrome.

Researchers have identified "impaired ability to inhibit" as a core problem in these hyperactive and impulsive symptoms of ADHD. Russell Barkley (1997) has argued that impairment of the ability to inhibit is *the* primary problem of persons with ADHD, and, of all the executive functions impaired in the disorder, is the one on which the development and effective functioning of all other executive functions depends.

For some individuals with ADD syndrome, like this six-year-old, impairment in the ability to inhibit action is the most basic problem. Until they can develop more age-appropriate control of their actions—that is, the ability to slow down and hold back so they can act carefully and do the right thing at the right time—these individuals continue to make a lot of trouble for themselves and those around them.

Yet to overemphasize inhibition as the central problem of ADHD is to ignore the essential connection between holding back actions and engaging in actions. It is to overlook the need to "go," which is as important as the need to hold back or stop. Certainly it is important for a person to be able to stop at the curb rather than impulsively running across a busy street. But it is also important for that person to be able to monitor the traffic on the street, to determine when it is safe to cross, and then to actually cross. Indeed, most behaviors require the ability to act, to "do it," as well as the ability to inhibit, to refrain from acting. And essential to one's success in this regard is the ability to monitor the context of action, in this case, the traffic, so that one can decide when to wait and when to cross the street.

Monitoring the context of action can be quite complex, even in the simple act of crossing a street. It involves looking both ways to notice oncoming vehicles, estimating their speed, and allowing for road conditions—for example, rain or ice that might affect their slowing down or stopping. It also includes consideration of factors that might affect drivers' ability to see the person attempting to cross, such as sun glaring toward the driver, fog, or darkness, as well as exceptional circumstances such as a car swerving as though out of control or a vehicle speeding with flashing lights and siren.

Crossing the street also requires one to take into account information about current personal circumstances that might affect the accuracy of one's perception or one's speed and efficiency of crossing. These variables might include one's having poor vision for judging vehicles' distance or speed; feeling tired or having an injured foot; being unfamiliar with local traffic patterns; or being constrained by carrying bulky packages or having to push a bicycle across the street.

To cross a street safely, or to do almost anything carefully, requires four coordinated functions: (1) inhibiting the action until the right moment, (2) monitoring one's self and the specific circumstances of the situation to decide how and when to act, (3) executing the appropriate actions when needed, and (4) monitoring one's self and the current situation while acting. Effective self-regulation of behavior involves simultaneous, often instantaneous, coordination of all these key functions.

Countless actions of daily life involve carrying out these components in an integrated way: interacting in a business meeting, participating in a classroom discussion, shopping in a supermarket, playing a game, attending a party, or driving a car.

> For me driving my car is a constant struggle. It really scares me because there are so many things to notice and think about, all at the same time you are propelling this huge, powerful machine along the highway or in the midst of heavy traffic and pedestrians. I've seen some car accidents where people got seriously hurt. I don't want that to happen to me. But it could.
>
> When I'm driving I have to be constantly watching what I am doing, what other drivers are doing, and what the pedestrians are doing. At the same time I have to monitor my speedometer so I don't go too fast and I have to keep watching the stop signs and traffic lights and lane changes. And I have to keep checking my rearview mirror and the side mirrors. If I'm trying to get to someplace I'm not familiar with I have to watch street signs and check addresses, all at the same time.

Driving is a complex task, but social situations are often among the most challenging for those with difficulties monitoring and self-regulating their actions. In those circumstances, one must quickly assess the expectations and perceptions of other persons in order to behave appropriately. When is it okay to tell this joke, or to complain about an injustice, or to confront one's boss, teacher, coworker, customer, parent, spouse, child, or friend? Because persons with ADD syndrome find it hard to monitor effectively the context in which they are operating, they report that they tend to be too random in what they notice, attending too much to some details and too little to others that may be equally or more important. Especially difficult for these persons are those situations where one has to monitor and gauge the emotions and intentions of other people with whom one is interacting. Indeed, often persons with ADD syndrome complain that they have gotten into trouble because they have failed to notice how others were reacting to them, or have been insufficiently aware of how they themselves were coming across to others. This monitoring is made even more difficult when one is simultaneously holding in check one's own reactions while interacting with others.

A forty-three-year-old man with ADD syndrome described his experience:

> I love getting into intense conversations with other people where it's not just small talk. I love sharing impressions and opinions between people about things that really matter. I think that's how people get to know each other and learn from one another. Usually it works out well, but sometimes I get too intense and turn other people off when I'm trying to find out what they think and why they think that way. Usually I don't notice it at the time; I just see that they drop out of the conversation or walk away.
>
> My wife says I just don't know how to keep my eyes open and notice when others are starting to act uptight or bored with what's being discussed. She says that most of the time I talk too much or ask too many questions without noticing how I am coming across and how others are reacting to what I'm saying. She says that most of the time I'm too much mouth and not enough eyes and ears when I'm in a conversation.

This man's self-description highlights his difficulty in self-monitoring and context-monitoring during conversation. He emphasizes that he wants to learn from others and share with others, but he frustrates himself, and probably others with whom he talks, because he is not sufficiently attentive to facial expressions, tone of voice, or subtle eye or body movements that signal tension, waning interest, or impatience. Careful attention to such cues is important for developing understanding and reciprocity in social interaction. Often people with ADD syndrome report chronic difficulty with this sort of social monitoring and self-control. They don't notice enough about themselves and others, and they have chronic problems in holding back or in keeping still, even for just a few moments.

Some other persons with ADD syndrome have a different problem with self-monitoring, contextual monitoring, and controlling their actions in social situations. They tend to be excessively focused on how others are reacting and are excessively self-conscious. They tend to be too constricted, too shy, too inhibited in their social actions. One thirty-five-year-old woman with ADD syndrome described her wish to be more sociable:

> I really wish I had more friends. Often I complain that nobody ever wants to talk with me, but I know that the problem is more with me than it is them. I'm not shy in my family or with a few people I know really well. But with everybody else I always feel like it is never the right time for me to say something or I just can't think of anything to say that would fit into the conversation. I'm always holding back, waiting until the right moment or until I can think of something to say.

Though these more cautious individuals with ADD syndrome may long for more reciprocity with others and may have many interesting ideas and feelings to share, they often get so caught up with intently monitoring that they are unable to engage themselves in social interactions. While they have no difficulty inhibiting their own actions and being very attentive in monitoring the social context, these persons often cannot bring themselves to act effectively in a group.

Although there are a variety of ways in which individuals experience difficulty in monitoring and regulating their actions, most with ADD syndrome report chronic difficulties in one of more aspects of inhibiting action, monitoring one's self, monitoring one's context, and taking action in an appropriate way. This cluster of ADD-related impairments extends far beyond simple excesses of hyperactive or impulsive behavior: these problems hamper one's ability to perform well in a wide variety of everyday tasks.

Snapshots of Complex Processes

This chapter began with a discussion about how snapshots can capture only very limited aspects of real experiences. These descriptions of six clusters of functions often impaired in persons with ADD syndrome are like those snapshots, showing only limited aspects of the rich and dynamic complexity of the cognitive processes described. In Chapters 4, 5, and 6 I elaborate on how these functions, which constitute the central components of the brain's executive functions, develop during childhood, adolescence, and adulthood. Here the main point is that persons with ADD syndrome report chronic impairments in a wide variety of cognitive functions that cause problems for most persons only occasionally.

Chapter 3   ADD Syndrome and the Working Brain

MYTH: Brains of persons with ADD are overactive and need medication to calm them down.

FACT: Underactivity of the brain's management networks is typical of persons with ADD. Effective medications increase alertness and improve communication in the brain's management system.

The executive functions impaired in ADD syndrome are not skills to be learned or aspects of willpower to be exercised, but natural activities of complex neural networks of the brain. Understanding these coordinated processes requires some grasp of how critical components of the brain work together. This chapter describes major circuits of the brain that sustain executive functions, the gradual process by which these functions normally develop, and how they are impaired in those who suffer from ADD syndrome.

The human brain weighs about three pounds and is composed of approximately 100 billion neurons, tiny cells only one millionth of an inch across. These neurons are the building blocks of the brain. Each neuron has a cell body on which develop tens of thousands of tiny branches called dendrites; these dendrites receive information from other neurons. Each neuron also has one extension, called an axon, for sending information out to other cells; these can range in length from less than a millimeter to over a meter long. Part A of Figure 2 shows a neuron and some of its dendrites emerging from the dense matrix of intertwined neurons in the brain.

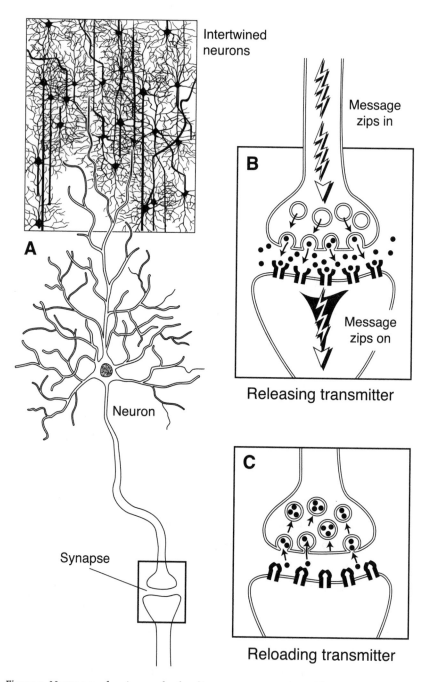

Intertwined neurons

A

Neuron

Synapse

B

Message zips in

Message zips on

Releasing transmitter

C

Reloading transmitter

Figure 2 Neurons releasing and reloading neurotransmitter. The neuron in (A) is shown emerging from its matrix of intertwined neurons. Its twiglike branches pick up information from other neurons and relay it through the synapse to another neuron. (B) shows the release of a transmitter chemical that helps the electrical message jump the gap to the adjoining neuron. (C) shows the transmitter chemical reloading back into the sending neuron.

Neurons make contact with other neurons at junctions called synapses. Every neuron makes from one thousand to ten thousand synapses with surrounding neurons. Some of these connections work as a chemical braking system, slowing down and inhibiting electrical connections at that juncture. Other connections act as a chemical accelerator, activating and intensifying electrical communication. The brain regulates itself and the entire body via the constant interaction among these many excitatory and inhibitory chemical processes. The information processing capacity packed into these networks of the brain is massive. V. S. Ramachandran (1998) observed that a piece of brain the size of a grain of sand would contain one hundred thousand neurons, two million axons, and one billion synapses, all talking to each other.

Imagine a skyscraper that is one hundred stories tall. Picture that massive tower covered from top to bottom and on all four sides with seventeen-inch illuminated TV screens. Paul Churchland (1995) pointed out that it would take all of the two hundred thousand pixels on each of those half million TV screens to amass as many pixels as the number of neurons in any one person's brain. Further, within the brain all these neurons are compacted into a wrinkled, layered mass only about the size of a large grapefruit.

Networks of Neurons

Inside the brain this enormous mass of microscopic neurons is organized into a large number of systems and subsystems that look like dense jungles of miniscule branches and twigs. These interacting networks have to communicate rapidly with one another moment to moment in order to manage the body, all mental functions, and the person's ongoing interactions with the world. Amazingly, these complex neural networks are not wired together; instead each of the trillions of connection points between neurons has a tiny gap between the back end of one neuron and the front end of the next. The whole system works on low-voltage electrical impulses. Each of the messages carried between neurons is a tiny electrical charge of about 0.1 volt. As this moving charge gets to each synapse it has to jump the gap, like in a spark plug. This jump across each synaptic gap is a chemical process.

Chemicals Facilitate the Transmission of Messages in the Brain

Chemicals manufactured in the brain manage the communication of messages from one neuron to another. Every neural network in the brain uses primarily one of about fifty different neurotransmitter chemicals. Each of these chemicals affects tiny receptors on adjoining neurons, receptors sensitive to that specific neurotransmitter and to no others. Receptors are like locks that will accept only one particular key.

Neurotransmitter chemicals are manufactured in the brain and stored in little bubbles, called vesicles, located near the back end of each neuron. Each time a message comes zipping along that neuron, the storage vesicles release very small amounts of the neurotransmitter chemical to carry the electrical charge of the message across the gap rapidly. The amount of transmitter chemical available for release varies according to how urgent or interesting the message appears to the brain at that moment. When a sufficient amount of the transmitter chemical contacts its specific receptors across the gap, the message is quickly sent on its way over the next segment, where the process is repeated (as long as there is sufficient transmitter to keep the message flowing). Part B of Figure 2 shows the release of neurotransmitter chemical and the movement of the message across the synapse.

As each message continues on its way, any neurotransmitter not used up or broken down in the signaling process is pumped back into the sending cell through specialized cells called transporters. This allows the system to reload for more action in fractions of a second. This chemical transmission system is quick: each molecule of transmitter stays on the receptor for only about 50 milliseconds. In one millisecond, one thousandth of a second, twelve messages can be carried across the synaptic gap. Part C of Figure 2 shows the reloading of the neurotransmitter chemical back into the side of the synapse that released it.

At any given moment, vast numbers of messages are surging through the countless shifting circuits of the brain. Some messages travel only short distances within the brain and then stop. Others are switched rapidly from one circuit to another, engaging additional subsystems or being pulled into ever more complex, more potent, and more complex aggregate networks.

Three Types of Processing Centers

Numerous centers process, organize, and regulate this constant flow of electrical communication within the brain. There are three basic types: local centers, which process only isolated fragments of information; regional centers, which put together these isolated local fragments from a given sensory modality; and integrative centers, which process increasingly large batches of information drawn from multiple centers.

Local centers, mostly in the posterior (rear) third of the brain, process only very specific types of information, for example, perceptions taken in from one particular sense: vision, hearing, smell, taste, or touch. Stimuli picked up by eyes, ears, nose, tongue, and skin are carried rapidly to the appropriate center at the back of the brain, creating a flow of fragmented images of what is seen, heard, smelled, touched, and so on in the outside world. These perceptual fragments might be compared to the fractured segments of a Picasso cubist painting, unrecognizable in isolation.

Regional centers pull together these information fragments to form more integrated and complex informational maps. For example, the visual cortex receives from the retina of each eye fragmentary images of objects and settings perceived by the eyes. These stimuli are then assembled by the visual association cortex into a more coherent and recognizable picture of what is being looked at, moment by moment.

Pulling together the steady flow of data from these specific association centers are numerous other centers that integrate. These integrative areas instantaneously assemble data from vision, smell, hearing, and so forth to create up-to-the-moment multimodality updates about our experience with the external world. Unlike the sensory modules in the back of the brain, these association centers are not isolated and encapsulated units; they are linked in many ways to allow for the rapid, progressive flow of information from one network to another.

Two Interconnected Halves

The various networks described thus far operate in both the left and right sides of the brain. Although similar, each of these two hemispheres is a bit different from the other in size, shape, and function. The two are connected by the corpus callosum, a dense band of 200 million fibers that runs front to back and integrates operations on the two sides of the brain. The corpus callosum is labeled in Figure 3.

In the past, the left hemisphere of the human brain was recognized as dealing primarily with language data, while the right hemisphere was seen as dealing primarily with visual and spatial operations. A different picture emerges from more recent studies. Robert Ornstein (1997) has reviewed research suggesting that the right hemisphere tends to deal more with getting the "big picture," the wider range of possible meanings, whereas the left hemisphere is better suited for dealing with more detailed and focused sequential information. In his view, these two hemispheres work together, with the right side more suited to recognizing the contextual forest while the left deals more with details of particular trees. Information flow in the brain thus involves not only circuits that pull together information from local and regional centers across modalities of perception, but also circuits that criss-cross the hemispheres to sort out and integrate constantly shifting details, sequences, and contexts.

Central Management Networks

Given the steady flow of complex information processed in the brain, a managerial system is essential. All neuronal networks are not created equal. Some networks monitor, coordinate, and manage other neural networks. Networks that manage these functions constitute the matrix that supports executive functions of the mind. These central cognitive management networks assess incoming information to establish and modify priorities. They start, stop, and integrate various functions, deploying from the brain's vast stores of memories the particular information needed to address the salient perceptions and tasks of each moment. These management networks are implicated in most of the impairments of ADD syndrome.

Circuits that support these executive functions are distributed throughout the brain. This chapter highlights three major centers in which executive functions are based. From these centers (and others), circuits controlling executive functions project widely throughout the brain's dense

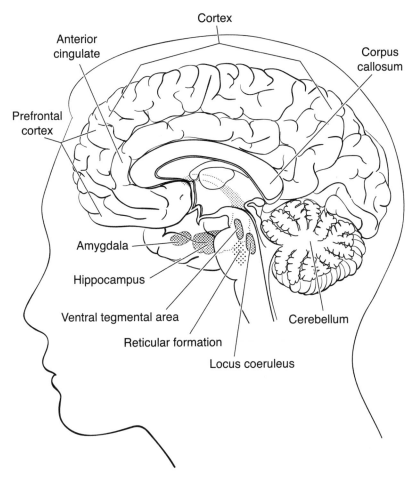

Figure 3 Primary brain structures involved in executive functions. Working memory circuits are located primarily in the prefrontal cortex; the hippocampus converts working memories into longer-term memories. Risks and rewards are identified primarily via the amygdala and dopamine circuits, which originate in the ventral tegmental area. Alertness is supported by circuits from the locus coeruleus and reticular formation, and circuits from the cerebellum drive the "fine-tuning" of cognition. These circuits all interact with many others.

matrix. Figure 3 shows these major centers of circuits for executive functions. One important center is the frontal region, particularly the prefrontal cortex, which is located just behind the forehead. Circuits important for assessing risks and rewards are located in the limbic regions deeper below the cortex. Centers that regulate alertness and vigilance are at the back of the brain, just above the spinal column.

In the Prefrontal Cortex: Working Memory Circuits

The prefrontal cortex is a relatively small component of the human brain; it takes up slightly less than one-third of the brain's total volume. This central management center is connected directly with every functional unit of the brain, those that:

receive sensory input,
control movement,
manage memory,
deal with emotion,
make decisions,
control activation, and
maintain stability of vital bodily functions.

The prefrontal cortex is the only segment of the brain so fully connected with other aspects of the brain and the neural pathways that link them.

Among the many specialized aspects of the prefrontal cortex are circuits managing central working memory functions. Many people think of memory as a self-contained function that, somewhat like a video recorder, captures pictures and sounds of each moment of personal experience, then files all of them in some cerebral vault for playback on demand. If that were the case, the brain would quickly be flooded with so much information that effective action would be impossible. Research suggests that the systems of memory are more efficient.

The brain has networks of neurons that very briefly hold in an active state the perceptions and thoughts of each moment, linking them with stored memories that allow the individual to string together experiences moment by moment to make sense of what is being perceived or thought and to act accordingly. This is working memory. Without it, an individual is perpetually locked into the present moment, unable to link what was seen, heard, or thought a moment ago with whatever is happening now. The importance of this function is painfully evident when one observes a patient with Alzheimer's dementia who asks someone a question and hears the answer, appears to register it, but then asks the same question of the same person again moments later, unaware of having just heard the response.

Specific cells that execute the functions of working memory have been identified in the living brain. For example, the late Patricia Goldman-Rakic (1987) found specific cells in the prefrontal cortex for spatial working memory—the ability to remember where something occurs—in a tiny region of the lateral prefrontal cortex. Her studies were done with monkeys, animals whose brains are organized almost identically to the human brain.

Researchers placed in front of a monkey two dishes that could be seen, but not touched. The experimenter placed a bit of food in one dish, covered both, then blocked the monkey's view of the dishes for several seconds. This made it necessary for the monkey to hold in mind the picture of which dish held the food; there was no other clue. After several seconds the experimenter removed the screen and the monkey was given one chance to grab the food. This was done with repeated trials that varied which dish held the food.

From electrodes placed in specific cells of the monkey's brain, researchers found that one particular set of cells was activated as the monkey watched the food placement. Another set of nearby cells lighted up while the monkey's view of the dishes was blocked; these were the working memory cells. These cells deactivated when the screen was removed and the monkey reached for a dish.

Repeated trials showed that those working memory cells played a crucial role. If they became activated during the task, the monkeys picked the correct dish, whereas if the working memory cells did not activate, the monkeys made many more mistakes. In monkeys with damaged working memory cells, performance was totally impaired.

This work by Goldman-Rakic identified specific cells with which the brain can transiently hold in mind and utilize information acquired just seconds earlier to guide current actions. Since these areas in the prefrontal cortex are intimately connected with other regions of the brain, working memory cells can guide our selection of incoming information, helping us to focus on what is needed to continue a task or to acquire more information.

For example, the brain of a person driving a car can notice and hold in mind the movement of a pedestrian stepping off a curb into the street, even if right afterward another car momentarily blocks the view of the pedestrian. By keeping the potential danger in mind, the driver can watch and be alert to the possibility that he might need to slow down, swerve, or stop to avoid an accident. All this can happen in an instant, without benefit of conscious thought, only to be forgotten moments later as the mind goes on to other tasks. The capacity to forget what is not needed is crucial; it prevents the brain from becoming gridlocked with excessive information.

Longer-Term Storage of Memories

While much of the data captured in working memory simply passes through in mere seconds, so as not to clutter up the brain's limited attentional resources, other information is held longer to be worked on and/or gradually shifted into longer-term memory storage. A chess player may hold in mind several moves made by an opponent, trying to discern the underlying strategy and plan countermoves. Or a listener may hold in mind several sentences of a funny story being told by a friend so he can grasp the punch line of his friend's joke. Sometimes the chess moves and the words of the joke may be retained; in other instances they are totally transient. Working memory functions like RAM on a computer; files are not saved after use unless they are converted to hard-drive data through a "save" function. The brain has a process for converting contents of working memory into longer-term memories.

Contents of working memory that are saved into long-term memory are usually routed through the hippocampus (identified in Figure 3). There the connections between the specific neurons that encoded the memory are "cemented" by development of specific proteins produced in the brain. This process of protein changes setting up a memory for longer-term storage is called LTP, which stands for long-term potentiation. If the hippocampus is seriously damaged by trauma or disease, this process of making new memories and holding them over the longer term is seriously disrupted, or even reduced to total amnesia. The individual with a damaged hippocampus may retain "how to do it" memories of certain limited skills newly learned, but cannot consciously remember and describe what they have learned. A more detailed description of how longer-term memories are formed is beyond the scope of this chapter, but Joseph LeDoux (2002) and Daniel Schacter (1996) have provided comprehensive and accessible descriptions of those processes.

Working Memory: Search Engine for the Brain

The processes of working memory are complicated. They involve not only briefly "holding onto" current information needed for current tasks, and transiently holding information to be encoded into longer-term memory, but also calling up those memories in longer-term storage needed for immediate tasks and experiences. Neuroscientists Stephen Kosslyn and Olivier Koenig (1995) described these complex functions:

> Working memory . . . corresponds to the activated information
> in long-term memories, the information in short-term memories, and the decision processes that manage which information
> is activated in the long-term memories and retained in short-term memories . . . an interplay between information that is
> stored temporarily and a larger body of stored knowledge.
> (p. 388)

This interplay between a current focus of attention, some task or idea that an individual is attending to, and that person's store of long-term memories is essential to countless functions in daily life where one must "pull out of the files" of memory information needed for answering a question or performing a task. This may involve recalling directions for driving to the local shopping center, remembering specific aspects of learned information to answer questions on an examination, or recalling events and characters encountered in earlier chapters of a novel when one resumes reading the book several days later. Joaquin Fuster (2003) emphasized the essential linkage between working memory and longer-term memory:

The content of working memory essentially consists of long-term memory that has been activated for the processing of actions . . . attention is inseparable from selective neural processing. (p. 155)

But not all new information activated in working memory for current tasks is held in lasting linkage with longer-term memories. What determines which information in working memory will be held onto and which will be allowed to fade out? And what determines which information encoded in longer-term memory will be called into conscious attention and working memory when it is needed? In short, what drives the "file manager" and "search engine" functions of working memory? One key element of these mechanisms is emotion.

Where the Brain Recognizes Risks and Possible Rewards

Circuits in the limbic region at the center of the brain beneath the cortex manage the critical task of assigning emotional importance and priorities to incoming perceptions and to internally generated thoughts and plans. These circuits instantaneously assess what may be attractive, dangerous, or rewarding.

Many think of emotion as a quality added to a perception or thought on the basis of conscious reflection—for example, "I smelled something burning and began to worry about whether there was a fire in the house." "I heard that song playing and began to feel sad; it reminded me of a girlfriend who left me." In these two examples something is noticed, thought about, and then reacted to with an emotion, in this case fear or sadness.

But the process by which the brain links perceptions or thoughts and emotions tends to be much quicker and less reflective. Usually the brain assigns emotion and thereby importance in ways that are instantaneous and automatic. Antonio Damasio described this process:

Emotion is critical for the appropriate direction of attention since it provides an *automated signal* about the organism's past experience with given objects and thus provides a basis for assigning or

withholding attention relative to a given object . . . first, processing of objects can take place; second, emotion can ensue; third,
further enhancement and focusing can occur, or not occur, under
the direction of emotion. (1999, p. 273, italics added)

The brain acts most quickly on perceptions that it judges as threatening. Joseph LeDoux (1996) and Elizabeth Phelps (2005) have described
how the amygdala, a tiny structure in the midbrain (see Figure 3), screens
incoming perceptions for any sign of potential danger. This structure, not
much larger than a walnut, receives constant input from all of the brain's
lobes, and rapidly screens incoming perceptions and thoughts to determine whether they present any threat. It functions something like an automatic missile-avoidance system on a military aircraft.

It is this mechanism that causes one quickly to jump aside to avoid a
car that suddenly speeds around the corner as one is crossing the street.
The unexpected car's approach, caught only in the periphery of vision, is reacted to with instantaneous movement before one is even aware of being
afraid. The brain reacts without delay to unexpected objects moving quickly
toward us, to objects touched that are too hot, to substances that taste rot-
ten; such self-protective reactions do not wait for conscious thought.

The brain's recognition of some situations as dangerous, to be avoided,
extends far wider than these simple examples of possible threats to physical safety. From earliest infancy the brain builds up a massive file of
memories that can signal possible danger, not only from speeding cars or
possibly poisonous foods, but also from situations that might elicit other
kinds of pain, for example, ridicule, disgust, anger, or rejection from others. The networks of the brain are such that the amygdala and its connections will react to these acquired warnings with instantaneous release of
chemicals that activate avoidance responses, often without awaiting reflection. It is these chemicals, quickly attached to the perception or thought,
that create the fear and mobilize appropriate action.

While some fear reactions are based on instinct, many more are based
on personal memories. Contents of these files used to identify potential
dangers are highly individualized, gradually accumulated from the earli-

est years and throughout each individual's life. In countless interactions with our physical and social world, each person acquires memories of what is considered dangerous or wrong. Interactions with parents, siblings, teachers, and friends, as well as exposure to stories and photos through various media, shape one's personal reactions about what is dangerous or wrong to look at, taste, touch, want, and do. Ongoing experiences continually update these mental files: some experiences reinforce previous understandings and others dramatically alter how a particular individual reacts to a particular perception, thought, or action.

On the basis of such files, the brain reacts automatically to some incoming perceptions with instantaneous signals that register discomfort ranging from mild unease to total repugnance or panic. In ensuing moments, hours, or days, one's emotional reactions may become more elaborated and more conscious, but the core emotional reaction, particularly to potential dangers, emerges usually in an instant via the brain's early warning mechanisms in the amygdala and associated systems.

Positive emotional reactions— interest, attraction, and desire—are also "automatically" assigned by the brain. One example is sexual attraction. Many have had the experience of feeling suddenly attracted to a person with a certain physical appearance, mannerisms, or more subtle qualities. Such attraction is often attributed to mysterious "forces of the heart," but in fact, the brain is in charge. Psychoanalysis has offered psychological explanations for how such experiences may be linked to unconscious aspects of life experiences, but ultimately all of our responses to experiences are carried out within the brain's neural networks. Mark Baxter and Elisabeth Murray (2002) presented evidence that the amygdala and related brain structures continuously scan the environment not only for dangers, but also for indications of something interesting or potentially rewarding.

The brain uses one specific transmitter chemical, dopamine, to highlight important stimuli. Numerous studies have demonstrated that dopamine release in the brain acts as a powerful signal to indicate important stimuli, particularly those that bring pleasure. Dopamine is produced deep in the midbrain at rates and in amounts that vary according to the brain's moment-by-moment perceptions. Figure 4 shows the origins of the dopa-

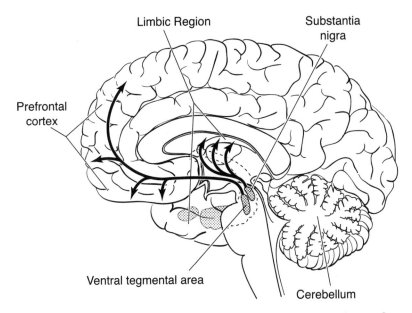

Figure 4 Main pathways of the dopamine system. Dopamine pathways for executive functions originate primarily in the ventral tegmental area. They extend throughout the prefrontal cortex and into limbic centers to release dopamine in response to perceived danger or reward.

mine system for executive functions, in the ventral tegmental area, and its major projections to other areas of the brain.

Once released by the ventral tegmental circuits, dopamine is carried through two primary pathways. One pathway feeds dopamine to the prefrontal cortex, where action plans are selected. The other carries dopamine to other regions that map and monitor the ongoing state of the organism to reflect comfort, displeasure, and so on (Pennington 2002; Damasio 2003). Dopamine provided through these circuits provides incentive for the brain to act when something important is noticed. This incentive is likely to be provided without much input of conscious thought. Selection and intensity of arousal, based on the individual's personal history, usually occurs as an aspect of perception—how this individual perceives any given stimulus or situation at a given moment.

When an individual perceives a situation that for him or her appears potentially rewarding, the brain suddenly releases more dopamine into specific circuits. If no signals of possible frustration or danger contravene, signs of interest are likely to appear very quickly and the individual's actions are likely to move toward seeking the anticipated pleasure.

These mechanisms apply to basic rewards such as food, social interaction, and sexual pleasure. They also extend to perceived opportunities for fulfilling desires such as getting money, power, or social status. Eric Nestler and Robert Malenka (2004) have described the complicated processes by which this reward system can be disrupted by addiction. They have shown that an individual with a history of cocaine or heroin addiction, even after protracted abstinence from using the drug, is likely to demonstrate measurable levels of arousal simply in response to entering a neighborhood where he previously had purchased or used the drug. When anyone notices or is reminded of something that may bring them pleasure, arousal is likely to be mediated by rapid release of increased dopamine into relevant circuits, even without any conscious thought.

Dopamine plays an important role not only in signaling possible reward situations, but also in registering reward as it is being experienced. As the brain registers an ongoing experience of pleasure, it responds with a further release of dopamine that helps to sustain the rewarding action. The dual dopamine circuits play a critical role in mobilizing and sustaining effort to get what the individual wants or needs. These are crucial elements in the chemistry of motivation.

If dopamine is not released in these critical areas, the brain tends not to experience motivation to work, even for rewards that might otherwise be pleasurable. Roy Wise (1989) and other researchers have shown that in rats, monkeys, and humans, when effects of dopamine are blocked in specific areas of the brain, motivation and pleasure are also blocked. Blocking of dopamine release in specific areas of the brains of rats can cause them to give up working for food or for sexual pleasure. And damage to dopamine-producing cells in relevant areas of the human brain can eliminate cocaine addicts' craving for the drug. Dopamine does not itself produce the pleasure, but it creates the conditions under which sensations are recognized as pleasurable. Lacking anticipation or awareness of getting a "payoff," the organism, whether mouse, monkey, or human, tends quickly to abandon working and to ignore the task, even when the task may be essential to life (Wise and Rompre 1989).

The brain's reaction to the possibility of reward and to the threat of negative consequences like loss or punishment is subtle and complex. John O'Doherty and colleagues (2001) used imaging studies to show that the brain registers differing intensities of reward and punishment, even when the rewards and punishment are merely symbolic. They focused on a region in the front of the brain because previous studies had shown that damage there causes humans to lose normal sensitivity to rewards and punishment, whether potential or actual. When this area is damaged, even persons who were previously cautious tend to become reckless gamblers oblivious to negative consequences, ignoring information that would allow them to switch to more rewarding actions.

In the O'Doherty study, the brain activity of adults was imaged during repeated trials of a gambling game. On each trial they were to bet which of two stimuli was the "correct" one. If they chose the "correct" one, they were given a simulated money reward; the wrong choice caused them to lose (in simulation) a portion of their accumulated rewards. Images showed that one specific brain section increased activation when each reward was given while a different section increased activation in response to each punishment. Not only was activation observed in differing regions under these conditions, it was found to vary in intensity, proportional to the magnitude of each reward or punishment.

If the brain can so sensitively react to different levels of simulated rewards and punishment in a gambling game that participants knew in advance would yield no actual gain or loss of actual money, how much more does it react to the multiple rewards and punishments that are a part of daily life? This mechanism by which the brain registers subtle levels of reward and punishment is crucial in many aspects of human living. These circuits create shifting "equations for motivation" that guide operation of those executive functions that activate people to work, help them sustain effort, and coordinate their monitoring and self-regulation.

Mary Phillips and colleagues (2003a, 2003b) have described how working memory depends on these processes of emotional weighting not only to figure out what stimuli are important enough to remember and act on, but also to facilitate activation of memories from longer-term storage. Phillips showed that emotional significance plays an important role in culling memories related to specific tasks and situations as the individual moves more or less seamlessly from one situation to another. The brain's processes of assigning emotional importance are crucial elements underlying multiple executive functions.

Brain Centers That Regulate Alertness and "Fine-Tune" Cognition

At the back of the brain are circuits that play important roles in regulating alertness and fine-tuning cognitive processes. Systems of the brain that control motivation, memory, and so forth are linked to the brain's alertness and to cycles of wakefulness and sleep. Aspects of the warning system for potential danger continue to operate during sleep so that, for example, a person might awaken from slumber to the smell of smoke or a sudden, unfamiliar sound. Yet for the most part, executive functions depend on the person being awake and not overly tired. Most aspects of the brain's executive functions require the brain to be "open for business."

Regulation of the stages of sleep and alertness, or vigilance, is influenced primarily by two structures in the brain (Parasuraman et al. 1998). One is the reticular formation in the middle of the brainstem near the back of the head. This structure (shown in Figure 3) has widespread connections to receive and dispatch messages throughout the brain and spinal cord. Antonio Damasio has described the complex connections from this region:

> The structures of the reticular formation, traditionally linked to the control of sleep-wakefulness cycles and attention, are also linked to emotion and feeling, as well as to the representation of internal milieu and visceral states and autonomic control.
> (1999, p. 259)

Another structure critically important in regulation of sleep and wakefulness is the locus coeruleus, located near the reticular formation. This tiny structure is composed of two segments, each of which has about twelve thousand neurons that fan out throughout the brain. Its connections are more diffuse than in any other neural pathway, covering like a hairnet not only the whole cerebral cortex, but also the cortex of the cerebellum, the "mini-brain" near the back of the head. These connections extend into the spinal cord and down through the rest of the body, where they affect muscle tone.

Recordings from rats and monkeys show that neurons of the locus coeruleus are most activated by novel stimuli in the environment and are least active when the animals are just sitting around digesting a meal or asleep. In multiple ways these cells are involved in regulation of attention, arousal, and sleep-wake cycles as well as learning and memory, anxiety and pain, and mood and brain metabolism (Bear, Connors, and Paradiso 1996).

Norepinephrine is the primary neurotransmitter chemical in the reticular system and the locus coeruleus. When the locus coeruleus fires, it distributes norepinephrine through its broad network of connections, alerting and increasing excitability in its diffuse neural networks. Lack of such firing and reduced distribution of norepinephrine is associated with inattention, increased drowsiness, and sleep (Marrocco and Davidson 1998). Effective operation of the executive functions "activating for tasks" and "regulating alertness" depends on the functioning of the reticular system and locus coeruleus, among others. Figure 5 shows the origins of the norepinephrine system in the locus coeruleus and its projections to other areas of the brain.

The cerebellum, another structure at the back of the brain, is connected to the brainstem. It makes up only about 10 percent of the total brain volume, yet it contains about half of all the neurons in the central nervous system (Feldman, Meyer, and Quezner 1997). Until about twenty years ago, scientists saw the cerebellum as a mechanism involved only in "fine-tuning" complex movements of the body. Its extensive loops of connection with virtually every portion of the brain allow it to make ongoing comparisons between intended actions and actions in progress, so that needed adjustments can be made to facilitate smooth bodily execution of intended actions (Leiner, Leiner, and Dow 1989; Feldman, Meyer, and Quenzer 1997). Without these continuing readjustments, physical movements would be uncoordinated and "jerky," like those of characters in very early motion pictures.

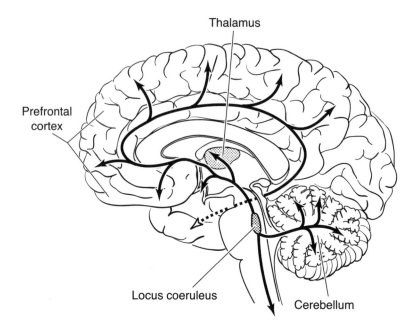

Figure 5 Main pathways of the norepinephrine system. Pathways for norepinephrine originate in the locus coeruleus and extend widely throughout the brain and down the spinal column. Norepinephrine initiates vigilance and sustains alertness; perhaps not surprisingly, sleep involves reduced levels of this transmitter chemical.

What has been recognized only in the past decade is that portions of the cerebellum provide similar "fine-tuning" for a wide variety of cognitive activities. Michael Posner and Marcus Raichle (1994) have demonstrated that the cerebellum plays an important role in selecting appropriate verbs to go with specific nouns. Antonio Damasio (2003) has reviewed research suggesting that portions of the cerebellum may also be involved in adjusting social behaviors, for example, laughing and crying, to specific situations. And Birgit Gottwald, with others (2003), has demonstrated that damage to specific areas of the cerebellum significantly impairs specific aspects of an individual's ability to divide attention between tasks and to utilize working memory. Apparently the cerebellum contributes to management of complex cognitive activities in a wide variety of ways.

Interacting Circuits Are Needed for Executive Functions

These various brain circuits that support executive functions do not work in isolation. For most tasks, their operations are closely linked and inter- dependent. For example, Jan de Fockert and others (2001) used imaging studies to demonstrate linkage of working memory with tasks of selective attention. Imaging by the labs of Helen Mayberg (1999) and Jean-Baptiste Pochon (2002) have demonstrated circuits in the brain that "gate" emo- tions. Florence Levy (2004) has explained the crucial role of dopamine in this gating process that allows most people to attenuate emotional reac- tions, such as anxiety or discouragement, when they are trying to deal with important concerns. Posner (1994) and Raichle did a series of imaging studies that showed linkages within the prefrontal cortex and with other brain regions; they found four different areas of the brain consistently lighting up when adults were asked to do simple verbal tasks.

All of the various circuits that support the brain's management func- tions repeatedly rearrange themselves in diverse connections as they deploy to manage constantly changing tasks and the brain's reactions to them. These multiple circuits integrate perceptions, assign importance, facili- tate memories, regulate alertness, and modulate emotion. They interact continuously to manage multiple events of daily life. These are the pri- mary neuronal networks that support executive functions.

The Development of Executive Functions in the Brain

These complex structures and neurochemical processes that facilitate ex- ecutive functions are not fully developed at birth. They are formed and gradually refined in a carefully timed sequence of events that begins early in fetal development, continues into infancy, and matures quite slowly throughout childhood and into adolescence and adulthood.

Although virtually all neurotransmitter systems are present in the cor- tex at birth, Francine Benes (2001) has shown that the systems for dopa- mine and norepinephrine are much slower to develop. These systems, crucial to executive functions, require much elaboration over the course of development, some of which continues at least into early adulthood and possibly beyond.

Another important but slowly evolving element is "myelination," the development of a protective surface coating that insulates the fibers that carry messages within the brain and elsewhere in the body. Myelin functions much as insulation around an electrical wire; it protects from "short circuits" and can enhance up to a hundredfold the speed with which messages can zip along the brain's networks, sometimes reaching transmission speeds of two hundred miles per hour. While most myelination of the human brain occurs before age two, the process continues well into the fourth decade of life. The more complex structures of the brain, those that exercise more central management functions, are not fully myelinated until considerably later than other brain structures that are less complex (Sampaio and Truwit 2001).

Although executive functions are slower to develop than many other aspects of brain function, foundations for their development are observable early in childhood. Adele Diamond and Colleen Taylor (1996) studied children three-and-a-half to seven years old who were asked to perform simple tasks that involved holding two pieces of information in mind at the same time while holding back or making a specific response. Results showed that between the ages of three-and-a-half and six years children improve significantly in their ability to hold two things in mind and in their ability to inhibit a strong response so that they can accomplish a task. Findings also showed that the older children were able to sustain their performance over more trials while many younger children who performed correctly at first were quick to give up following the directions. The foundation for executive functions is laid early, but full development of these linked abilities to regulate action, sustain attention, and modulate one's emotions takes many years.

Not all children of the same age are at the same point of development in their executive functions and not all reach the same point over the course of their overall development. The reasons for these differences, linked to aspects of the individual often referred to as "temperament," may rely on aspects of body chemistry that are variable across persons of the same age, though they tend to be relatively stable in any given individual across time.

In a similar manner, individuals differ in their inborn baseline levels of sensitivity to change and stress. Studies by Jerome Kagan and colleagues (1994, 2004) showed that in a sample of infants about 20 percent are born with a very low threshold for anxiety; they tend from the earliest months of life to respond with obvious distress and excessive behavioral inhibition when confronted with novel or stressful situations. These individuals are likely to be seen by others as exceptionally "sensitive" or "overly fearful" well into childhood and beyond. Work by Louis Schmidt and others (1999) indicates that these more socially reticent and anxious children tend to be less successful than age-mates at tasks requiring use of working memory and are more often off task. This may be due to these children being flooded with anxious emotions in ways that interfere with their attending to other stimuli and tasks.

In contrast, Nathan Fox and colleagues (2001) have reported on exuberant infants who are highly reactive and display positive emotions in response to novel situations and mild stress. These children are quicker to interact socially with others, are more active in exploring their environment, and show less fear in new situations. These temperamental characteristics, which are present in infancy and differ considerably from one individual to another, suggest what most parents of more than one child are quick to notice: infants seem to arrive in this world with neurochemical "wiring" that lays a foundation for how they respond to people and situations. Even within the same family, individual children can differ considerably along these dimensions. These individual differences in basic physiology, sensitivity to stress, intensity of engagement and of effort, and so on are likely to have considerable influence on the development of what will eventually become executive functions of the brain.

Environmental Influences on Executive Function Development

Development of the brain circuits that support executive functions is strongly influenced by genetic factors, but environmental factors also play an important role. Patterns of interaction between the developing infant and its caretakers actually influence the physical development of the neural networks.

Daniel Siegel (1999) described the pivotal role of interpersonal attachment in shaping neural networks throughout life, particularly during infancy and early childhood when the youngster is least able to regulate the intensity of his own emotions. When a parent or other caretaker responds to an infant's distress with soothing comfort, the disorganizing effects of the infant's stress are reduced and networks for self-calming are strengthened. In addition, when the caretaker echoes the infant's pleasurable reactions to daily events with warmth and enthusiasm, these more positive emotions are amplified and networks for pleasure are strengthened. Siegel refers to this emotional interaction of infant and caretaker as "attunement." He sees it as the foundation for the emotional attachment of the infant to caregivers.

Siegel argues that this process of attunement between infant and caregiver has a direct effect on the physical development of the infant's brain. He notes that those neural networks used most, especially in the earliest years, have the greatest probability of further development and subsequent use, whereas those less used are more likely to atrophy.

> The brain's development is an "experience-dependent" process, in which experience activates certain pathways in the brain, strengthening existing connections and creating new ones. Lack of experience can lead to cell death, called "pruning." . . . Genes contain the information for general organization of the brain's structure, but experience determines which genes become expressed, how and when. . . . Experience—the activation of specific neural pathways—therefore directly shapes gene expression and leads to the maintenance, creation and strengthening of the connections that form the neural substrate of the mind. (p. 14)

The experience of an infant during its first years of life is powerfully shaped by emotional exchanges with caretakers. Recurrent patterns of these interactions mold not only the content of the individual's experience, but also the structures of the brain within which subsequent experience will be processed and understood. Unlike a television that remains unchanged by the visual and auditory content displayed on its screen, the actual circuits of the infant's brain are shaped by the quality of the infant's early emotional experience.

When one or several caretakers for an infant closely monitors the child's emotional reactions, sharing in moments of pleasure and providing a buffer of comfort at times of distress (such as when the baby is hungry, cold, in pain, or overstimulated), this "attunement" can provide a structure of support and facilitate development of brain circuits more adequate for self-regulation. When such nurturing responses are relatively consistent over time, the infant is likely to form an attachment to that caretaker, who becomes a source of emotional security, a "secure base" from which the growing child can gradually learn to move into the wider world.

When caretakers do not provide a reasonably secure base for attachment, when they are excessively distant, inconsistent, rejecting, or disorganized, the growing child is likely still to become attached to the caretaker, but that child's subsequent development, especially in interpersonal interactions, is more likely to be avoidant, highly ambivalent, or disorganized. These less-secure attachments, for better and for worse, provide not only the foundation for mental models, crystallized sets of default assumptions about self and others, but also a complex set of neural networks less adequate for self-regulation.

Mary Ainsworth and colleagues (1978), as well as subsequent researchers, have found that different patterns of attachment observed at age one year are associated with varying styles of peer relationships, emotional maturity, academic performance, and capacities for self-regulation in adolescence. According to Siegel, these behavioral patterns develop from those neural networks preferentially developed in the brain during the earliest years of development. Siegel (1999) noted that an individual's patterns for attachment are not inalterably established during the first year; they may be improved or damaged by subsequent life experiences. This process continues throughout childhood and into adolescence, a time when a massive surge of brain development occurs along with rapid changes in the maturing child's social outlook.

Executive Functions and Adolescence

Adolescence is a time of dramatic changes in brain development, many of which are likely to have a significant influence on the individual's executive functions. Jay Giedd and others (Giedd, Snell, et al. 1996; Giedd, Blumenthal, et al. 1999) conducted imaging studies of the brains of teenagers, taking MRI images of each teenager's brain at six different times during adolescence. He found a pattern in early adolescence, around puberty, where brain volume rapidly increased, with a massive jump in the size and number of neural networks, particularly in the frontal lobes and in the cerebellum, two regions particularly important for executive functions. Subsequent images of the each individual's brain showed a pattern where this rapid proliferation of brain cells was followed by a period of rapid pruning of neural networks, allowing far more efficient operation of the overall system.

This rapid, massive growth and pruning of the brain during adolescence is accompanied by equally massive increases in the myelination of brain cells during the same period of development. Frances Benes (1994) has demonstrated that myelin increases by 100 percent during the teenage years, particularly in connections important for integrating emotional reactions with cognitive processes that involve accessing stored memories. Benes has suggested that as these connections are developed more fully during adolescence, the teenager may become less impulsive and better able to integrate feelings with important memories and thought processes.

The corpus callosum, the structure that connects and integrates operations in the brain's two hemispheres, is another region that has been found to undergo a burst of increased myelination during early adolescence. Paul Thompson and colleagues (2000) have shown that this adolescent increase in myelination of the corpus callosum improves connections between areas crucial for both the more complex, emotionally sensitive use of language and for logical thinking.

Taken together, these recent findings of widespread advances in development of the brain during adolescence—large increases in brain volume followed by greatly increased pruning of neural networks and dramatically accelerated rates of myelination—provide substantial evidence that the circuits that support executive functions of the human brain are not fully developed until after puberty. This is consistent with cultural expectations that defer until some time after puberty those important responsibilities that require mature executive functions—for example, driving a car, managing one's own finances, making contracts, and achieving more freedom from parental control.

The Decline of Executive Functions in Later Years

Once developed, executive functions do not remain static over the lifetime. They may be refined further during early and middle adult years, and in later adulthood, for many, they begin to decline. Monica Fabiani and Emily Wee (2001) have shown that impairment in frontal lobe functioning is characteristic of elderly adults on many cognitive tasks, especially those involving working memory; but they emphasize that individual differences tend to increase with age. Lifestyle, general health, and other factors greatly contribute to the effects of age on executive functions.

Although there is considerable variability among elderly persons in the quality of their cognitive functioning, many manifest impairments in working memory as they age, even without any disease processes or dementias. Some suggest that the increasing inefficiency of working memory in the elderly is due to specific impairments in memory; other researchers, for example, Timothy Salthouse (1991), suggest that the apparent memory problem is really a result of a more generalized slowing of information processing functions.

In contrast, Michael Milham and others (2002) demonstrated that the problems of working memory in the elderly result from impairments in the brain's mechanisms for controlling attention. These researchers used imaging studies to compare attentional control in younger (21- to 27-year-old) versus older (60- to 75-year-old) people during a task requiring careful attention. Results suggested that aging compromises the brain's ability to exercise attentional control, allowing excessive distractibility and causing decreasing efficiency in working memory.

This decline in working memory that often occurs in later years is not necessarily global. Robert West and colleagues (2002) compared young adults (ages nineteen to twenty-nine) with older adults (ages sixty-five to eighty-three) on repeated administrations of a working memory task that was adjusted for low demand and higher demand. West found that young and older groups did equally well on the memory task when there was little demand on executive functions. As the need for use of executive functions increased, however, requiring one to hold one item in mind while checking others, members of the older group showed much greater variability in their performance. Sometimes they got it; often they did not.

For many, then, normal aging causes an increasing impairment of executive functions, for example, working memory, sustained attention, and processing speed. Practice of the specific skills can reduce some of the impairment, and individuals with higher intelligence tend to show less of a falloff overall. Nevertheless, multiple studies argue that these impairments are due to an age-related decline in the functional integrity of the prefrontal cortex, where many executive functions are localized.

One cause of the decline of this region is thought to be an age-related weakening of the brain's dopamine system. Lars Backman and colleagues (2000) used imaging to demonstrate that age-related reductions in the brain's transmission of dopamine play an important role in age-related decline on cognitive tests. Nora Volkow and others (2000) have shown that even healthy older persons tend to suffer age-related losses of dopamine receptors in areas of the brain (for example, the prefrontal cortex and cingulate shown in Figure 3) that are crucial for executive functions, though similar declines were not found in some other regions of the brain less involved with executive functions. She found that individuals tend to lose about 5 percent of their dopamine receptors during each decade of life. Apparently networks that support executive functions are not only slower to develop than other brain networks; they also tend to suffer an earlier decline.

Only a Glimpse: The Complexity of the Human Brain

This chapter provides just a tiny sample of the complexity of the variegated structures and chemical functions that flexibly, often creatively, manage the ongoing functions of the human brain. The massive scope of the brain's ability to make connections within itself boggles the mind. Paul

Churchland (1995) described the staggering range of possible ways in which the brain's synaptic connections can be arranged and rearranged, moment by moment. He notes that the 100 billion neurons of the brain form over 100 trillion synaptic connections with one another, each of which can vary in intensity from very weak to very strong. Each individual's unique and changing configuration of these vast and intricate networks of 100 trillion connections determines how that person's brain

> reacts to the sensory information it receives, how it responds to the emotional states it encounters, and how it plots its future behavior. We already know how many different Bridge hands can be dealt from a standard deck of merely 52 playing cards. . . . Think how many more "hands" might be dealt from the brain's much larger "deck" of 100 trillion modifiable synaptic connections.
>
> If we assume, conservatively, that each synaptic connection might have any one of ten different strengths, then the total number of distinct possible configurations that the brain might assume is, very roughly, ten raised to the 100 trillionth power, or $10^{100,\,000,000,000,000}$. (p. 5)

The amazing capacities of the human brain to operate with such wide variability are all the more incredible when one considers that no two brains are exactly alike. Gerald Edelman and Giulio Tononi (2000) have emphasized how each brain is much more flexible in its capacities, and more individualized than the most advanced computer ever made.

> Each individual's brain is continually changing. Variations extend over all levels of brain organization, from biochemistry to gross morphology, and the strengths of myriad individual synapses are constantly altered by experience. The extent of this enormous variability argues strongly against the notion that the brain is organized like a computer with fixed codes and registers. (p. 81)

We are just beginning to learn about the brain mechanisms that support executive functions across the lifespan.

Executive Networks Differ in Those with ADHD

The complex cognitive processes I have described thus far are not specific to persons with ADD syndrome; these structures and neurochemicals manage brain functions in all of us. Over recent years researchers have begun to accumulate evidence, especially from brain imaging studies, of some differences in brain development and functioning in those who suffer from ADD syndrome.

One of the earliest studies of differences in brain functioning of persons with ADHD was provided in 1990 by Alan Zametkin and colleagues. They used imaging to compare levels of chemical activity in the brains of adults with and without a history of hyperactivity since childhood. Results indicated that when adults with ADHD did a task that required sustained concentration, they demonstrated a lower rate of chemical activity, both globally and in specific regions of the brain, than did normal controls. Brains of those with ADHD were less "turned on" while doing the concentration task than were the matched controls.

Monique Ernst and others (1999) did an imaging study that compared brains of children with ADHD to normal controls. These images showed that children with ADHD had an abnormality in the processing of dopamine in their midbrain regions. Sarah Durston (2003) used a different imaging method to study self-control systems in children with ADHD compared to normal children. While in the scanner, each child was asked to press a button each time a particular Pokémon cartoon character appeared on a screen and to avoid pushing the button each time another Pokémon character appeared. Children with ADHD had great difficulty in holding back their button press in the "avoid pushing" situation if it was preceded by even just one "push" signal. The brain scans showed that while doing this task children with ADHD also showed a more immature pattern of brain activation; their brain activity was more characteristic of patterns in younger children.

Imaging studies have also shown that many with ADHD use different, less efficient circuits of the brain to do certain cognitive tasks. George Bush and colleagues (1999) observed brain activity in a specific area, the anterior cingulate (shown in Figure 3), in adults with ADHD while they were doing a simple task that required resolving conflicting information. When the brain activity of the ADHD adults on this task was compared with that of a matched sample of non-ADHD adults, there was a significant difference when distracters were present. Non-ADHD adults showed significant activation of the anterior cingulate region most persons use for resolving such conflicts. By contrast, those with ADHD showed almost no activation anywhere in the anterior cingulate when confronted with distracters while doing this task; instead, totally separate circuits were employed and the result was a significantly slower response. It is as though the ADHD adults, when they were being distracted, had to use a slower, detour circuit to accomplish the task.

Ernst and others (2003) showed another difference between the brain functioning of individuals with ADHD and those without. They used imaging scans to observe brains of adults with ADHD and age-matched healthy volunteers as they were making decisions about the relative importance of alternative rewards. These adults were asked to make a series of choices that involved weighing short-term gains against long-term losses. Results showed that while both groups utilized similar regions of the prefrontal cortex for making the decisions, the brains of the ADHD adults were markedly less active in regions that facilitate evaluation of the emotional attributes of stimuli. The researchers suggested that cognitive deficits in ADHD adults might interfere with their "coding of motivation," that is, their ability to assess the relative importance of one object or situation over another.

Although there are currently only a few relevant imaging studies, their results thus far suggest that there are demonstrable differences in the functioning of executive function brain circuits between persons with and without ADD syndrome. As imaging technology and understanding of this disorder improve, more refined studies should become possible. Meanwhile, however, the response of persons with ADHD to specific medications has been consistently demonstrated in many studies.

Chemicals That Alleviate Impairments of ADD Syndrome
Since Dr. Charles Bradley's accidental discovery in 1937 of the benefits of stimulants for hyperactivity, discussed earlier, there have been over two

hundred scientifically controlled research studies consistently indicating that 70 to 80 percent of persons with ADHD show significantly less impairment from their ADHD symptoms when they are treated with appropriate doses of specific medications. The improvements produced by these medications cure nothing; impairments return to baseline levels immediately after the medication wears off. Moreover, not all medications have this effect; only those that facilitate the release of and/or slow the reloading of dopamine, norepinephrine, or both at the synapses are helpful.

Virtually all of the important circuit centers in neural networks for executive functions operate primarily on one of these two neurotransmitter chemicals: dopamine or norepinephrine. These particular transmitter chemicals are not equally distributed throughout the brain; they are heavily concentrated in areas of brain discussed here as important to executive functions.

Research suggests that persons diagnosed with ADHD manufacture dopamine and norepinephrine in their brains just as everyone else does. The primary problem seems to be that their brains simply do not release and reload these neurotransmitters, dopamine and norepinephrine, effectively in areas crucial for executive functions. At these junctions not enough transmitter is released or the amount released is too quickly reloaded, taken back into the sending cell, before the message is fully carried across. As a result, many messages that need to get carried along these management networks are not consistently transmitted in an adequate and timely way.

These medications allow the two crucial neurotransmitters, dopamine and norepinephrine, to be more available in the hundreds of thousands of synaptic junctions where and when they are needed for the central management functions of the brain. Medications for ADD do not create the dopamine or norepinephrine, and they do not increase the overall amount of these transmitter chemicals in the brain, as a chef might put more salt in the soup. Instead, at countless junctures of the management networks, these medications facilitate the release and slow the reuptake of these two critically important transmitter chemicals, sequentially unlocking a series of chemical gates so that transmission along these crucially important circuits can be facilitated.

After administration of such medications, dramatic increases in chemical activity can be observed in images of the prefrontal cortex, specific subcortical regions, and the cerebellum, important centers for management functions of the brain (Volkow, Wang, et al. 1997; Voeller 2001; Anderson, Polcari, et al. 2002). And these changes last only as long as the medication is on board, thus confirming self-reports and observations of persons with ADHD.

The results from these many medication studies clearly indicate that ADD syndrome is essentially a chemical problem, specifically an impairment in the chemical system that supports rapid and efficient communication in the brain's management system. Just as diabetes is a disease that reflects impairments in the body's processing of insulin, ADD syndrome is a disorder that reflects impairments in the brain's processing of dopamine and norepinephrine. I discuss implications of these findings for the treatment of ADD syndrome in Chapter 9.

At this point, we know that the structures and physiological processes of the brain that develop and sustain executive functions are vast, subtle, and amazingly complex. It is also clear that these structures and functions develop rather slowly compared to other aspects of the brain, and that in most cases they gradually decline in efficiency as individuals approach old age. The next three chapters describe the interplay of developing executive functions and the changing demands of development and daily life during childhood, adolescence, and adulthood.

Chapter 4   Childhood: Struggling with Self-Management

MYTH: ADD is simply a label for behavior problems; children with ADD just refuse to sit still and are unwilling to listen to teachers or parents.

FACT: Many with ADD have few behavior problems. Chronic inattention symptoms cause more severe and longer-lasting problems for learning and relationships for those with ADD.

Many, but not all, who suffer from ADD syndrome have noticeable problems during childhood. The child with ADD syndrome often needs much more assistance and many more directions or reminders to behave appropriately and to accomplish tasks readily managed by most children of the same age. Parents and others become progressively puzzled and frustrated as the child lags ever further behind in learning to manage daily routines and interactions.

More than a specific skill is involved; the child tends to have trouble with many aspects of self-management. Because children vary widely in their speed of development, it is sometimes not clear whether a child is just a bit slower developmentally or significantly impaired. At first, the child just doesn't seem able to understand and to do what is generally expected of children that age, or may show extraordinary inconsistency in behavior. For a time, concerned adults may assume that this particular child just needs a little longer to mature before he or she will master these tasks.

For children with ADD syndrome, the delay is often very protracted and the difference from expected development becomes increasingly worrisome. But for a small percentage of children eventually diagnosed with

ADD syndrome, problems emerge very early in development, when young children are expected to show only the most basic elements of self-control.

Behaving Carefully

As a result of their impulsive and hyperactive behavior, children with ADD syndrome tend to get injured more often than most others of the same age. Stephen Hinshaw (2002a) reviewed studies of accidental injuries in children diagnosed with ADHD. There are strong indications that accidental poisonings, broken limbs, head injuries, and other accidents requiring hospitalization occur at much higher rates among children with ADHD compared with others of the same age. Benjamin Lahey and colleagues (1998) reported that these elevated injury rates apply to young children aged four to six years, as well as older children, who meet the diagnostic criteria for ADHD. One mother described her difficulties in keeping her daughter safe:

> Our daughter is only four years old and she has been impossible for us to control ever since she started to walk. I've had to quit my job so I can stay home to take care of her because she has been kicked out of three day care programs for being uncontrollable and too aggressive with other children and staff. We try to get relatives or babysitters to take care of her, but none of them will ever come back for a second time; she is just too much for them to handle. She has to be watched every minute or she could do something that could really hurt her or do some serious damage.
>
> Last week while I was in the bathroom for just a few minutes she went into my purse and took the car keys. She went out and unlocked our car that was parked in the driveway. She got in and stood up behind the steering wheel, got it started, put it into gear, and drove it through the garage door. She wasn't hurt, but she could have been killed! And repairs on the car and replacing the garage door are not going to be cheap. Regardless of how much we try to teach her how to be careful, she doesn't understand.

Fortunately, not many children with ADD syndrome are so dangerously out of control as this preschool girl. Her difficulties illustrate an extreme variant of frustrations and risks encountered by parents of young children with early onset ADD syndrome.

More common are children who are far more restless and reckless than average. Even when most other children of the same age can generally be relied on to wait a moment for help from an adult or to heed a warning, some children with ADD syndrome are chronically too quick to grab things that may be dangerously hot or sharp, unwilling to wait for help in crossing a busy street, or determined to climb into dangerously high places. They are extremely impulsive and resistant to adult control. Regardless of how many times they are cautioned and shown how to "be careful," these hyperactive and impulsive children move too fast and too heedlessly, sometimes at considerable risk.

Far more than most others of comparable age, these children depend on parents, older siblings, teachers, and other caregivers to protect them with constant vigilance and quick responses. Those who care for such children need to be on high alert, always trying to anticipate and protect against whatever dangerous move the child might try next. Compensating for the inability of these children to be careful is a demanding and exhausting responsibility—and one that babysitters, grandparents, and other adults who might otherwise assist with childcare are understandably reluctant to share.

Cooperating with Adults and Peers

Injury to children from ADD syndrome is not limited to the physical. Many who are careful enough to avoid breaking their bones or being jolted from placing metal into an electrical socket behave chronically in ways that can provoke frustrated and angry reactions from peers, siblings, teachers, and parents. These children's problematic behavior can cause serious damage to relationships and sometimes elicits hostile or abusive treatment. One mother described the pressures of caring for her son:

> My eight-year-old, Joey, is not a bad kid; often he is charming
> and funny. But he really is a handful for everyday stuff! Every

night, bedtime is a nightmare for at least an hour or two. Joey never feels tired and is always arguing to stay up. Even when he is really tired, it's tough to get him to quit whatever he is doing, to get him in pj's and into bed. He gets loud and stirs up the little ones. In the morning he gets up okay, but he is incredibly slow about getting himself dressed and ready for school. I set out his clothes and ask him to get dressed while I'm dressing myself and my two younger kids, so we can get out too. But if I don't stay on Joey constantly, talking him through every step of the morning routine, he'll never make his bus. His five-year-old brother is more independent!

Joey always gets involved in playing with his transformer toys and forgets what he is supposed to be doing. He'll still be sitting on the floor in just his underpants with one sock on when he needs to be walking out the door to catch his bus. Then when he finally hears me telling him it's too late, he gets upset, crying and blaming everyone else because he's going to miss his bus. It's the same routine every day! We've tried star charts and all kinds of rewards and punishments. He just hasn't learned how to be careful about time and getting things done so he won't make all of us late.

Doing this every morning and every night with him is exhausting, especially for a single parent like me. I never get any rest. And more than that, he's made me late to work so many times that I've gotten two warnings. I'm worried that I might get fired because of this. I can't afford to have that happen.

Joey's mother's feeling of exhaustion from her struggles with her son at the beginning of most every day is shared by many parents of young children with ADD syndrome, especially those who must manage child-rearing tasks alone. Preparing breakfast and lunches, as well as waking, feeding, dressing, and launching several children and oneself each morning—under pressure of tight deadlines for school buses and getting off to one's own job—is stressful enough when children cooperate, but when

one or more of the children frequently becomes sidetracked and is uncooperative, frustration can become intense and tempers can flare.

For many parents like Joey's mother, these challenges are repeated at
the end of each day when the parent and children return home tired and
hungry, all with very low thresholds for frustration. From late afternoon to
bedtime the parent may often be forced to fight recurrent brushfires of
conflict among siblings while trying to monitor the activities of each child,
initiate and supervise completion of homework, prepare and clean up
after dinner, spend some "quality time" with the kids, and get everyone
bathed, into pajamas, and settled into bed while doing housework like
laundry.

Provocative Oppositional Behavior

Some children with ADD syndrome are not only uncooperative; they are
intensely oppositional—often mouthy, argumentative, and extremely demanding. Many are quick to mount a protracted temper tantrum if, say,
they are not allowed to eat what they want when they want it, to watch a
particular program on television even if it is their sister's turn to choose,
or to play a video game on the family computer even though an older
brother is using it for a homework assignment.

Some of these children are also outrageously presumptuous and
brazen with parents and siblings alike, acting as though their every wish
must immediately be fulfilled. For any parent, coping every morning and
every evening with the emotional intensity of frequent, protracted temper
tantrums, as well as whining or recurrent and intense sibling battles, all
while struggling to accomplish necessary tasks and daily routines, would
be an extreme challenge; for some parents it is totally unmanageable.

Some readers, when learning about such difficulties in eliciting cooperation from children, might argue that more effective parenting strategies are needed. It is true that some parents, especially those who are very
inexperienced and highly stressed in many areas of life, have never
learned how to effectively guide their children. Often their efforts to direct
and intervene unwittingly throw gasoline on the fire. But there are many
parents of children with ADD syndrome, some of whom have successfully

raised other children, who have worked very hard with multiple strategies to elicit cooperation from their child, only to find that even carefully executed advice from experts fails to help.

Regardless of the reasons for such problems, chronic and severe lack of cooperation between parents and children can cause serious difficulties for the child as well as for parents and other members of the family. George DuPaul and others (2001) studied a group of children aged three to five years, some of whom had been diagnosed with ADHD (the others were a comparison group of normal children). Direct observations were made of these children in a play situation where the parent was asked to help the child do a task, and in a situation where the parent was asked to have the child pick up toys in a playroom.

Children with ADHD exhibited more than twice the level of noncompliance and greater than five times the level of inappropriate behavior displayed by the normal comparison children when asked by their parents to complete the assigned tasks. When parents in both groups were queried about the level of stress they routinely experience in dealing with their children, parents of the ADHD children reported higher levels of chronic stress than 83 percent of the other parents; there was a very large difference (two standard deviations) between scores for their reports and those of parents of non-ADHD children.

In this study observers noted that parents of children with ADHD tended to behave in a more negative way toward their children than did parents of children who did not have ADHD. It is difficult to know how much of their more negative interaction was due to their daily frustration in trying to get their children to cooperate, possibly exacerbated by the demands of being observed. Alternatively it is possible that some of these parents tend generally to be impatient and irritable, and had been very negative and controlling with their young children from their earliest days. In that case, the child's lack of cooperation might be a reaction to the parent's problematic temperament or parenting style.

DuPaul's study demonstrated that these preschool children with ADHD were much less cooperative not only with their parents, but also with their peers and teachers. When observed in a free-play situation in their preschool classrooms, these young ADHD children exhibited very significantly higher levels (three standard deviations) of negative social behavior with their peers. Teachers rated the ADHD children as having markedly lower levels of social cooperation and markedly higher levels of behavior problems, as well as elevated levels of inattention, hyperactivity, and impulsivity.

The problems that young ADHD children have with peers are important. Susan Campbell (2002) has emphasized that despite the importance of family life in shaping a child's ability to deal with other people,

> It is also clear that children learn much about the rules of social exchange in the peer group. Turn-taking, sharing, control of aggression, empathy, helping, sex-role learning, role taking, strategies of conflict resolution and moral reasoning all develop within the peer group as well as within the family, and appear to be central components of the ability to establish reciprocal friendships and maintain relationships with others in the larger peer group. (p. 177)

In her long-term research on hard-to-manage preschoolers, Campbell found that children with early behavior problems at home varied considerably in the quality of their relationships with peers. Some wanted to play with others, but were too aggressive and too forcefully dominating of other children while playing; this resulted in their being actively avoided by peers. Others who had considerable difficulty at home were able to function in age-appropriate ways with other children; they derived considerable pleasure and support from being with peers. Still others, though oppositional and hard to manage at home, were unassertive and wary of other children. As a result, they isolated themselves, and because they avoided peer contacts, they developed lower peer competence and continuing reticence with other children.

Campbell (2002) found that children who showed severe peer problems at ages two to three years, and had peer relationships that worsened with development, tended to have significantly poorer outcomes six to seven years later. She noted that "early peer problems may be interpreted as contributing, in a sort of snowball effect, to the persistence of general difficulties at school and at home" (p. 198).

One mother described her worry about the peer relationships of her daughter with ADD syndrome:

> Our daughter is ten years old now. Her ADHD didn't get diagnosed until she was in third grade, probably because she is pretty smart and not really a big troublemaker for the teachers. She does okay with most of her schoolwork because it hasn't started to get very challenging yet, but she's had trouble in getting along with other kids and in making and keeping friends ever since she was in preschool.
>
> Lots of kids just don't like her. It breaks my heart to see how disappointed she gets when all the other girls get invitations to one another's birthday parties and she is never invited. Once in a while I can get another girl's mother to have her daughter come over for a playdate, but most of them don't want to come back a second time and they never seem to reciprocate. I think my daughter just isn't very good at joining in with them in the things they like to do. She gets too bossy and doesn't know how to cooperate with other kids her age.

Darna Blachman and Stephen Hinshaw (2002) studied girls with ADHD aged six to twelve years during summer camp programs. They found that even in the camp situation, where they could make a fresh start with peers they had not previously known, girls with ADHD developed fewer friendships than girls without ADHD. They were more likely to be disliked and have no friends, and less likely to have more than one friend than were girls without ADHD. Social problems of these ADHD girls seemed to result from their tendency to be intrusive and noncompliant. Some were able to attract friends initially, but then had great difficulty in maintaining the engagement, focus, and persistence needed to develop friendships at camp.

Boys who suffer from this disorder also tend to experience elevated levels of rejection from their peers. Sharon Melnick and Stephen Hinshaw (1996) studied six- to twelve-year-old boys with ADHD in comparison to age-mates without ADHD, all of whom were participating in a summer camp program. They used ratings from adult observers, self-ratings, and friendship choice ratings by the groups of boys to assess how much each boy was liked by the others and what behaviors were associated with more or less group acceptance. They found that many ADHD boys were rejected quickly by the group because of excessive aggression, pushing too much to get attention for themselves, and not sharing their peers' concerns for fairness.

In a similar summer camp study, Drew Erhardt and Stephen Hinshaw (1994) demonstrated that boys with ADHD were rejected very quickly by their peers. Their negative status in the peer group was quick to form; they were rejected on the first day of camp, four times faster than comparison boys. And this negative peer status persisted, for most, until the end of the camp session weeks later.

These data suggest that both boys and girls with ADHD tend to have significant problems in cooperating with peers just as they tend to have significant impairments in cooperating with their parents and other adults. Some might consider this simply a problem of misbehavior, but, as I discuss later, these behavioral problems may be complicated, if not caused, by less obvious problems with language development and/or impairments of executive functions.

Communicating Effectively with Others

One important aspect of cooperating with others is learning to communicate effectively. This reciprocal process involves far more than simply understanding the meanings of specific words that are heard and stringing words together in an appropriate way to speak to others. Careful examination of the processes involved in interpersonal communication shows it to be a complex interaction that often places heavy demands on the executive functions impaired in individuals with ADHD.

> Our son, Phil, is now twelve years old. We have always thought
> of him as a really difficult child to raise. From his preschool
> years he has always been stubborn. We've always had trouble

getting him to follow directions at home. And his teachers have complained that he doesn't listen or follow directions at school. He's always been quick to get into arguments with family members and with other kids; sometimes the fights actually get physical. And when he gets into arguments he often just keeps repeating himself and doesn't really listen to what the other person is trying to say.

Last month we found out from a school evaluation that Phil has ADHD and a pretty serious language problem that none of us had ever recognized. The school did a comprehensive evaluation that included assessment by a speech and language specialist. She gave Phil some tests and found out that he has serious problems with both receptive and expressive language. We always noticed that he often jumps to wrong conclusions and sometimes didn't say things quite right, but we never realized that he often doesn't really understand what others are saying and often can't come up with the right words to say what he is thinking or feeling.

Unrecognized language problems are not uncommon. Nancy Cohen (1996) and Cohen and colleagues (1993, 1996) studied a group of children aged four to twelve years who had been referred for psychiatric outpatient treatment for a variety of behavioral and emotional problems. They evaluated language development in the entire group and found that 62 percent of those children who had emotional and/or behavioral problems met diagnostic criteria for language impairment. In the general population of school-aged children, only about 3 percent have such deficits.

There are two basic categories of language disorders: understanding what others are trying to communicate (receptive language) and expressing one's own thoughts and feelings (expressive language). While these basic problems in language processing are not usually seen as a component of the ADD syndrome, they are present in a disproportionately high percentage of children with this disorder. This increased incidence is likely to be due to the heavy demands of interpersonal communication on executive functions.

In addition to basic problems in receptive and expressive language, speech and language specialists also check for "pragmatic deficits." These involve problems in using language appropriately within social situations— to join a conversation, to clarify or correct misunderstandings, and so on. Pragmatics also involves many nonverbal aspects, for example, facial expressions, tone of voice, body language, as well as use of words.

Rosemary Tannock and Russell Schachar (1996) reviewed studies that compared children with ADHD to normal children in their use of pragmatics. They found multiple studies indicating that ADHD children tend to exhibit:

> excessive verbal output during spontaneous conversations . . .
>
> decreased verbal output . . . when confronted with tasks which require planning and organization of verbal responses, as in story retelling or giving directions . . .
>
> difficulties in introducing, maintaining and changing topics appropriately and in negotiating smooth interchanges or turn-taking during conversation
>
> problems in being specific, accurate and concise in selection and use of words to convey information
>
> difficulties in adjusting language to the listener and specific contexts. (p. 139)

ADHD children often have combined problems in listening, speaking, and pragmatics. Each of these communication activities involves executive functions. Listening is not a simple or passive skill. It involves actively receiving and organizing verbal and nonverbal information: words spoken, tone of voice, facial expressions, and gestures presented by the speaker. Listening also involves grasping elements of the other's message that are implicit, or that refer to facts or experiences linked only indirectly to the present moment or topic. Also involved are processes of "putting the pieces together" to understand what the other person is saying, sorting out the important facts, ideas, and feelings, as well as monitoring the interpersonal interaction. These tasks all involve use of executive functions.

Speaking involves actively choosing words, assembling the words in phrases and sentences, speaking them at a rate, volume, and tone that others can grasp, and utilizing facial expressions and gestures to emphasize or clarify meaning—all while monitoring one's output for accuracy and coherence (Am I saying what I mean in a way that the other person will "get it"?). Simultaneously the speaker needs to monitor reactions of the listener for clues about whether one's message is being received and accurately understood. When it appears that the listener is not attending, has not heard, is puzzled, has misunderstood, or is reacting in another unwanted way, the speaker usually needs to stop and try to find ways to gain, or regain, the listener's attention and understanding. Executive functions are involved in many aspects of communication.

Karen Purvis and Rosemary Tannock (1997) studied story retelling abilities of seven- to eleven-year-old children with ADHD and compared both (1) to children diagnosed with reading disorders (including some who also had ADHD) and (2) to children who had neither ADHD nor a reading disorder. Each of these children was asked to listen to a story that continued for three minutes and involved multiple characters and a detailed series of events. Immediately after hearing this narrative, the child was asked to recall and retell the story.

Children with ADHD made significantly more errors in organizing their stories, in accurately retelling story details, and in correctly reporting the sequence of events in the story. ADHD children also had a higher incidence of ambiguous references and other failures to take into account the needs of their listener. Purvis and Tannock concluded that these problems of the ADHD children in understanding and retelling the story were due not primarily to language impairments, but to difficulties with their executive functions: the processes that mobilize attention and help one organize and monitor information both coming in and remembered.

Impairments of communication in children with ADHD often are not recognized in the way that behavioral problems are, but they can be a powerfully damaging manifestation of executive function impairments. These impairments can create many difficulties in a child's efforts to communicate effectively with peers as well as with adults, with family and playmates as well as with teachers and others less familiar. And when effective communication fails, misunderstandings often arise and conflicts between persons tend to escalate.

Learning to Read and Write

Reading and writing are additional modes of communication that become increasingly important from early childhood on. Both of these involve considerable work to develop needed skills. One mother described problems in motivating her son to work at learning.

> Our son Wally is a very bright boy, but he just won't work in school. When they do things that interest him, he will join in the conversation and contribute some good ideas, but he has never had any patience for when the teachers or assignments are boring. His father and I think the problem is that he is so bright. Most of the teachers are not very inspiring and a lot of the work they assign is a waste of time.
>
> Wally is in sixth grade now and he doesn't get many good grades on his report card. He is just not a worker. In class he spends a lot of time daydreaming and drawing cartoon characters or racing cars. At home he spends hours every day surfing the internet and concentrating on video games, but we just can't get him to work in school. His teacher says he just doesn't seem motivated. We are starting to wonder how we can get him to work on things that he really needs to do.

This mother is beginning to realize that her twelve-year-old son will have significant problems if he doesn't learn soon to work on school tasks, even when they are not very interesting to him. He may be very intelligent and she may be right that his teachers are not very inspiring and that they give him a lot of boring work, but this boy is currently lacking a willingness to *work at learning* content and skills set before him by others.

In the field studies used to develop the *DSM-IV* diagnostic criteria for ADHD, one survey item was "Seems unmotivated to do schoolwork or homework." This descriptor fit many children with ADHD, but it was not ultimately included in the published diagnostic criteria, presumably because of a concern that the cause of the motivation problem might be misunderstood as a simple obstinance. Yet motivation to work is a major problem for many who suffer from ADD syndrome.

Over three decades ago, Erik Erikson (1968) wrote about the importance of children developing the capacity to work at learning the skills they need to get along in life.

> When they reach school age, children in all cultures receive some systematic instruction. While all children at times need to be left alone in solitary play and . . . hours and days of make-believe in games, they all, sooner or later become dissatisfied and disgruntled without a sense of being able to make things and make them well and even perfectly. It is this that I have called the *sense of industry* . . .
>
> [The child] learns to win recognition by producing things. He develops perseverance and adjusts himself to . . . become an eager and absorbed unit of a productive situation. The danger at this stage is the development of an estrangement from himself and his tasks . . . the sense of inferiority . . .
>
> Children at this age like to be mildly but firmly coerced into the adventure of finding out that one can learn to accomplish things which one would never have thought of oneself, things which owe their attractiveness to the very fact that they are not the product of play and fantasy but the product of reality, practicality, and logic; things which thus provide a token sense of participation in the real world of adults. (pp. 123–127)

Erikson's point here is that it is important for children to be helped to develop skills and attitudes that can lead to productive work. He noted that in literate societies, where careers are more specialized, each child needs first to be given a basic education that will prepare him or her for a wide range of possible careers. This education is likely to involve activities and skills that the child would not spontaneously choose for pleasure, though the child may find pleasure in mastering the skills at progressing levels of difficulty. But useful skills alone are not enough. Erikson emphasizes also the importance to the child of developing a work ethic, "a sense of industry," an ability "to win recognition by producing things," an idea of "the pleasure of work completion by steady attention and persevering diligence" (p. 259).

Studies have shown that many persons with ADD syndrome have considerable difficulty developing this "pleasure of work completion by steady attention and persevering diligence." Because of their chronic problems with executive functions, individuals with ADD syndrome are at high risk for chronic academic underachievement and school failure.

Stephen Faraone and others (1996) compared children aged six to seventeen years diagnosed with ADHD to normal controls. Results indicated that at some point in their schooling, 56 percent of the ADHD children had needed academic tutoring, 30 percent had repeated a grade, and 35 percent had been placed in a special class. Comparable numbers for normal controls were much lower: 25 percent had received academic tutoring, 13 percent had repeated a grade, and 2 percent had been placed in a special class.

Inattention Interferes with Learning to Read and Do Math

Such high rates of academic underachievement and failure among children with ADHD may result from a number of causes, one of which is likely to be chronic inattention. David Rabiner and colleagues (2000) reported on a large study of children monitored from kindergarten through fifth grade. They found that children identified by their teachers in kindergarten as being more inattentive than most others in their class had significantly lower reading achievement when they reached fifth grade. The problems of these low-achieving children were based on their significant impairments in sustaining attention, not on behavioral difficulties, IQ, or prior reading achievement. From their six-year study the researchers concluded:

> About one third of the children who were reading in the normal range after kindergarten, but who were highly inattentive during first grade, had fifth grade reading outcomes more than one SD

[standard deviation] below their peer group. . . . Because first
grade is a critical time for the acquisition of early reading skills,
one plausible hypothesis is that attention problems interfere
with the acquisition of these skills and that it is difficult for children to "catch up." (p. 866)

There are several ways in which learning to read can be problematic
for a child. One is a persisting difficulty in recognizing words on the page
as words one has heard in conversation. This involves the ability to break
down unfamiliar words into their component parts. There are just forty-
four of these components, phonemes, in the English language; these combinations of letters that represent a specific sound are the building blocks
for all spoken and written words in the language. Sally Shaywitz (2003)
has described the fundamental importance of phoneme processing in
reading:

Before words can be identified, understood, stored in memory,
or retrieved from it, they must first be broken down into
phonemes by the neural machinery of the brain. . . . Language is
a code, and the only code that can be recognized by the language
system and activate its machinery is the phonologic code. . . .
Overall the child must come to know that the letters he sees on
the page represent, or map onto, the sounds he hears when the
same word is spoken. (pp. 41–44)

Shaywitz points out that virtually all humans acquire spoken language
simply by consistent exposure to their mother tongue, that learning spoken
language is relatively effortless and natural, while reading is not. "Reading
is an acquired act, an invention of man that must be learned at a conscious
level. . . . The key to unraveling it is not so readily apparent and can only
be accessed with effort on the part of the beginning reader" (p. 50).

About 80 percent of American children learn how to transform
printed symbols into phonetic code without much difficulty, but for the remaining 20 percent, this code-cracking task is much more difficult. These
are the individuals who, in varying degrees, are dyslexic. Many of them

can be taught to read, but this usually requires alternative approaches and more intensive instruction and practice than is required for most others.

Among individuals with ADHD there is a markedly elevated incidence of dyslexia (Tannock and Brown 2000). As was shown in the Rabiner study, attentional problems and other impairments of the ADD syndrome can severely impair an individual's ability to read.

Yet phonemic decoding is not the only element involved in reading; gradually the child needs also to develop fluency and comprehension of longer stretches of text. Virginia Berninger and Todd Richards (2002) described the development of two types of fluency:

> The first kind is oral reading fluency in which children not only become faster in recognizing words, but their oral reading begins to reflect the melody or intonation of the spoken language. The second kind is silent reading fluency in which children quickly and automatically access . . . word forms . . . thereby freeing up limited working memory resources for reading comprehension. (pp. 162–163)

Children who suffer from chronic impairments in their ability to sustain attention and effort, to utilize working memory, and to employ other executive functions usually impaired by ADD syndrome, are likely to have continuing difficulty in these more advanced aspects of reading comprehension.

In our Yale Clinic for Attention and Related Disorders, Donald Quinlan and I administered reading tests to older adolescents and adults diagnosed with ADHD. Their ability to recognize and correctly pronounce lists of words on the Woodcock Johnson Achievement Test was in the high average range. But their scores for demonstrating comprehension of passages several paragraphs long on the Nelson-Denny Reading Test were significantly (1.5 standard deviations) lower. They were also significantly slower at reading the passages. These preliminary findings suggest that adolescents and adults with ADHD are likely to have persisting problems with reading fluency and comprehension that are not explained by poor decoding skills. These findings also indicate that reading problems associated with ADD syndrome do not disappear over time.

Children with significant attention impairments during their early school years are likely to experience difficulties not only in reading, but also in learning mathematics. Elizabeth Benedetto-Nasho and Rosemary Tannock (1999) studied students aged seven to eleven years, half of them with an ADHD diagnosis, half without. The two groups of students were matched for equal math skills and none had any learning disability. When asked to complete sets of math problems appropriate for their ability level, the ADHD students attempted fewer problems, were three times less effective in solving the problems, and made six times as many errors when doing subtraction problems. Errors in subtraction were mostly errors in borrowing; for example, 120 − 9. Such difficulties are likely to involve not only attention to details (for example, noticing whether one is supposed to add, subtract, multiply, or divide), but also working memory functions (such as keeping in mind that one has "borrowed" from the tens column when one subtracts from the ones column).

ADD Syndrome Impairs Written Expression

Skills of written expression, the ability to put thoughts into sentences and paragraphs that others will be able to read and understand, are also problematic for many children with ADHD. Written expression is a more demanding task than is talking, reading, or doing basic math computations. To write one's thoughts places much heavier demands on learned skills and executive functions. Virginia Berninger and Todd Richards (2002) described some of these demands:

> Writing, especially expository writing, is not talk written down—
> it requires self-generated language without social supports during the initial planning and text generation processes. Thus,
> writing is not the inverse of reading or aural/oral language . . .
> in the sense that division is the inverse of multiplication.
> (pp. 168–170)

Put another way, writing lacks the scaffolding—the support—of having a partner in conversation. And a blank page does not offer the structure of other words to read. It therefore is much more demanding on executive functions than is reading or conversation. Berninger and Todd noted that

> both writing and reading draw on . . . memory, executive processes, and thinking processes—but in different ways. Because the reading system [of the brain] can refer to written text at any time, the memory burden is greatly reduced. In contrast, the writing system . . . may place a greater burden on working memory than does reading comprehension. Writing is an immense juggling act, with more jobs to do than reading. The writing jobs include planning (generating ideas and setting goals), translating those ideas into text, transcribing that text, and reviewing and revising it. . . . Control processes for extracting meaning from a finished text (reading) are not as taxing as the executive processes that go into generating and repairing a text until it is deemed a final product (writing). (pp. 172–174)

Relatively few studies have assessed impairments of written expression in individuals with ADHD. Susan Mayes and colleagues (2000) studied children with ADHD in comparison to children who had other emotional or behavioral problems without ADHD; all of these children were eight to sixteen years old and had been referred to a child psychiatric treatment clinic. Each child was given individually administered tests for IQ and academic achievement. Of the children with ADHD, 65 percent had a score for written expression that was significantly lower than that predicted by their IQ test score; only 27 percent of the clinic-referred children without ADHD had such a discrepancy.

Taken together, these several studies and others not described here show that significant percentages of students with ADHD demonstrate substantial basic impairments in reading, math, and/or written expression, often from their earliest years in learning these skills. These academic impairments suggest that many children with ADD syndrome have a weak foundation of basic academic skills on which to build their education. Such impairments are also important because they tend to demoralize children early in their educational careers and deprive them of "the sense of being able to make things and make them well," which Erikson claimed was the foundation for a "sense of industry."

Many children with ADD syndrome are not able to "win recognition by producing things" in their elementary school classrooms. Rather, they tend to be recognized by teachers and peers as the ones who didn't get the assigned task completed, missed the main point of it, or did it too hastily or with too many errors. When a child encounters such defeats frequently, especially in the early years of schooling, it doesn't take long to become discouraged with academic work, and to develop a sense of inferiority that undermines one's attempts to learn. Shortly before his evaluation for ADHD, a six-year-old boy in kindergarten was asked to try tracing the shape of the letter "H." He told his mother, "I don't even want to try doing that. I'm just going to mess it all up like everything else I do."

Faced with repeated early failures and frustration in trying to learn basic verbal and mathematical skills, many children with ADD syndrome give up on truly learning academic tasks. They may be forced to continue to do their lessons, prepare their papers, and take the tests, but their motivation to invest themselves in such learning, to work at learning, is likely to be markedly diminished. They may continue so as to avoid getting into trouble with the teacher or parents, but they may not anticipate feeling satisfied in having done a task well. Sometimes such discouraged children develop alternative skills that bring other kinds of recognition: clowning to get classmates to laugh, challenging the teacher with defiance, or bullying other children.

But academic weakness is not the only reason that many children with ADD syndrome seem relatively unmotivated. Sometimes parents unwittingly sabotage the motivation of their children to work at learning. Sometimes parents of bright children, like the underachieving Wally described earlier, do not adequately appreciate the importance of teaching their child to work at a task and learn to do it well, even if it is not especially interesting or challenging.

Much of what children are required to do in school is not very interesting to them and much of it may not even be directly useful in later years. But the experiences of accepting an assignment and working to learn a new skill, practicing and refining the skill, applying it to assigned tasks, and working to get it done well can all contribute substantially to a child's developing a sense of industry. If the child finds that recognition is given for significant effort, and if his work or developing skill is acknowledged by others, especially the parents, as having importance and value, then the child is likely to develop some pride and satisfaction in doing the work.

Some parents overlook the value of nurturing the child's developing academic competence, but are quick to give such recognition to their child's efforts in sports, art, music, mechanical tasks, or other nonacademic pursuits. Often this results in the child's becoming strongly motivated to improve those skills while neglecting academic challenges.

> Sarah has never been much of a student, but she has always been a good athlete. She says she tries hard to do her schoolwork, but she never does it very well. Her father and I are both very athletic and we have ADHD like she does; she has to have gotten it from us. But we noticed from when she was just a toddler how much she loves physical activities. She was pretty good at dribbling a soccer ball when she was just five years old. We've spent a lot of time coaching and practicing with her and we've paid for her to get private lessons in ice skating and tennis and skiing. She's been on soccer and Little League teams since she became old enough to sign on. And she's already earned all of the figure skating badges.
>
> Sarah has always worked very hard to improve her performance. Coaches all tell us that she is one of hardest working kids they have ever seen. Her natural talents and hard work pay off. She's always a star! We attend all her games and competitions. We stay in close touch with her coaches and we take her to see the pros in her sports whenever we can. We have a display of all her ribbons and trophies in our dining room. Our only worry now is that her sixth-grade teacher is saying she is failing and

may have to repeat the grade. If she can't get all passing grades, she won't be eligible to play on the school teams next term. That would ruin everything. She's never been very interested in working on schoolwork, at school or at home. We are getting worried about that.

It may be true that Sarah is naturally much more talented in athletics than in academics, and thus more motivated to work consistently at learning to improve her athletic abilities. But it is difficult to know how much of Sarah's lopsided motivation is due to her parents' strong enthusiasm for her efforts in sports and their years of relatively weak interest in her academic work. If her parents had invested more effort and interest in encouraging Sarah's academic learning, it is possible that she would have learned to work productively at learning in school, just as she has learned to do in sports. She may never have become as competent and interested in schoolwork as she has become with sports, but she might have developed that aspect of herself well enough that she would not need to repeat her grade. Given her ADHD diagnosis, it is unlikely that her difficulties in school are due solely to the attitudes and behavior of her parents, but these may be contributing to the problem.

Sarah is a good example of someone with situation-specific ADD syndrome impairments. She demonstrates that she is able and willing to work hard at learning and practicing skills that interest her, while she complains that she is unable to sustain enough interest and effort to do the schoolwork that may eventually determine whether she will be eligible to play on school sports teams.

Executive Functions and the Tasks of Childhood

This chapter has described examples of four developmental tasks or challenges faced by most children during childhood:

Behaving carefully,
Cooperating with adults and peers,
Communicating effectively, and
Learning to read and write

The child's performance on each of these tasks is initially micromanaged on behalf of the child by parents, older siblings, or other caregivers, until the child is able to perform the tasks alone. Each of these tasks involves many steps and depends on some combination of those executive functions described in Chapter 2.

Some situations require only the simple exercise of very basic functions: waiting a moment, heeding a warning to stop, saying a few words, or noticing the lighted color on a stoplight. Others are more complex and require more refined executive abilities. For example, in many situations behaving carefully requires attending to details that may signal risk; it also requires working memory to keep in mind what one is doing, for example, avoiding distractions and attending to traffic while trying to cross a street. It also requires calling to mind information relevant to the present moment, such as remembering cautions one has been given to avoid certain potentially risky situations. And it requires monitoring and self-regulating actions so that one is not completely dependent on others to protect and control what one is doing.

For very young children, executive functions are performed by parents, older siblings, or other caregivers in virtually every situation. These guardians, present almost constantly during the young child's waking hours, protect and guide the child until, gradually, the child learns to manage an increasing range of situations for herself. Seeing this, most caretakers allow and encourage the child to do more for herself while they continue to provide support for those more challenging situations that may exceed the child's present abilities. Assessing the child's readiness to handle new situations usually requires gauging the child's competence in using the needed executive functions.

All four of the developmental tasks I discuss in this chapter are important for all children. And none of these tasks is ever fully completed. As the child gets older there will be new tasks to master and new settings where one must learn more about how to behave carefully, cooperate with adults and peers, communicate effectively, and work to learn. Task demands become more complex and required skills become more subtle. While there may be considerable truth in Robert Fulghum's assertion that everything he ever needed to know he learned in kindergarten, few would argue that later childhood, adolescence, and adulthood do not require refinement of those most basic skills.

In early years the child learns to be careful to wait at the curb until he can hold the adult's hand while crossing the street. Later he learns how to look carefully both ways, judging the movement of traffic so he can safely cross himself. Still later he learns to ride his bicycle safely in the traffic, and when older he will learn to be careful in driving a car. As an adult he may need to learn how to be careful when accompanying a young child, remembering to anticipate the child's moves and to be sure to hold the child's hand.

Even in the early years of preschool, some children demonstrate significant delays or impairments in development of certain capacities of working memory, planning, cognitive flexibility, and capacity to tolerate delay—all of which are foundational to the development of executive functions. These delays or impairments have been documented by Edmund Sonuga-Barke and colleagues (2003), who tested children between three and five-and-a-half years old on measures of executive function and capacity to tolerate delay. He selected 70 percent of the children randomly from community nursery schools and compared them with 30 percent who had been identified as showing ADHD impairments in school, at home, or both. Impairments of executive function measures, including the capacity to tolerate delay, were strongly correlated with the level of ADHD symptoms in both boys and girls. The author concluded that

> these data add substance to claims that preschool and school-aged children with ADHD symptoms share similar neuro-psychological characteristics . . . and [provide] evidence for an association between preschool ADHD symptoms and more general executive deficits. (pp. 1339–1340)

During childhood, then, most individuals who suffer from ADD syndrome tend to have considerable difficulty achieving basic and important tasks of self-management. In addition, the difficulties such children have performing these tasks are due largely to impairments in executive functions of the brain. All children with ADD syndrome do not have equal impairment in each of the four self-management tasks. Some may be quite impaired in being careful while generally being able to communicate rather effectively. Others may be reasonably careful and generally cooperative with others, though they tend to struggle to communicate well and to work to learn. Despite this variability, however, relative to their peers, most of those diagnosed with ADHD during childhood tend to demonstrate significant impairments across all of the clusters of executive function impairments that constitute ADD syndrome.

Chapter 5   Adolescence: Greater Independence
Brings New Challenges

MYTH: Those who have ADD as children usually outgrow it as they enter their teens.

FACT: Often ADD impairments are not very noticeable until the teen years, when more self-management is required in school and elsewhere. And ADD may be subtle but more disabling during adolescence than in childhood.

While many with ADD syndrome suffer impairments that become apparent sometime during childhood, for some, these difficulties are not evident until adolescence. In addition, among those children whose ADD syndrome is obvious in childhood, most experience increased difficulty as they are forced to meet growing challenges to their executive functioning in school, at home, and in social relationships. For most individuals with ADD syndrome, the years between junior high school and their early twenties are the most frustrating. It is during this period, from adolescence to early adulthood, that one faces the widest range of tasks challenging executive functions, but has the least opportunity to escape from those tasks at which one is not very competent.

One point at which ADD syndrome impairments often become more noticeable is the transition from elementary to secondary school. In elementary school, students are usually in the care of one teacher most of each day. This allows the teacher to become familiar with every student in the class, developing personal relationships with each one and helping to manage any interpersonal conflicts. In addition, the elementary school-teacher provides a continuity of structure and organization for students throughout each school day, helping them to set priorities, reminding them of upcoming deadlines, and monitoring all aspects of their work, learning, and social interactions. When the students move to secondary school, most of this nurturing structure and supportive continuity is lost; instead, they must rely much more extensively on their own executive functions.

Managing Time and Homework

Secondary school generally requires much more complex self-management than does elementary school. Schedules for secondary school usually involve seven to nine class periods, each of which is held in a different room with a different group of students and a different adult in charge. Instead of working closely with twenty to twenty-five students all day, each teacher is likely to encounter 125 to 150 students daily, each for just one class period. Without one teacher to provide coherence and structure, students themselves need to be much more organized, managing by themselves their schoolwork, school activities, and school relationships.

In many schools class schedules are not consistent; they rotate from day to day so the student must keep in mind which schedule is in place for a particular day. Each class period usually requires different materials and tools—for example, textbooks, notebooks, writing implements, calculators, gym uniform, and so on—that the student must carry from class to class, getting them out of or into a locker or backpack as needed. Many students with ADD syndrome have a lot of trouble keeping track of these belongings, remembering which items to bring to which class period and then remembering to collect and reorganize everything in the few minutes allotted between classes.

Rotation from one class to another seven to nine times daily also increases the complexity of social interactions for adolescent students. This frequent reshuffling typically involves many social interchanges, some of which may be pleasant conversation fragments with friends. But walking the hallways and entering into each classroom also exposes the student to a constantly changing mix of other students, some of whom may be aloof, taunting, provocative, or threatening. Interactions and anticipated interactions with other students may stir up many unsettling thoughts and feelings in students that may linger even after the teacher begins organized instruction.

Teacher-student interactions also vary from class to class. Each teacher has a unique personality, a different style of interacting with students, and personalized ways of managing a class. Some teachers are highly structured and demanding of students, quick to confront anyone slow to comply. Others are more casual, less willing to control the class. Some teachers are very supportive and encouraging of students, whereas others may be condescending or hostile. In more extreme cases, students can get caught up in power struggles with a teacher or suffer verbal taunts or embarrassing criticisms from a teacher whom they cannot safely confront.

Thoughts and feelings about social interactions with classmates and teachers may consume a large portion of a student's energy and time during school. Mihaly Csikszentmihalyi and Reed Larson (1984) studied adolescents who were asked to carry beepers each day and to record in detail what they were doing, thinking, and feeling each time the beeper alerted them. Students in this study reported that they were thinking of schoolwork only 40 percent of all occasions in class when they were randomly beeped. This study also reported that

> compared to other contexts in their lives, time in class is associated with lower-than-average states on nearly every self-report dimension. Most notably, students report feeling sad, irritable and bored; concentration is difficult; they feel self-conscious and strongly wish they were doing something else. (p. 204)

From intensive study of these students, selected from the general population of a suburban high school, these researchers concluded, "Even in a very good high school such as the one studied here . . . students are probably absorbing only a fraction of the information being presented." They found that "classic academic subjects such as mathematics, foreign language and English showed the lowest levels of intrinsic motivation, coupled with low affect and activation" (p. 206). If students in the general population commonly experience such difficulties in the classroom, it is not surprising that individuals with ADD syndrome report significant problems managing their time and effort at school.

The work of school does not all happen at school. Secondary school usually brings substantial increases in the quantity and complexity of homework that students are expected to manage, complete outside of school, and then hand in to the appropriate teacher at a designated time. Many adolescents have great difficulty keeping track of what homework has been assigned and when it is due. Many also have problems getting the work done on time. Some even have trouble remembering to hand in completed assignments at the designated time so they can receive credit. For students with ADD syndrome, these escalating demands of homework may become overwhelming.

> We never got any complaints about Emily when she was in the elementary grades. Teachers generally had good things to say about her. Once in a while the teacher would alert me about her needing help in completing a project or longer-term assignment, but usually she got her work done without much difficulty. Trouble started when she got into junior high and had six different teachers each day instead of just one. That's when homework became a really big problem.
>
> Often she would forget to write the assignments down so when she came home she didn't know what she was supposed to be doing for homework or when the quiz or test would be. Things started to snowball. She would get behind in a couple of classes and we would get a note from the teacher that she had failed a test and owed a bunch of homework assignments. We would get on her to complete that work and then she would fall behind in another class or two. Every year it was constant brush fires of late or incomplete work. None of the teachers seemed to know what was going on with her in any of her other classes and she just couldn't keep the whole picture in mind.

"Keeping the whole picture in mind" is a task that many individuals with ADD syndrome find quite difficult, particularly when the picture is as complex as in secondary school. When a student spends most of the school day with one teacher who knows her well, that teacher can monitor the assigned schoolwork, suggesting priorities and reminding about deadlines. If a student is not writing down assignments, the teacher may notice this and prompt the student to do so. Teachers in lower grades are aware of how much work they are assigning for each day and can adjust this when needed so that students are not overwhelmed with too many quizzes, tests, or papers on the same day. In junior high and high school, by contrast, teachers usually do not coordinate assignments or test dates with other teachers. Often this results in several major assignments needing to be turned in at one time or several long reading assignments, quizzes, or tests being due on the same day.

Homework is not the only demand on an adolescent student's time. Many students are also active in sports teams that have frequent practices and games, all of which require substantial time and energy. Others take lessons in music or dance that require daily practice. Some also belong to clubs or take religious instruction after school, which may mean that they need to set aside time for study, projects, or group activities. Others have part-time jobs that may require many hours of after-school and weekend time. Homework and study requirements compete against these other structured activities for the time, energy, and attention of adolescents.

Another domain of activity that looms large in the life of many teenagers is making and maintaining contact with friends. This often involves large amounts of time spent each day talking with peers during the school day while changing classes, on the bus to and from school, at the lunch table, or in the locker room—or after school as small groups of friends gather on a corner, at the home of a classmate, or at the local mall.

Sometimes conversations are not face-to-face. Many adolescents spend literally hours on the telephone each day talking with one or several friends. Modern telephone connections even make possible "conference calls" that link multiple simultaneous connections between several callers. Another mode of communication in heavy use among many adolescents is email, particularly instant messaging. In this modality many computer-savvy adolescents can carry on lengthy conversations by sending a few instantly delivered sentences at a time. These messages, short or long, may be forwarded to other friends as a way of sharing information or comparing notes.

Regardless of how they communicate, the act of comparing views—checking to see how friends describe or react to the clothing, comments, interactions, or alliances of peers—serves a crucially important role for most adolescents as they make and repeatedly revise their own perspectives. In similar ways many adolescents compare complaints about parents, siblings, and teachers as well as swap enthusiasms and complaints about music, movies, sporting events, music videos, or television shows. Exchange of such information provides a continuing opportunity for adolescents to experiment with various attitudes and viewpoints, thus defining themselves vis-à-vis others and learning what elicits agreement, enthusiasm, or rejection from valued friends. But for some adolescents, these activities become virtually incessant, crowding out other activities that are also important.

> Jim used to spend hours every day riding his bike or shooting baskets with his friends. Over the past couple of years, since he started high school, he holes up every day in his bedroom, always on the phone or on his computer. He and his buddies exchange more emails every day than I usually get at work in a full week. Most of it is just each one checking out the other's opinion about who was acting "cool" or not and who said that this friend likes that one.
>
> What worries me is that he seems to get too caught up in this. We've tried to set some limits on how much time he is allowed to be on the phone or computer each day because often he is not getting his homework done. All of his time is spent talking with this one or emailing that one. He says everybody is doing it just as much as he is, but I don't see everybody getting warnings of possible failure in three different courses because they haven't been getting their homework done and haven't studied enough for tests. His father and I are talking about taking away his use of the phone and computer until his grades get better. But we

both work and it's almost impossible for us to enforce what we think is right.

This mother is concerned about the excessive amount of time her son spends exchanging phone calls and emails with his friends, realizing that he is ignoring homework to the extent that he is failing courses. Yet she also notes another problem faced by many parents of adolescents: There are limits to how effectively parents can control how their adolescents spend their time. Especially when both parents are working, it is very difficult for parents to force their adolescents to invest time and significant effort on their homework. They may remove a computer from the adolescent's room or disconnect his phone or access to internet service, only to find that alternative connections are found during the many after-school hours when they are not at home. And even if these distractions are effectively taken away, it does not guarantee that the adolescent will invest more time and effort in serious study.

An adolescent's daily communications with friends can be an important way of making, maintaining, modifying, and shifting alliances; protecting oneself from possible embarrassment, ridicule, or isolation; assessing one's one status and performance; and shaping one's self-definition. But waking hours not consumed by school are limited, and adolescents are faced daily with decisions as to how that time will be spent. Multiple executive functions are involved in the daily process of estimating, organizing, prioritizing, monitoring, starting, and stopping daily tasks and activities. These are not easy for any adolescent, but they are very difficult for many adolescents with ADD syndrome, and overwhelming for some.

Sexual Feelings and Relationships

Although most adolescents, especially those with ADD syndrome, are challenged by the self-management required for school and daily activities, a greater challenge is often the management of their thoughts, feelings, and imaginings about themselves. For most adolescents, each day is filled with many minutes or hours of thinking about their physical and social appearance: how they look, how they are seen by others, and how they compare with their peers. Some of this preoccupation is linked to experiencing the physical changes of puberty and to an emerging sense of themselves as sexual beings. One fifteen-year-old boy described his daily struggles:

> I don't know what's the matter with me. My brain is always stuck on thinking about sex and it gets me into trouble. Maybe it's because I hit puberty earlier than most of the other guys in my grade. I'm always horny in school and then I'm thinking about "Will I jerk off when I get home or will I be able to resist it?" Some days I can resist, but usually I have to do it as soon as I get home from school. Then I take a nap. At night I try to do my homework, but usually I go on line to IM with my friends and then I spend an hour or two surfing the porn sites and getting myself off again. Afterwards I feel stupid for being so messed up and then I just don't feel like doing any homework, so I just listen to some music and go to sleep.
>
> Lots of days I have a hard-on all the way through English class. There is this one girl who sits across from me. She's really hot. I'm always looking at her and thinking about what I'd like to do with her even though I've never done anything with anybody yet. Last week after school I was instant-messaging with one of my buddies and told him some of the stuff I was thinking about her. He emailed that to his girlfriend and then she emailed it to the girl herself and then I got an email from her saying that I'm a pervert. Next day she spread a bunch of rumors about me to her friends. All week I couldn't even go to school. I was so embarrassed!

This high school student with ADD syndrome described several painful dilemmas that are not specific to adolescents with ADD syndrome, but his problems in coping with his difficulties were exacerbated by his ADD impairments. He described how he is distracted throughout much of most school days with internal struggles over his wish to masturbate versus his guilt and shame about doing so. Though many adolescents have similar struggles that occasionally intrude into their work at school, this young man reported that his inability to block these preoccupations significantly intruded on his ability to pay attention and take adequate notes during most classes. Similarly, he left many homework assignments undone because he could not delay his wish to surf pornographic web sites and masturbate. His problem was not simply the time involved in these activities. He also was unable to block the self-criticism that left him feeling "messed up" after each time he masturbated. He illustrates the continuing truth of the observation of John Gagnon and William Simon (1973) that

> there is little evidence that there has been any reduction in the
> anxiety associated with masturbatory practices by the young who
> are beginning their sexual lives . . . it is the existence of this anx-
> iety about masturbation that supports our experiential belief that
> the sexual drive is one of extreme potency. We presume that we
> are experiencing a biologically powerful experience when in fact
> it is the guilt and the anxiety associated with arousal identified
> as sexual which is provoking our sense of intensity. (p. 56)

Many adolescents (and adults) struggle with sexual preoccupations and with feelings of guilt over their actual or imagined sexual activities, but those with ADD syndrome often report much more difficulty in managing these thoughts and emotions than do most of their age-mates. It seems to be more difficult for them to compartmentalize them and to focus on necessary tasks than it is for many others of the same age.

This boy's report also highlights the social risks associated with sexual development in adolescents. Impulsively, while instant-messaging, he had shared with a friend details of his fantasies about the girl he was attracted to in his English class. Equally impulsively, the friend, who also had ADD syndrome, pushed a button to share this electronically transmitted confession with his girlfriend, who quickly sent it to the girl who was the object of the boy's fantasies. The resulting embarrassment and shame caused the boy who had shared too much information to avoid attending school for a full week.

Two aspects of the revelation caused the student to feel humiliated. First, he expected, rightly, that peers would ridicule him for confessing to masturbating, an activity in which most adolescents engage, though few acknowledge. Second, he was very ashamed to have his classmates know that his exciting fantasies sharply contrasted with his total lack of sexual experience with any other person. While many adults worry about adolescents becoming too aggressive sexually, many do not understand how difficult it is for many adolescents to get started sharing sexual intimacies with any partner. The vulnerability of adolescents to fears of rejection by a potential partner and risk of humiliation if a partner reports one's sexual uncertainty or ineptness to others would be difficult to overestimate. For those with ADD syndrome, managing fears of peer ridicule and uncertainties about who to ask out and how to act when dating or during sexually charged social interactions can be very difficult, even more than for most others of the same age.

For some adolescents with ADD syndrome, developing sexual relationships can become a way to compensate for frustrations in their academic work and other aspects of life. One very attractive girl with ADD syndrome reported:

> My parents sent me to this private high school for ninth grade because they knew that I'm smart, but had a lot of trouble in school. They thought it would be better for me because the classes are smaller, but they didn't know the work there is a lot harder than in public school. Lots more homework and lots more tests. My grades in eighth grade weren't good, but my ninth grade report card was loaded with D's and F's even though I was working pretty hard. In the third quarter of my first year there I got caught cheating on a history test and they kicked me out, so I had to go to public high school. At first I just hated it, but then I met Mike, a senior. He was easy on the eyes and captain of the football team and co-captain of the baseball team. He was no honor student, but he did OK on grades. And he had a car with an amazing sound system. When I started going out with him, everybody started to be my friend.
>
> I had gone out with some other guys before, but never with somebody so much older. My parents said he was too old for me and didn't want me to see him, but I kept going out with him

anyway. He just didn't come to the house. I would tell them I was going to my girlfriend's house and then I would go out with him. At first I wasn't too comfortable with the marijuana and beers; I hadn't done that before. But then it relaxed me and I really enjoyed partying with Mike and his friends. Then that summer I got pregnant. I found out just before Mike was going off to college. I had been on the pill, but sometimes I forgot to take it.

At the time of this incident, this girl's ADD syndrome had not been recognized. Like many other students with ADD syndrome, she had struggled with her schoolwork and found that even when she worked hard, her grades were disappointing to her and to her parents, who were spending a lot of money to provide a better education. In such a competitive setting, students who do poorly in their studies often face daily humiliation as classmates and teachers witness their inability to keep pace with burdensome homework assignments, lively class discussions, and challenging tests. When she got caught cheating, this girl was further humiliated by the expulsion that resulted from her desperate but misguided efforts to get a better grade. She was then faced with the embarrassing task of having to answer seemingly countless friends, acquaintances, relatives, and neighbors who wanted to know why she was transferring mid-semester from a prestigious private school to the local public school. She reported,

> I feel like I have a big "C" for "cheater" or "R" for "reject"
> stamped on my forehead. Kids at the new school keep asking
> me why I'm coming here now. I can't say I just moved to town,
> because some of them already know me from elementary
> school. I try to tell them I just didn't like the other school, but
> they all know it has to be because I got kicked out.

Faced with many weeks of multiple daily reminders of her failure to find success at the more prestigious school, of her inability to satisfy her own aspirations and those of her parents who struggled to continue to pay the high tuition that had to be forfeited when she was expelled, this girl was exceptionally vulnerable as she tried to work her way into the established social networks of the public high school. Being attractive, she caught the eye of an older boy whose attentions both helped her feel valued and brought her recognition by classmates who liked and respected him. When her parents, fearful of her associating with an older boy, forbade her to see him, she resorted to deceit so she could continue the relationship.

The significance of this new relationship was complicated. Not only did the girl gain status among peers for being chosen by this popular older boy, she also was welcomed into his peer group and included in their frequent gatherings. Because she was bright, empathic, and articulate, she was someone her new boyfriend could confide in as he was struggling to cope with the recent death of his father. Repeatedly she was told by his mother and friends that her support had lifted him out of his grief; she felt needed and valued by her boyfriend, his mother, and many of his friends. Their warmth and gratitude served as an antidote to her strong feelings of failure and shame; it also intensified her resistance to her parents' continuing demands that she stay at home more and study harder to succeed at school.

As she spent more time with her older boyfriend and his friends, the girl also joined in the beer drinking and marijuana smoking that often occurred at their weekend parties. Joseph Biederman, Timothy Wilens, and others (1998) have shown that individuals with ADHD not only have a twofold increased lifetime risk of substance use disorders than those without ADHD, but also tend to begin substance abuse earlier and continue it longer. Elizabeth Disney and colleagues (1999) found that girls with ADHD often begin substance abuse earlier than boys with ADHD, possibly because they tend to associate with older boys whose patterns of substance abuse may be more fully developed.

This girl reported that despite her initial discomfort with drinking beer and smoking marijuana, she soon came to enjoy its relaxing properties as well as the concomitant social interaction. She said she also appreciated her boyfriend's gentle sexual attentions that gradually developed into an active sexual relationship enjoyed by both of them. Her failure to take regularly the contraceptive pills she had obtained from a clinic was probably due to the effects of her ADD-related working memory problems combined with her dimly sensed hope that if she were accidentally to become pregnant he might abandon his plans to go off to college the following autumn, choosing instead to remain at home to intensify his relationship with her while attending a college in the community.

This girl's early adolescent coital experience and premarital pregnancy are consistent with a pattern reported from the Milwaukee longitudinal study of hyperactive children by Russell Barkley (1998). His group followed 158 hyperactive children and 81 matched controls for more than fourteen years. During this period the children with ADHD started having sexual intercourse earlier than the controls (at fifteen years rather than sixteen years), had many more sexual partners in their lives (nineteen versus seven), were less likely to employ birth control methods, were more likely to have contracted a sexually transmitted disease, and were much more likely to have conceived a pregnancy (38 percent versus 4 percent). These findings related to adolescents who had been hyperactive as children; most of the hyperactive subjects met *DSM-III-R* criteria for ADHD. Since this pattern of high-risk behaviors has not been reported for adolescents with ADHD who lacked a history of hyperactivity, these findings should not be taken as applicable to all adolescents with ADHD. The pattern reported for the hyperactive subjects in Milwaukee did, however, fit closely with the experience of this particular girl.

It would be too simplistic to argue that this girl's school failure, debased self-esteem, cheating, alienation from her parents, and premarital pregnancy and subsequent problems were all a direct result of her ADD syndrome. Multiple influences were at work in this complex situation. Yet it is hard to avoid the conclusion that this girl's life might have been much less painful if her ADD syndrome had been recognized and treated early in her school career. As it was, she was not evaluated, diagnosed, and treated until after she had aborted the pregnancy and her boyfriend had gone off to college. She responded well to medication for ADD syndrome and completed her high school education with very high grades. Two years later she wondered aloud:

> Seeing how much this medication helps me focus, and seeing
> how good my grades are now in advanced classes with only
> about 60 percent of the effort I was putting into getting those

lousy grades before, I really wonder. I wonder how things might have been different if my ADD had been picked up when I was in junior high. I bet I would have been just as good as most of the other kids at that prep school if only I had this medication then. I wonder where I would be today if that had happened.

Another question that might be raised is: "Where might this girl have ended up if her ADD syndrome had not been identified and treated when it was?" She came for evaluation because she was severely depressed and a heavy abuser of alcohol and marijuana. She did not come for treatment immediately after she had aborted the pregnancy with support from her boyfriend, but months later, after her boyfriend had gone off to college. To some her substance abuse might have appeared as simply a grief reaction to the abortion. Others might have seen it simply as a typical depressive reaction in an adolescent high school student whose older boyfriend has left for college. It was only after detailed inquiry that the long history of failure due to untreated ADD syndrome emerged as a major contributor to this girl's painful experiences of loss and as a persistent impediment to her future success. Linkages between ADD syndrome, academic achievement, family relationships, emerging sexuality, dating relationships, substance abuse, and self-esteem are often subtle and complex, though quite powerful.

Working for Money and Driving a Car

An eighteen-year-old boy and his mother came for consultation. He was a senior in a technical high school, referred by the school because he was in danger of being unable to graduate due to failing grades in the theory portion of his shop course, where he majored in culinary arts. The school reported that for the past two-and-a-half years this boy had been consistently described by his shop teacher as "the best culinary arts student I've ever had. He is a master in the kitchen, but he never does any homework and doesn't study for the tests on the textbook. I can't pass him unless he does that work."

At the outset of his evaluation interview the boy proudly handed me a thick stack of paycheck stubs from his work in a local restaurant over the past three years. He said,

Regardless of what they tell you in those reports from school, I want you to know that I'm a really good worker and a really good cook. I work thirty hours a week in the kitchen at this restaurant; I'm there every day. When there is no school, I work even more. I started as a dishwasher and then I was a prep cook and now I'm one of the chefs. I know more about cooking than anybody else in our shop class except for our teacher.

My boss will tell you. I'm one of his best workers. Always on time; often I stay late. I like my work and I'm good at it. It pays pretty well too. You can see it from those pay stubs and you can see it right out the window in your parking lot. I bought that pickup truck completely from my own money that I earned at the restaurant! Now they say I can't graduate from high school just because I don't do those Mickey Mouse assignments and tests from the book. That has nothing to do with knowing about cooking and nothing to do with the real world.

After their five-year study of one thousand adolescents in transition from school to work, Mihaly Csikszentmihalyi and Barbara Schneider (2000) reported that although most teenagers by the end of high school have done some paid work as babysitters, lifeguards, or fast-food servers, very few gain experience in jobs around which vocations are built. This exceptional young man took well-deserved pride in his demonstrated ability to function well in the world of work. Unlike most in his peer group he had already developed and refined many practical skills directly applicable to employment. And he proudly drove around in his self-bought vehicle that served not only as a means of transport, but also as enviable evidence of his earnings-relevant accomplishments. Yet though his work experience yielded him money and considerable self-esteem, it also had costly effects on his academic work and his attitude toward school.

Evaluation indicated that this young cook had solidly average intelligence, but fully met diagnostic criteria for ADHD. He had been frustrated throughout his schooling by chronic difficulties in sustaining attention to assignments requiring reading and writing. Although he was very competent at organizing his work in the kitchen and in sustaining attention to countless details involved in preparing and serving multiple meals simultaneously, he had great difficulty organizing his academic work, attending to details of reading-based or math problems, and recalling what he had read. His part-time work had served for many years to compensate for the frustration and embarrassment he chronically felt in the classroom. Yet a few months before his scheduled graduation, his demonstrated success in practical skills of the kitchen could not alter the fact that he would be denied a high school diploma if he did not successfully complete enough of the reading and written work required for graduation from this technical high school. To accomplish this he needed treatment for his longstanding ADD syndrome.

For most adolescents, employment is not so productive as it was for this young cook. Ellen Greenberger and Laurence Steinberg (1986) studied tenth- and eleventh-grade students who were employed part-time and a comparison sample of adolescents who had never held a steady job. They concluded that

> adolescent work is now, for the most part, totally different from the type of work youngsters will do in the future. Once motivated by the economic needs of the family and the community, most adolescent work today represents "luxury" employment, of which adolescents themselves are the chief beneficiaries. And the workplace, once an area where the generations were united in common tasks, is now an age-segregated adolescent stronghold . . . excessive commitment to a job may pose an impediment to development by causing adolescents to spend too much time and energy in a role that is too constraining and involves tasks that are too simple, unchallenging and irrelevant to their future. (pp. 6–7)

The young cook was an exception to these observations in some ways. His work did place him in an apprentice-like situation where he learned skills of his trade by working collaboratively with an experienced chef. As it had evolved, his part-time employment had led him to become immersed in work that held the promise of becoming a satisfying career. Such work is far different from that of most adolescents, who serve burgers in fast-food outlets or check in videotapes and DVDs at the local rental center. Yet the many hours spent at work did take away considerable time and energy needed for aspects of his schoolwork that were challenging to him and necessary for graduation.

The pickup truck that the young cook had bought with his earnings was a source of great pride to him, but it also had a negative effect on his schooling in several different ways. First, the truck cost a lot of money not only for its initial purchase, but also for insurance, fuel, desired improvements, and unanticipated repairs. Even while he was feeling desperate to fend off the threat of failing to graduate, this young cook initially argued that he could not reduce his long hours at work even temporarily because he needed to get more money to pay for new tires he had already bought and for imminently needed repair of the truck's transmission.

Second, having his own vehicle diminished contact between him and his parents. He was rarely home for meals, he drove himself to and from both school and work, and he used his truck during his spare time to drive around and look for friends with whom to socialize. His mother reported that she saw very little of her son and had little opportunity to talk with him about school, work, or anything else. She commented, "Since he's been getting his own paycheck and paying his own bills, and not needing to borrow my car, he feels independent, that he should be able to do pretty much whatever he pleases. I don't have much control over him anymore."

Even for adolescents who are not employed and do not have their own car, parents often feel a substantial loss of control over their adolescent sons and daughters after they get their license to drive. This is one of many reasons that most adolescents long for the day when they are able to obtain that little plastic-covered document that certifies them legally to drive a car. The driver's license becomes a badge of having left behind the constraints of childhood and of entering the privileged world of adults. But for most parents this transition is fraught with much worry and feelings of helplessness.

Parents may continue to exercise power over whether and when the adolescent is able to use their car, but whenever the teenager gets behind the wheel to drive unaccompanied by a parent, control of the driving is squarely on the shoulders of the adolescent himself. Some teenagers are careful and very competent drivers, but many are not. Escalated insurance rates for drivers under the age of twenty-five reflect the fact that, as a group, these less experienced adolescents and young adults have more accidents with more costly consequences than do most drivers older than twenty-six.

For adolescents and young adults who suffer from ADD syndrome, driving a car presents not only the same challenges and satisfactions as for anyone else of the same age, but also additional obstacles. In a series of studies of driving in young adults with ADHD, Russell Barkley (1993) and colleagues (1996, 2002) found that those with ADHD demonstrated numerous problems in operating a motor vehicle. In a study comparing adolescents and young adults with ADHD to matched controls, all of whom had comparable years of experience in driving, Barkley found that those in his ADHD sample did not differ significantly in their driving skills and experience by gender or by ADHD subtype, but they clearly differed from the non-ADHD control group. Official records showed that the individuals with ADHD had significantly more total traffic citations, license suspensions and revocations, and speeding tickets.

Further, while most members of both the ADHD and control groups had received at least one speeding ticket and had been involved in at least one motor vehicle accident while they were driving, there were significant differences between the two groups in the degree of their driving problems. Significantly more of the ADHD group reported that they had driven illegally before being licensed to drive; had been ticketed for twelve or more driving offenses; had received five or more speeding tickets; had their license suspended or revoked during their driving careers; and had been involved in three or more crashes. Similar findings have been reported by Shyamala Nada-Raja and colleagues (1997) from their epidemiological study of 916 adolescents in New Zealand. That study also found that females with ADHD were as much at risk of impaired driving and serious crashes as were males.

These data indicating that adolescents and young adults are at greater risk of driving violations and motor vehicle accidents are not surprising when one considers the great demands that driving places on executive functions, demands outlined in the opening pages of the Introduction.

Leaving Home

While getting a license and driving a car are important steps in an adolescent's journey toward independence from the parents, a far greater step occurs when the adolescent moves away from home to live at a university or in his own apartment. It would be hard to overstate the magnitude of change that this transition requires from any adolescent, but for those with ADHD, this massive separation from day-to-day contact with parents is even more challenging. At no point in life does the average individual face so many changes in so many aspects of life at one time with so few precedents to provide guidance.

> Like most of my friends, I really looked forward to college. All during senior year and through graduation everyone always talked about how we could hardly wait to get out of high school with those boring classes and ridiculous rules; and we were desperate to get away from our nosey parents who were always checking up on us—"Have you done your homework?" "Were you drinking last night at the party?"—and making stupid curfews even for weekend nights. For us, college meant freedom, a place where you can take care of yourself and where there is nobody checking up on you.
>
> When I actually got on campus it felt good, but kind of strange. Nobody really cared when I went to bed or when I got up or whether I ever went to class. Most nights I went out for beers with some guys from my dorm and smoked some weed on our way back. Back in my room I could stay on the Internet as late as I wanted and then I would crash about three or four in the morning. That left me too tired to get up for morning classes. Usually I slept until about noon. I missed a lot of classes and never really got most of the reading done. When I got up I would smoke a little more. Then lots of times I felt too tired to get to my afternoon classes. After a while I just gave up on going

to classes. I was hopelessly behind. That's how I failed all my
classes and got kicked out of the university at the end of the year.
It was all kind of a shock to my parents, because they never got
to see my grades and until the letter with bad news came in June
I kept telling them how it was hard, but I was doing OK.

This boy had been an honor student in a very competitive high school.
He had taken two advanced placement courses during senior year, scoring
well in both of them. He was a good high school athlete, earning varsity
letters in soccer and swimming. Although a bit shy, he had some friends
in high school and in the youth group at his church. While in sixth grade
this bright boy had encountered academic difficulties that led to his being
diagnosed with ADHD and placed on appropriate medication, which he
continued to take throughout high school because he and his parents
agreed it was helpful to him. He took a supply of his ADHD medication
to college, but rarely remembered to take it. He explained, "I guess I was
just used to my mother setting it out for me every morning. When I had
to remember for myself, it almost never happened."

This young man had been dependent on his parents in many unacknowledged ways, not only for taking medication. Throughout his schooling, despite his complaints, he depended on his parents to limit his tendency to stay up too late using the Internet, and to urge him to get to bed
early enough that he would be able to get up for classes the next day. He
said that his parents sometimes guided him explicitly, for example, by
chiding him when he stayed up too late or reminding him of the need to
get up on the many mornings when he slept through his alarm clock. But
he noted that his parents' influence on his behavior was more often indirect, without their actually intervening.

Even if they didn't say anything to me, I knew how they felt about
what I should be doing. Just knowing that they were there living
in the house with me, and that they would be worried if I just
slept and didn't go to school one day. Or that they would be really disappointed if they got a call from a teacher saying I hadn't
turned in some important term project.

It's not that they had any real power over me or would punish me. It's more that their presence, and their knowing what I was doing or possibly finding out pretty soon if I messed up, that would usually push me to do what I knew I really ought to be doing. It's like just their being around made this pressure inside me to "do the right thing." When I was away at school, I wasn't able to make myself do what I needed to do when I had to do it. I was completely by myself where nobody else around really knew or cared what I was doing.

For some adolescents, their primary source of emotional and social support is not their parents, but a dating partner, an older sibling, or a close friend. As they approach graduation, many high school students, with and without ADD syndrome, feel great worry and grief about the loss of their network of high school friends and others on whom they depend for daily commiseration, encouragement, study support, advice, and companionship. They are aware that they can stay in touch with each other via email, telephone, and occasional visits, but departing students also know that after high school graduation it won't be the same. While some high school seniors clearly anticipate and talk about the difficulty of leaving home, others are eventually surprised to realize the intensity of their feelings about leaving their "home" in this broader sense.

One high school senior in treatment for ADD syndrome was surprised in this way. He sought consultation soon after going by ambulance to the emergency room because of terrifying chest pains that had made him fear he was having a heart attack.

My girlfriend and I were with a few other seniors at this one kid's house. We'd gotten a pizza and Cokes to celebrate that all of us had finally finished up our college applications. It was the last day for us to hand them in to the guidance counselor for mailing. Just after we got to the house with the pizza I got this huge pain in my chest and couldn't catch my breath. I'm a good athlete in good condition and I've pushed hard in tough competition, but I'd never had anything like this. I felt like I was going to die. My friends got the ambulance and they took me to the hospital. I was there for about five hours having tests. After all that the doctors said I was just having a panic attack, not a heart attack. I don't know how that could be because I didn't feel worried about anything.

After a series of conversations, the precipitants of this young athlete's panic attack became less mysterious. Although he was not consciously aware of any specific worries, he gradually realized that the act of completing his college applications and sending them off was a milestone that had triggered many hidden fears. Most of all, he was afraid to leave his girlfriend.

I just can't imagine being without her. We've been going together for almost three years and we do everything together. All of the colleges I have applied to are just a couple of hours away, but she is just a junior so she'll still be here after I go. Even though we say we will never break up, I've seen a lot of other junior-senior couples at our school say that and then they ended it before Thanksgiving because they couldn't handle being apart in two worlds that are so separate. I just couldn't take the idea of her dating anyone else.

Besides, I don't know if I can get my work done without her. She's smarter than I am and she's always helping me study for tests and helping me write my papers and reminding me to get my reading done. She gets mad at me if I don't get decent grades on everything. And every night I talk to her on the phone for at least an hour while I'm at home in bed, even if we have been together all the time from when practice ended until we have to get home. It's almost like we're married.

This boy was taking medication that was helpful for his ADD syndrome, but he was not a strong student and he was very dependent on his girlfriend's daily support to help him organize his work and get it done. She quizzed him to prepare for tests and she nurtured his motivation to work hard at his sports, even when he felt discouraged about the team's performance. For several years he had spent far more waking hours with her than with his parents or anyone else. The prospect of living away from her, even just a couple of hours away, and having to function without her constant support, was frightening to him in many ways that he sensed only dimly until he began to explore the reasons for his panic attack.

Although many students with ADD syndrome face difficulties in making the transition to college because they are more dependent on their parents, dating partners, or others for daily support than are many of their friends, some have difficulty making the transition because others are dependent on them. One high school senior had been very successful in her academic work since junior high school when her ADD syndrome had been first diagnosed. Since that time she had been on a regimen of medication that worked well for her. She was very bright and worked hard on her studies, which included several honors-level classes each semester. It was a great shock to her and to her teachers when this girl's grades dropped in all of her classes during the first semester of her senior year of high school. She lamented,

> I don't know what's wrong with me. Ever since the second quarter of this senior year I just haven't been keeping up with my work. I still read a lot, but none of it is what is assigned. I've fallen behind in my homework in every class, even with a couple of big projects. Some tests I do OK on because I still listen in class, but if the test requires any real preparation, I don't do well because I'm not prepared. All my teachers are puzzled and some of them are really mad at me. Every night I go home intending to get my work done and every night I end up putting it off and doing just part of it or sometimes none of it at all. Same thing with my college applications. They all have to be done in less than a month and I haven't even started on one. Maybe I'm just not ready for college yet.

In talking further about her dilemma, this extraordinarily bright girl described a family situation that played an important role in her uncertainty about whether she was ready to go to college. Her father's work required frequent traveling, often for several nights at a time. Her mother had a long history of depression for which she had once been hospitalized after a suicide attempt. As an only child, this young girl felt an unspoken responsibility to provide daily companionship and support for her mother.

Each evening the girl helped her mother to prepare dinner. Later she spent an hour or more with her mother after supper while they watched and then discussed the television news. Just before retiring the girl would sit again with her mother, telling her about events at school or about the novels she was reading. These interactions brought much pleasure to the mother, who rarely smiled except when she was with her daughter. As the girl began her senior year of high school and began to talk about plans for college, the mother appeared to her daughter to be getting increasingly depressed.

Although the mother was explicitly encouraging her daughter to go forward with plans for college, her undercurrent of depression left her daughter fearful that going off to college might leave her mother feeling so lonely and sad that she might again become suicidal. This girl felt enormous guilt for disappointing her parents and teachers with declining academic work, but she felt even more fear about abandoning her needy mother. Her unwitting compromise was to fail at school and remain at home. Although adolescents with ADD syndrome often depend on others for support more do than many of their friends, sometimes they are also an important source of support for others, their family or friends. These are not mutually exclusive possibilities.

Executive Functions Involved in the Tasks of Adolescence

The developmental challenges described in this chapter are only a few of the many that adolescents face. Yet even in these simple examples, it is clear that adolescents are confronted with many complex tasks that require extensive use and further refinement of multiple executive functions. Moreover, the teenage years are when much of the support provided by teachers, parents, and others is diminished or withdrawn.

Sometimes the transitions are abrupt, like the move in school from having just one teacher in a single classroom for most of the day to having six or seven teachers daily (with rapidly escalated requirements for self-management of time, materials, and effort), or the move away from home and community to go to college. Sometimes the changes are more gradual. Either way, adolescence usually brings an escalation in the magnitude and complexity of task demands and social relationships, at a time when the teenager's physical and social development make peer interactions more complicated and introduce sexual overtones to social relationships. At this time the individual is required to manage not only concrete tasks, but also more complex social interactions, all while taking on much more planning for both the immediate future of the next few days or weeks and the longer-term future of graduation and beyond.

This longer-term future planning challenges an aspect of working memory that has not been discussed much in the neuropsychological literature thus far. Paul Eslinger (1996) observes:

> Executive functions importantly include diverse goal-directed behaviors over a period of time that extends beyond a few minutes and even to different spatial settings. For example, completing a graduate degree requires constant vigilance to both short-term and long-term goals. Development and maintenance of important social relationships . . . also requires persistent attention to immediate, short-term, and long-term goals.
>
> This type of prospective archival memory is not well-defined in current models. . . . It qualifies as a type of working memory because it implies prospective memory-guided responding rather than sensory-guided responding. It is frequently changing yet enduring over a long period of time. Does the influence of future goals reside in some form of longer-term working memory that is kept alive by daily activities such as the behaviors that alter future consequences? (p. 385)

It is during adolescence that this ability to relate the choices of the moment and of the day to longer-term aims and goals becomes increasingly important. This aspect of working memory is often significantly impaired in adolescents with ADD syndrome. As the scaffolding of earlier years is

gradually removed and, further, as the individual encounters the cata-
clysmic changes of moving out of the family home to live in a university
dormitory or one's own apartment, the effect of impaired executive functions is likely to become increasingly powerful, though it may not be recognized as causing impaired functioning. Eslinger (1996) emphasized,

> Executive function impairments have a particularly insidious
> effect on child, adolescent and even adult development and may
> underlie difficulties in many poor learners and workers as well
> as poorly adjusted parents and citizens. Throughout life phases,
> there is increasing demand for complexity and organization of
> psychological processing as well as control of powerful emotions
> and potentially destructive behaviors.
>
>   With development, most settings also provide only partial in-
> formation pertinent to long-term goals and require greater inhi-
> bition of prepotent responses and longer delays before rewards
> are to occur. Hence, unlike content-specific deficiencies in read-
> ing and spelling, developmental executive function impairments
> are much more difficult to observe, identify and manage. (p. 387)

As described in Chapter 3, Jay Giedd and others (1999) used longitudinal imaging to study brains of teenagers to demonstrate that, contrary
to earlier assumptions, adolescence is a time of amazingly rapid and extensive brain growth followed by extensive pruning of neurons to make
the adolescent's brain more efficient. Despite this growth, for many adolescents there is not a good fit between their developing capacities and the
demands of their environment. Their ability to negotiate the increasingly
complex demands of adolescence is inconsistent and sometimes wildly erratic. For most adolescents who suffer from ADD syndrome, this process
of major transitions is even more difficult; for some, it is overwhelming.

Chapter 6 Adulthood: Managing Responsibilities, Finding a Niche

MYTH: Unless you have been diagnosed with ADD as a child, you can't have it as an adult.

FACT: Many adults have struggled all of their lives with unrecognized ADD. They haven't received help because they have assumed that their chronic difficulties were caused by character faults such as laziness or lack of motivation.

During the adult years, especially the early adult years, most individuals are faced with many new adjustments and important choices that will shape their future in both the short and longer term. For those who suffer from ADD syndrome, these challenges are especially difficult. One twenty-six-year-old man with ADD syndrome described his difficulties with selecting options and working productively:

> I've always had a hard time making choices. I switched my major five times in the three years I was in college. I keep trying things out and then I get bored and feel like something else would be better, so I switch. Finally I dropped out to try getting a job. Figured I'd go back to school after I knew better what I want. That was four years ago and since then I've had seven different jobs. All of them seemed OK for a while. I came in on time and worked hard to learn the job and do it right. Then I always started getting bored and coming in late and slacking off. And sometimes I'd get in trouble for being too mouthy with the boss. Once I got fired for that. The rest of the jobs I just left because I had an idea of something else that might be better.

I do the same thing with everything. When I'm watching TV I have to hold the remote because I always have to keep changing channels to see what else is on. Same with girlfriends. For a while I like this one, then I see someone else who looks better. So I drop the first one and then hook up with the other one for a while, until someone else comes along. Recently though I've been remembering something one of my professors said: "As we grow up, life has to be a succession of amputations of possibilities." I always like to keep all my possibilities open, but I don't know where I'll end up when I'm forty if I keep doing this.

This young man was very bright. His tested IQ was in the very superior range. He had perfect scores for both the verbal and math portions of the SAT. His grades in college courses varied widely, usually between "A" and "F" with not many in between. He explained, "It all depended on whether I was interested in the course." Professors in a variety of subjects often commented that his papers were "brilliant" and encouraged him to follow through with more advanced studies. This "hyper" man was also very creative: he was skilled at playing many musical instruments and had won awards for photographs he had taken. He had an appealing manner and a quick wit. But he was also very impulsive, hyperactive, and restless, both cognitively and behaviorally.

Like many others treated for ADD syndrome during their elementary and secondary schooling, this young man had decided to stop taking medication for ADD when he entered college. Though he was very bright, his untreated ADD symptoms seriously interfered with his attending classes regularly and completing assignments for his courses. He invested himself energetically in courses that appealed to him; those were the courses in which he earned A's. But if he felt the professor was not a sufficiently lively lecturer, he avoided attending. If he found some of the assigned readings uninteresting, he simply did not read them. Many short papers and major projects were not completed. By the end of his third year, this student had developed a smattering of interest in several areas, but was not able to invest himself enough in any one field of study to create a major. This is when he dropped out of school.

It is not unusual for individuals with ADD syndrome to drop out or fail out of college. At our clinic for attention and related disorders at Yale, we studied 103 adults with high IQ scores who had sought treatment for attentional problems. Each person entering the clinic who scored 120 or above on the IQ test, within the top 9 percent of the general population, was invited to be in the study. All agreed. We found that 42 percent of these extremely bright men and women had dropped out of postsecondary schooling at least once. Many eventually returned to complete their education and some later did quite well. Academic problems of these high-IQ adults were not due to any lack of intelligence, nor were these adults uninterested in learning. Like the young man described earlier, many of them did extremely well in a small number of courses where they found the instructor especially stimulating or where they had a strong personal interest in the subject.

These bright individuals dropped out or were kicked out of university because they were not able to manage themselves well enough to meet minimal requirements for university study. With just a few exceptions, they did not leave because of substance abuse; they failed out because they were unable to make themselves go to classes regularly, take decent notes, complete the assigned readings, study adequately for tests, and finish enough written assignments on time. Most reported that they realized at the time what needed to be done, and tried to push themselves to do it, but just did not have enough "willpower" to make it happen.

Many reported that while in university they often became distracted by issues or topics outside the curriculum, while ignoring the courses they had signed up for. Or they would invest all their efforts and energy in one course they found stimulating, while totally ignoring several others that they also needed to pass. In their earlier years of schooling they might have gazed out the window excessively during class or have been slow to complete homework assignments, yet they still met most of the basic requirements. As adults, distractibility might mean that they stayed away from the classroom altogether and avoided any or all assignments. Many of these high-IQ students spoke of how when they first arrived at college they wandered about from one interest to another, with no sense of where they were headed or how their activities day-to-day and week-to-week were linked to any longer-term goal like completing course requirements, earning a degree, or preparing for a career.

The young man's comment "I've always had difficulty making choices" reflects a problem with "omnipotentiality"—a fantasy-based attitude, common among adolescents, that all things are possible, all choices are open. Usually this attitude is dispelled during mid- to late adolescence as most individuals are forced to confront the reality that some doors are not open to them. They discover that they cannot get into a particular college they want to attend or enroll in a specific course that sounds interesting or be hired for a specific job that they would like to do. Sometimes these impediments to fulfilling a particular aspiration come from lack of ability, sometimes from not having met educational prerequisites, sometimes simply because there are many more qualified applicants than there are available openings.

As they experience such disappointments and frustrations, most young adults reconcile themselves to the need to make choices and to abandon some interests, "amputating" some possibilities in order to invest themselves in others. Usually they also come to recognize that choosing a career is not simply a matter of making a decision about what one wants, but about trying to make an acceptable fit between what one wants and is able to do with opportunities that are actually available. Many young adults with ADD syndrome take longer to learn this lesson. With a persisting sense of omnipotentiality, they experience themselves as being on a protracted shopping trip for life options—interested in multiple possibilities, but unable to invest in any one choice enough to put up with the inevitable frustrations of getting started and becoming established.

In 1978 Daniel Levinson and colleagues published a study of adult development reporting results of in-depth interviews with a sample of men aged thirty-five to forty-five, some blue collar, some white collar. He found that despite their diversity of employment and social class, these men all experienced predictable phases in their adult development. In particular, most of the men found choosing an occupation to be a long, difficult process.

It is often assumed that by his early twenties a man normally ought to have a firm occupational choice and be launched in a well-defined line of work. This assumption is erroneous. It reflects the prevailing view that development is normally complete by the end of adolescence. We have found that the sequence is longer and more difficult. . . . An initial serious choice is usually made . . . sometime between 17 and 29. Even when the first choice seems to be very definite, it usually turns out to represent a preliminary definition of interests and values. . . . A young man may struggle for several years to sort out his multiple interests, to discover what occupations, if any, may serve as a vehicle for living out his interests, and to commit himself to a particular line of work. (p. 101)

Among young adults with ADD syndrome, this lengthy process of developing commitment to a particular line of work appears often to be more protracted than for most of their peers. Many of these men and women find themselves having a hard time not only with making occupational choices, but also in dealing with the usual frustrations of getting started in a job. Their chronic impulsivity may lead to a long series of quick and sometimes unwise decisions to pursue other jobs that seem more interesting, have fewer frustrations, or offer greater potential rewards. Russell Barkley and colleagues (1996) compared young adults with ADHD to others of similar ages from the same community. They found that the average time on the job for the ADHD group was 9.3 months, compared to 21.5 months for controls.

The experience of the twenty-six-year-old man profiled at the beginning of the chapter illustrates how job problems may involve interpersonal conflicts with coworkers, supervisors, or employers. One source of such conflict reported by many adults with ADD syndrome is failure to comply with deadlines or to get to work on time. Sometimes their lateness is a result of not being able to fall asleep at a reasonable hour and thus having difficulty getting up early enough in the morning. For some, the cause is a chronic difficulty in waking up, regardless of how much sleep they have had. For still others, the fault lies in chronically poor planning: they fail to allow enough time for showering, getting dressed, eating breakfast, and driving to work.

Many of these young adults have a long history of missing their school bus and being tardy to school, even when parents have been very active in trying to awaken and prompt them. It is not surprising that they continue to experience such difficulties, especially when no one living with them will take on the frustrating task of getting them started each morning. Yet research suggests that the problems of adults with ADD syndrome in regulating their time stem not simply from failing to learn how to manage a morning routine. Chronic difficulties in fitting actions into segments of time appear to be an aspect of the ADD syndrome.

Russell Barkley and others (2001a) studied time perception and reproduction in adults with ADHD compared to normal controls. Each was asked to estimate the duration of various short intervals of time, from two to sixty seconds, presented to them by an examiner. They were also asked to reproduce time intervals by telling the examiner when to start and stop a stopwatch to make intervals of twelve, forty-five, and sixty seconds. Regardless of ADHD subtype or gender, the adults with ADHD were able to estimate time duration as accurately as controls, but they reproduced the time intervals significantly less accurately than did the control subjects, by making them longer than they were supposed to be. Barkley commented, "The problem is not so much one of inaccurate sense of time as inadequate behavioral performance relative to it (p.357)." The intervals that these adults were being asked to stipulate were only sixty seconds or less. This is but a miniature of the problem experienced by many adults with ADD syndrome when they need to allocate time for longer tasks with multiple variables, for example, driving to work in rush-hour traffic. Their difficulties with such tasks cause many adults with ADD syndrome chronically to arrive late for work or for meetings with colleagues or customers.

Often these adults also have chronic difficulties with deadlines. One young salesman was shocked when his employer threatened to fire him for failing to submit expense-account reports in a timely fashion. This occurred after he had ignored repeated requests and reminders, then submitted six months' worth of expense reports totaling over seventeen thousand dollars just after the small company had closed its books on the fiscal year. He was confident that his very successful record in sales for the company would cause his employer to overlook his delinquency in filing the reports. He assumed that his boss would make allowances just as most of his high school teachers had given him high grades because he wrote very good papers, even though he usually handed his papers in late. He assumed too much.

Like the young man described at the beginning of the chapter, this salesman got mouthy with his boss when confronted about his negligence. He did not adequately modulate his emotions. Rather than accepting the correction and promising to improve his performance, he impulsively talked back to his boss, angrily pointing out shortcomings he saw in the boss and in other colleagues. His emotional outburst exacerbated the conflict and got him fired from a position in which he had made a very promising start. Further, this result affected subsequent efforts to seek another position. His reference letter from the job he lost indicated strong sales ability, but also significant problems with record keeping, meeting deadlines, and insubordination.

Some individuals take longer than others to recognize such problems in themselves and to begin an effort to change. In the case of the college dropout described earlier, what caused him to seek treatment was not his failure to complete his university studies, nor his difficulty in sustaining a job. He came seeking help because he was close to losing a relationship that had become important to him. His girlfriend had threatened to dump him because he was unable to sustain a serious relationship with her. Only then did he begin to realize that he was setting himself up for long-term frustration if he continued to switch girlfriends and jobs as rapidly and impulsively as he switched channels on the TV.

His girlfriend had told him that she loved him, but could not continue the relationship because she was at a point in her life where she wanted and needed someone more ready "to quit jumping around and more ready to start investing himself in one job and one long-term relationship." He described her as "very special in a different way" than any other woman he had ever dated and said tearfully that he didn't want to lose her.

Yet he was very uncertain about whether he could make and sustain the kind of commitments she was asking for.

The young man's primary motive for seeking consultation was that he wanted to resume taking medication that had been helpful in alleviating his ADD syndrome impairments earlier in life. He had been diagnosed as "hyperactive" and was given medication for these symptoms from third grade until the end of high school, when he had decided to stop taking it. "When I was on that stuff I was still pretty hyper, but it seemed like I could stick with things a lot better. I'm wondering if something like that could help me now so I could settle down at my job and in my relationship with her, and maybe even go back to school."

After this consultation at age twenty-six, he resumed taking a medication for ADD syndrome, an improved version of the same medication he had stopped taking ten years earlier. With this support he was able to sustain the relationship with his girlfriend and stay in his job long enough to get promoted twice.

Some adults with ADD syndrome can negotiate the frustrations of their early adult years without too much difficulty. Many successfully complete their education and find that their ADD symptoms do not impair them so much after they get into more advanced stages of education, where they can specialize in studies that interest them. In later years of schooling and as they enter the world of employment, some are able to specialize in work that "turns them on," avoiding tasks that were very difficult and burdensome when they were in school full-time. Some are even able to find employment that for them is much like getting paid to play an enjoyable game. This fortunate outcome would be equivalent to Larry, the inattentive goalie of Chapter 1, successfully finishing college and then developing a career as a professional hockey player. Many others, however, are not so fortunate.

Managing a Household and Finances

Regardless of their work situation, most adults eventually need to manage their own household. For many young adults, the tasks of household management are initially frustrating and somewhat difficult, but mostly mastered without serious problems. For young adults with ADD syndrome, however, these tasks often tax their impaired executive function abilities in ways that can become highly problematic.

One twenty-seven-year-old junior high school teacher sought treatment after studying about ADHD in a graduate course she was taking to fulfill requirements for a master's degree. Arriving thirty minutes late for her first appointment because she had lost the directions mailed to her, she apologized and then explained:

> I need to get evaluated for ADD because I know I have it and it's really messing me up. Maybe if I get the right medication, things will get better. In this graduate course we just studied about ADD and every symptom on the list is something that has been a problem for me all my life. I'm terrible about planning and organizing. I can't stay focused when I read. I never remember what I've read. I've got a great memory for things from a long time ago, but my short-term memory has never been any good. I'm the world's biggest procrastinator, always late with everything. I got through my undergraduate degree, just barely, but now I'm really struggling with this graduate course. I can't keep up with the reading and the tests are really hard. I haven't even started yet on a big paper that is due in three days.
>
> I need to pass this course because I need more graduate credits to earn more money. And I desperately need more money because my financial situation is a mess. I just got an eviction notice from my landlord because I'm three months behind in my rent. And the leasing company is threatening to repossess my car if I don't pay up on three back payments I owe them. On top of that, I'm driving now with no insurance on my car because I haven't kept up with paying that either. I've lost two department store charge cards because of late payments and I'm up to my neck in credit card debt. Oh, and I haven't filed income tax for the past two years, even though I want to get it done because I should be getting a refund.

I hope I don't have to move because I like my apartment. Besides, my place is such a mess, I could never get it all packed up. I'm totally disorganized with piles of stuff all over the floor and the tables and the chairs. There's barely enough clear space for two people to sit and eat a meal or watch TV. I always take good care of my appearance, but at home I'm such a slob. My sink is always full of dirty dishes and I never do laundry until everything I own is dirty and I have nothing left to wear. Sometimes I just go out and buy some new clothes so I can put off doing the laundry for just a little longer.

This intelligent, witty, vivacious teacher was well liked by her students and respected by her colleagues, but she had great difficulty meeting the demands of her graduate-level course and in managing her household routines and finances. Her parents had provided "loans" to bail her out of several financial scrapes, but their resources were limited and she recognized that she needed to manage her own money, time, and stuff in a much better planned and more responsible way.

During our evaluation, this teacher described her repeated efforts to plan a budget so she could meet her expenses in a systematic way. Always she found herself sabotaging her good intentions by impulsively buying new clothes or choosing to go with friends on expensive vacations she could not afford. Both her apartment and her leased car had been selected too much on the basis of how desirable they were without enough attention to the high monthly payments required. She had calculated her expenses for these items on the basis of her total monthly paycheck without taking into account the amount needed for utilities, groceries, gas, and other recurrent expenses.

The results of her evaluation indicated severe ADHD, which responded well to appropriate medication treatment. With that treatment she was able to organize her household more effectively, though it took her two years to stabilize her finances. She did this by implementing plans she had drawn up much earlier, but hadn't been able consistently to follow. Her problem had not been a failure to understand what she needed to do. It was that she could not consistently do it.

Managing Work While Nurturing Relationships

The challenges of adult life do not all come in the earliest adult years. Some with ADD syndrome report that they encounter problems from their executive-function impairments later, in unexpected ways. One thirty-three-year-old woman with ADD syndrome sought treatment after working successfully for ten years as an intensive care nurse in a large hospital. She had been diagnosed with ADHD during high school and had benefited from medication treatment for this throughout high school and college.

> My ADHD is kicking up again. With the medicine I was taking for it during high school and college I did very well. I stopped taking it after I graduated and got into full-time nursing. I didn't seem to need it anymore. The excitement of working in the ICU kept me plenty focused. I'm good at my work and I love the challenge of caring for these really sick patients. Now things are getting bad again for me. I'm having that same frustration and feeling of helplessness and stupidity that I had for so many years before I got diagnosed.
>
> The trouble started after I gave birth to our son three years ago; he's our second kid. We wanted two kids and they're both a lot of fun. But they're also a lot of work, and he's an especially lively handful. Since he started walking and getting into things, it has been a real struggle for me at home. My husband helps a lot and my mother-in-law provides day care for him when I work. That's all good, but the two kids together exhaust me. And then two months ago I got promoted to be nurse manager for our ICU. That's been a disaster. I can't keep up with all the work of scheduling staff, ordering supplies, and attending meetings. It's worse than it ever was for me when I was doing just direct patient care. I can't go on this way.

This woman speaks of her ADHD "kicking up again" as though it were a recurrence of a disease that had been in remission. But ADHD is not a disease; instead it is a disorder that is closely tied to daily experiences. The woman's problem resulted from the escalating demands of her new job as a nurse manager, along with the exhausting responsibilities of caring for her two young children. So long as she had only one child to care for and was doing only direct nursing care, she felt competent and was successful, so much so that she was offered and accepted the promotion. The trouble emerged when she was faced daily with increasing challenges to her executive functions both on the job and at home with her family.

The administrative burdens of her manager's job included setting up the work schedules for three shifts, finding coverage for nurses calling in sick, keeping track of supplies that needed to be ordered, filing required reports, representing the interests of her unit in administrative meetings, and arbitrating disputes among staff members. Unlike direct patient care, which was intensive and complex but limited to dealing with just a few patients within the limits of eight-hour shifts, this administrative position required much planning, thought, and discussion over both the short and longer terms. It required her to keep in mind countless requests, complaints, and tasks that carried over from one day to the next, sometimes over weeks and months. In short, these management tasks severely challenged this nurse's chronic executive-function impairments in organizing and prioritizing, in sustaining attention, and in utilizing working memory.

At home too this woman encountered increasing demands on her executive functions. When her son became old enough to walk, talk, and actively engage with his sister and the rest of his environment, the task of caring for him became much more demanding. He was a very lively little boy who turned out to have a fairly severe case of ADHD (this was not surprising, since parents with ADHD have a markedly elevated risk of having a child with ADHD). His energetic, sometimes wild temperament intensified the mother's already substantial job of parenting, given that the two children were only two years apart in age.

The woman's challenges at home included not just twice as many loads of laundry to fold, baths to give, and plates to prepare at each mealtime. She was also faced daily with repeated hassles between the children, each one often complaining to her about the other and persistently demanding that she resolve their dispute of the moment. Her son presented special problems with his fearless impulsivity. He required extremely close monitoring virtually every moment; often quick interventions were needed to protect him from unanticipated dangers. In addition, like many children with ADHD, her son had chronic difficulty falling asleep. This resulted in his making numerous curtain calls well past his bedtime; often it also brought two or three interruptions to her sleep each night as she was asked to calm him after a nightmare or to change wet sheets on his bed.

These and countless other demands by her children on her energy, efforts, patience, and management skills were exhausting to this mother. Some of the problems she faced at home were common to caring for any pair of young children; others were more typical of families that include a young child with severe ADHD. Even though she had support and assistance from her husband and mother-in-law, this mother felt chronically fatigued and frustrated, with an increasing feeling of incompetence at home and at work. The gap between her executive-function capacities and the expanded demands on these capacities from her family and new job had become too wide.

After his intensive interview study of life-course development in men, described earlier, Daniel Levinson similarly studied three groups of women: homemakers, women with corporate-financial careers, and women with academic careers. Levinson died just after completing the first draft of the manuscript reporting their results. His wife, Judy Levinson, a coworker in the study, completed the project and brought the book to publication in 1996. In summarizing reports from women who were attempting to balance both marriage and a demanding career, they observed:

> By their late thirties most of these career women came to understand the illusory nature of the image of Superwoman who could "do it all" with grace and flair. Their self-image was more that of the Juggler, who kept many spheres in the air without dropping any or losing a step in the perpetual forward motion. While continually seeking balance, most women found it impossible to give anything like equal priority to the various components of the life structure. In general, occupation was the first priority, motherhood second, marriage a poor third, leisure and friendship a rare luxury, and with all the external tasks to be

done, almost no time for the self. The women's lives were usually hectic, at times chaotic and exhausting. . . . It would get better in time, they hoped, as the children grew older and the career stabilized. (p. 349)

The nurse described in this case example faced the same draining pressures that Levinson found characteristic of many career women, most of whom, presumably, did not have ADD syndrome. In her case, these pressures were intensified by the special needs of her son who suffered from ADHD, at that time untreated. The combination of these increased demands on her executive functions and her chronic impairments of ADD syndrome caused her to seek treatment.

During treatment, this nurse recognized her dilemma and clarified her priorities. She spoke most of her painful awareness that she was not providing for her children the quality of care that she wanted to give them. She said,

I'm usually doing OK at getting them the basics, but I know that I'm just not there enough for them emotionally. I'm always disorganized and frazzled and tired and too frustrated. Half the time when I lie down beside them at night to read a story, I fall asleep before they do and during the day, so much of the time I'm just too impatient. I'm not expecting to give perfection; no parent can do that. But I know they need me to be there to talk with them and to listen, to explain things to them, and to be there for them emotionally. I want to do that for them. That's an important part of my helping them to grow up. I don't want to miss out on it.

After some psychotherapy and talking at length with her husband, this woman decided that she wanted not only to resume medication treatment for her ADD syndrome, but also to resign from her manager's position and return to direct nursing care. She felt this would be more satisfying for her and that it would allow her to engage more fully in caring for her children.

Any parent's task in providing good scaffolding for a child is complex, requiring daily changes and heavy demands on executive functions. It includes anticipation, planning, and actions—doing tasks to care for the child and gradually teaching the child how to do these tasks alone. It includes modeling and explaining—showing the child in countless examples how to act and react in multiple practical and social situations of daily life. Scaffolding also includes attitudes and expectations, some overt and explicit, others more implicit and subtle, that help the child to form a personal picture of what ought to be, of what ought to be expected from one's self and others. Perhaps most important in this aspect of scaffolding is the parent's communicating to the child a sense of being cared for not only as one who is valued as a precious being, but also as one from whom certain attitudes, behaviors, and outcomes are expected—showing throughout the changes of each month and year that what this growing child feels and does each day really matters to this loving and beloved parent.

Providing this scaffolding is the process in which this nurse and mother wanted to be more fully involved. The disruption of her life that she had experienced after her promotion had created a crisis that helped her both to redefine her priorities and to find a more effective way to cope with her ADD syndrome.

Parenting and Sustaining Partnerships

It is not only women who find that ADD syndrome can unexpectedly disrupt life in the middle adult years. One man with unrecognized ADD sought consultation at age forty-three when his wife shocked him by announcing that she wanted to end their sixteen-year marriage. When the couple came for consultation together, the wife quietly presented her long pent-up frustration and her reasons for wanting to leave:

> I've just reached a point where I am fed up with too much giv-
> ing and not enough getting back. I feel like I've been raising not
> just two children, but three. My husband does a good enough
> job at work, and he's a good provider, but at home he's just like
> one of the kids. I have to struggle with him to get him up and
> off to work every morning and I have to remind him to get off

the computer every night so he won't stay up playing games until 2 or 3 a.m. I've given up on his taking care of the monthly bills because he never remembers to pay them on time. We were getting threatening letters and calls from creditors because he forgot to pay. There was enough money in the bank and he had said he would take care of it.

Once in a while he'll start a project at home, but then he never finishes it. For two years we've had bare two-by-fours in our bedroom where he keeps saying he's going to put in new plasterboard. Mostly when he's home, he's on the computer or watching sports on TV. He never remembers anybody's birthday or our anniversary and he says he'll come to the kids' sports events, but then forgets to show up. When I try to talk with him, he listens for maybe a minute or two and then he's drifting off talking about something else. Even in those times when he starts to say something to me, he gets off the point before his third sentence. He's not a heavy drinker and he's not abusive, but he is neglectful. I've been married to him for sixteen years, but all that time I've felt neglected by this man. He seems to need a mother to take care of him day by day more than he needs or wants a wife.

The husband did not dispute his wife's complaints. He cried. He acknowledged his recurrent forgetfulness and his frequent neglect of tasks, events, and concerns that were important to his wife and to his children.

You're right! I make a lot of promises to you and the kids that I don't follow through on. And I do depend on you to keep me organized and to remind me about what needs to be done and when to do it. I've never been good at stuff like that. When I was a kid, even all the way through high school, my mother had to hassle me every day to get up in the morning. If she didn't, I would sleep through school. I've never been able to get myself up with an alarm clock. And she had to keep pressuring and reminding me to get my homework and chores done. Even though

I wanted to, I just couldn't manage that stuff myself. You help
me with so much, and you're not even mean about it. I just
don't know if I can change the way I've been for so many years.
I don't know if it's something that can be changed.

The complicated causes of the crisis in this marriage had been fester-
ing for many years before they erupted in the wife's threat to separate. Initially the husband claimed and believed that he had not been unhappy in
the marital relationship. Later he gradually recognized that his wife's frequent reminders and supports were frustrating and sometimes very irri-
tating to him, even though they were also helpful protection against his
own tendencies to live too much in the moment.

As they talked further about their mutual frustrations, this couple saw
that they had become trapped in maladaptive efforts to cope with the husband's unrecognized ADD syndrome. During childhood and adolescence
his mother had provided intensive support and structure without which
this man probably never would have finished high school. Shortly after
high school he met and quickly married his wife, who gradually took over
his mother's caretaking role, supporting him through his college studies,
maintaining a household, and eventually carrying most of the responsibility for caring for their two children.

Both partners agreed that they had shared many satisfactions and
good times in their sixteen years of marriage, but they also recognized that
their relationship could not continue without major changes. The change
most urgently needed was for the husband to begin treatment for the
ADD syndrome that had plagued him since childhood; it had never been
recognized in school or at home, probably because he had never been hyperactive or disruptive. As they learned about the nature of ADD, the
couple recognized that symptoms of this syndrome had contributed substantially to the husband's serious underachievement in school, his very
marginal performance in college, and his continuing erratic performance
on the job.

When he began appropriate medication treatment, the husband experienced dramatic, rapid improvement in many of his ADD symptoms.
This did not suddenly resolve all the couple's marital problems, but it cre-

ated and sustained conditions under which they were able gradually to work out a very different, more reciprocal style of relationship. In the process they also recognized that the increasing underachievement of their fourteen-year-old son in high school was virtually a carbon copy of his father's problems at that time in his own life. Both father and son benefited from ADD treatment in ways that produced a much more satisfying life for the entire family.

In looking at the development of this family, one might wonder how this particular husband and wife happened to find each other. How did this man so early in life find a partner so willing and able to provide him the scaffolding previously created and sustained by his mother? Why would this woman choose to attach herself so early in her life to this man with such great needs for a parent-like partner? Why did she continue so long in this pattern? And why did she then become so frustrated with their established patterns of interaction after sixteen years of married life together? Adequate answers to these questions are beyond the scope of this book, but the questions highlight factors that are relevant and important to the experience of many adults with ADD syndrome.

Most individuals do not choose a life partner or other important voluntary relationships at random. People tend to seek out and pursue relationships with others to whom they feel attracted and with whom they feel comfortable. When discussing their choice of marriage partners, people often describe the attractions of physical appearance, but usually far more important are mutual attractions due to many complicated, unrecognized features of personality and interpersonal style. Such elements can have a powerful effect on interpersonal attraction and/or conflict, often in ways that are noticeable only over time as the attachment develops more fully.

John Bowlby (1978), a pioneer developer of attachment theory, wrote about the persistence of early experience in such choices throughout the lifespan. He used the term "representational models" to refer to individuals' persisting personal views of self and others—their aggregated expectations, complex and only partly conscious, of persons to whom they are attached, which includes their image of who a person is and of what that person wants, intends, and will do.

Whatever representational models of attachment figures and of self an individual builds during childhood and adolescence tend to persist relatively unchanged into and throughout adult life. As a result one tends to assimilate any new person with whom he may form a bond—a spouse, child, employer or therapist—to an existing model and often to continue to do so despite repeated evidence that the model is inappropriate. Similarly, one expects to be perceived and treated by others in ways that would be appropriate to his self-model and to continue with such expectations despite contrary evidence. Such biased perceptions and expectations lead to various misconceived beliefs about other people, to false expectations about the way they will behave, and to inappropriate actions intended to forestall their expected behavior. (p. 16)

In this passage Bowlby emphasizes problematic ways in which expectations from earlier relationships can carry over into formation of adult relationships. But the same processes sometimes bring a good fit, or at least, a mixed bag. A person may unwittingly seek out and develop a relationship with another person amazingly well-suited and motivated to continue, at least up to some point, patterns of interaction familiar from early family life.

In this couple, the man found a woman who was attracted to him for many reasons, one of which was that he needed and wanted the nurturance and support that she was motivated by her earlier life experiences to provide. He was strongly motivated to become bonded to a caring person who would provide the scaffolding earlier provided by his mother to compensate for persisting impairments of his ADD syndrome. And she found and joined herself to this man whose need and wish for her to provide such intensive scaffolding was, at least initially, appealing and rewarding to her. Over the many years of their marriage, the wishes and needs of each partner changed, resulting in the conflict that threatened to disrupt their marriage.

One primary source of change in most marital relationships is the birth and development of a child. Usually each new member added to a family profoundly changes the routines and dynamics of the family. The newborn infant's very survival depends on the parents adequately arranging their schedule and activities to see that the child is carefully watched over, fed, comforted, rested, played with, and cared for throughout each day and night. Usually this involves not only a rearrangement of schedules, but also massive sacrifices of time, energy, and freedom by the parents, often far more from one parent than from the other. And when a new child arrives in a family that already includes one or more children, sacrifices are inevitably forced on the older children as well.

The entry of a new child into a family does not only mean sacrifice, however; it also enriches the lives of parents and any siblings. Donald Winnicott, the extraordinary British pediatrician (1965), put it this way:

> The parents, in their efforts to build a family, benefit from . . .
> the integrative tendencies of the individual children. It is not
> simply the loveableness of the infant or child; there is some-
> thing more than that, for children are not always sweet. The in-
> fant and child flatter us by *expecting a degree of reliability and
> availability* to which we respond. . . . In this way, our own capaci-
> ties are strengthened and brought out, developed, by what is ex-
> pected of us from our children. In innumerable and very subtle
> ways, as well as in obvious ways, infants and children produce a
> family around them, perhaps by needing something, something
> which we give. (p. 47)

Since the needs of children are not static, but change dramatically as the child grows older, the effects of the child's needs and of his giving to the parents continually evolve, causing ongoing change in the parents, both in themselves and in their interactions with one another. In the couple described earlier, the wife's frustrations with her husband escalated as their children entered adolescence. As the children appropriately became less engaged at home and developed more independent adolescent lives, the mother acutely felt the loss of the precious satisfactions of providing a competent and caring scaffolding for them. And as her children became more private and more independent from the family, this mother felt

more intensely the lopsidedness, frustrations, and loneliness in her marriage. Consequently, she began increasingly to resent the continuing lack
of mature reciprocity in her relationship with her husband.

Changes in the life situation outside of the family can also alter the
effects of ADD symptoms on adult lives. A fifty-seven-year-old man, chief
executive officer of a multinational corporation, brought his son for consultation after the boy had failed out of university. The boy had done fairly
well in an exclusive prep school where his daily routine had been tightly
organized for classes, sports, and supervised homework. In the very competitive college that enrolled him, however, he failed miserably during his
first year. At the suggestion of a perceptive professor, the father brought
his son to be evaluated for a possible attention disorder.

The boy fully met diagnostic criteria for ADHD and responded well to
appropriate medication treatment as he took courses in a local college. He
returned to the university on probationary status and was quite successful
with the support of continuing treatment. A few months later, the boy's father called me, requesting an appointment to be evaluated himself. When
we met, he explained his motivation.

> I've been very successful in my career for several reasons. First,
> I'm a good idea man: I can envision how things can be devel-
> oped in a creative way. I'm also a good troubleshooter, identify-
> ing problems and finding effective ways to fix them. But most
> important, I know how to pick good lieutenants.
>
> I have several very competent administrative assistants who
> keep me organized and help me do my job. They keep my calen-
> dar and remind me of what needs to be done when. They help to
> organize and prioritize my work. They track my correspondence
> and edit my dictation. Without them I could never stay on top of
> all I have to do. If my son had someone like that to assist him in
> college, he never would have flunked out.
>
> Not many people know this, but I never finished university.
> I flunked out at the end of my third year. I lasted a little longer
> than my son did in his college studies, but mine was an easier
> school. We both failed for very similar problems.

I want this evaluation for ADD because I know I still have the same problems my son has. I could see that when I was here as you asked him all those questions in his evaluation. I've made all the money I need and I'm planning to take early retirement next year. My goal for retirement is to return to university and finish the degree I wasn't able to complete before. But I know I can't take any administrative assistants into courses with me, and there is just no way I will be able to do that work unless my attention and memory problems are fixed. I want you to evaluate me and see if you agree that I have ADHD too. If so, I'd like to arrange to get the same medication my son is being helped by. I believe, no—I *know*—that the medication will be helpful to me. I've already tried it.

This very successful executive did, in fact, fully meet diagnostic criteria for the predominantly inattentive type of ADHD, and he did respond well to treatment as well as finally complete a university degree. His story illustrates how some fortunate individuals with untreated ADD syndrome can achieve extraordinary success, even in very demanding and responsible positions, when they have sufficient help to compensate for their executive function impairments.

In this case, the administrative assistants in the corporation supported this talented man in leading his massive corporation to international success. While rising to the top of his corporation's administrative ladder, he had also benefited from the work of many other secretaries and subordinates who helped him to do tasks that he continued to find very difficult. But when he anticipated his early retirement, he realized that his persisting problems with executive functions would prevent him from completing a degree, just as they had thirty-six years earlier, unless they were alleviated.

Not every adult with untreated ADD syndrome is fortunate enough to have salaried assistants to help compensate for executive function impairments. But many do have coworkers, spouses, or others from whom they obtain needed assistance. Sometimes help comes in the form of a simple redivision of labor, whereby an employer allows a worker with ADD syndrome to be responsible for aspects of the job in which that worker has strong interest and talent, while assigning other parts of the usual portfolio to another worker with complementary gifts and limitations. Sometimes a spouse without ADD syndrome takes responsibility for managing the family's financial affairs, while the spouse with those impairments takes on other household responsibilities.

The value of such supports often is not recognized until, for some reason, they are withdrawn. One interior decorator with untreated ADD syndrome had a flourishing business until his junior partner suddenly died from a heart attack. The business began to collapse after the younger man's death as the senior partner failed to monitor income and expenditures, did not follow up promptly on inquiries from prospective clients, did not write up and send his estimates, failed to collect on accounts receivable, invested in excessive inventory, and mistreated his office assistants.

For twenty years these partners had thrived in a business where the senior partner employed his strengths in imaginative use of color, design, and arrangement while the junior partner provided steady management of their business finances, guided the flow of inventory, oversaw interaction with clients, and provided guidance and support for their office assistants. After the loss of his partner, the decorator received useful advice from his office staff, but his problematic personality style and ADD impairments, accentuated by his grief, caused him to ignore their advice and drove them and several successors to resign. Only after the business had virtually collapsed did the decorator finally recognize limitations from his ADD syndrome and seek appropriate treatment.

Executive Functions Used in Adulthood

Examples in this chapter highlight four types of developmental challenges of adulthood in which executive functions play an important role:

Selecting options and working productively,
Managing a household and finances,
Managing work while nurturing relationships, and
Parenting and sustaining partnerships.

Each of these developmental challenges is ongoing and multifaceted, often changing and evolving in complex ways over the adult years. Some adults invest most of their efforts and interest in their job. They may labor through a long career in one setting, or they may make a series of lateral or vertical moves, some or all of which involve new demands on executive functions. For others, paid work is much less important. For them time with a partner or family remains of primary importance throughout their adult years. Still others may have few long-term relationships or stay mostly to themselves. For many of these adults, there is a continuing struggle to balance somewhat equally the demands and satisfaction of work or personal interests with the challenges and rewards of family and friends.

Regardless of the weighting of vocational and social interests, few maintain a static life situation over their adult years. Satisfactions and frustrations ebb and flow in work, in family life, and in social relationships. As one's children grow, each developmental stage brings new challenges, new pleasures, and new worries. One's parents get older and eventually die, a process long or short that can present multiple challenges as one struggles to simultaneously earn a living and, perhaps, raise children and sustain a marriage or other close relationship. For many, separation or divorce disrupts an established relationship, causing emotional, social, and financial upheaval. For some, health problems intervene in occasional or persistent ways that limit physical or mental capacities and may throw off balance relationships, work, and routines of daily life in ways never anticipated.

Throughout the vicissitudes of adult life, executive functions remain critically important. Those fortunate enough to enjoy generally effective executive functions are not likely to be always happy, but they are likely to have less difficulty in playing the cards that life deals them than are those whose executive functions are impaired by ADD syndrome.

Chapter 7   How ADD Syndrome Differs
from Normal Inattention

MYTH: Everybody has the symptoms of ADD, and anyone with adequate intelligence can overcome these difficulties.

FACT: ADD affects persons at all levels of intelligence. And although everyone sometimes has symptoms of ADD, only those with chronic impairments from these symptoms warrant an ADD diagnosis.

Most people who hear about the symptoms of ADD syndrome respond by commenting, "Oh, I have those problems too. Doesn't everybody?" This reaction is understandable because symptoms in this syndrome occur from time to time in all children, adolescents, and adults, especially when they are overtired or stressed. The difference between persons legitimately diagnosed as having ADHD and those who do not warrant this diagnosis is essentially one of degree. How severely are these problems interfering with their lives? And are they impaired just briefly once in a while or consistently over an extended time?

There is no single measure, no blood test or brain scan, no rating scale or computer task that can make or rule out an ADHD diagnosis. The most effective instrument for assessing ADHD is an intensive interview conducted by a clinician who understands what ADHD looks like, and who can differentiate ADHD from other disorders that may cause similar problems. In this chapter I explain some things I try to keep in mind when doing an assessment, and I describe tools and specific questions useful in trying to determine when a diagnosis of ADHD is appropriate.

Failure or Success Is Not a Good Measure

An attorney once came seeking evaluation and treatment for ADHD after partners of his law firm decided that he would not himself become partner, a promotion he very much wanted and felt that he deserved. Here is his explanation:

> I've decided that I have ADHD. I am a bright guy and I work hard and I earned very good grades in law school, but I'm not getting the success I should have by now. Each year the senior partners promote a couple of attorneys from our firm to junior partner. That's a signal that they really like you and your work and that they want you to stay in the firm. If you don't get picked after a while you need to start looking somewhere else or just accept that you are going to stay stuck in associate status without a very promising future.
>
> There has to be some reason that I'm not getting moved up. I read an article about ADHD and how it can cause even very bright people to underachieve and not reach their potential. I looked at the list of symptoms: difficulty staying focused, being forgetful, and not getting things done on time. I have all those problems sometimes.
>
> And I read that some medicine can help to improve those problems. Probably that's what I need to get myself promoted.

When I questioned this attorney about his experiences in the law firm, I learned that the senior partners had already explained their reasons for not promoting him. They had told him that his written work was of high quality, and they had no complaints about his organizational abilities, his use of time, his level of effort, or his understanding of the law.

Apparently several of the senior partners simply did not like him. They had complained that he was too worried about insignificant details and too domineering in conversations with coworkers and clients. Colleagues and secretaries found him self-centered and annoying; clients had complained about his reluctance to consider others' viewpoints. As we discussed these criticisms, the attorney reluctantly acknowledged his having heard similar complaints from his wife as well as from colleagues in law school and at a previous job.

When I inquired in detail about specific ADHD symptoms, the attorney identified very few of them as applying to his experience. He had not been significantly impaired by ADHD symptoms during his years in school, and he was not currently experiencing more difficulties from these symptoms than most other adults. His lack of success in his goal of becoming a partner in his law firm was not due to his having ADHD. It appeared to be due more to his chronic anxiety and some personality problems. Not all lack of success is due to ADHD; countless other variables may be involved, including luck.

Further, some individuals attain impressively high goals while suffering significant impairments in executive functions needed for many other aspects of daily life. One example is an emergency room physician who was almost apologetic in seeking an evaluation for himself.

> Most people wouldn't ever believe it, but I think I have ADHD. It's true that I graduated from college and from medical school and that I'm licensed to practice medicine. I can be really on top of my game when I'm in the ER and managing six or eight patients with serious trauma. I can remember current vital signs and what we are doing for every one of them. I'm good at directing multiple treatments and I'm good at talking with patients. Nurses and patients all like me. But the rest of my life is a mess!
>
> I'm in constant trouble with my supervisors for not paying attention to their directions and for not doing adequate charting. I try to study for my board exams, but can't remember what I've read. I've already failed them twice. I've never been good at studying and just barely graduated from a second-rate medical school. My finances are a total mess because I spend too impulsively and can't keep track of my bills. I've had three speeding tickets in the past six months and my wife is threatening divorce because she says I never listen to her, I'm irresponsible, and I procrastinate on too many things that need to be done. I've al-

ways been this way, but it's worse now that I'm out of residency and have to do so much more on my own.

Like the high school hockey player described in the Chapter 1, this physician is able to perform well under intense, immediate pressures that are exciting and interesting to him. But despite the talents that brought him a college degree, a medical degree, and a license to practice medicine, he suffers from longstanding problems with executive functioning. When not under the immediate pressures of treating critically injured patients, he has great difficulty organizing and prioritizing his work, his time, and his money. He can't sustain focus on important tasks like keeping adequate patient records and communicating with his supervisors and his wife. He can't hold in mind what he has studied to prepare for an important exam. And his impulsive style of spending and driving is currently threatening him with bankruptcy and possible loss of his driver's license. His difficulties were not due to substance abuse or any other psychiatric problem; they were the consequence of unrecognized and untreated ADHD.

Many factors contribute to a person's success or failure in specific areas. Presence or absence of the impairments of ADD syndrome can't be determined simply by whether a person does or does not achieve a specific goal.

Many with ADHD Are Not "Hyper"

For decades the primary marker used to identify individuals with ADHD impairments was hyperactivity. Children who were very obviously hyperactive were considered candidates for evaluation for ADHD, especially if they were being disruptive or making trouble for their teachers. ADHD diagnosis was not even considered for those who were not hyperactive and not disruptive in school. An elementary-school janitor described this as he came seeking evaluation for his ten-year-old daughter:

> I could always spot the kids with the hyper. They were the ones always sent out to sit in the hall because they were making too much trouble in class. Some of them were actually pretty funny in their antics. Usually these were the same kids who would be running down the hall with the teacher calling after them to

slow down and walk quietly. They were the ones on the play-
ground who were always getting into arguments and fights with
other kids or the last ones to come back in after lunch or recess.

It was never the kids who kept the rules who got picked as
having ADD and it was never the quiet kids or the girls. That's
why I never thought ADD could be my daughter's problem.
She's always been kind of quiet and a little shy. Never made any
trouble in class. Teachers have always liked her and said she was
really bright. She loves to read and to learn. She's got insatiable
curiosity and lots of good ideas, but she's not getting her work
done and her grades have been dropping more every year. She's
losing interest in school.

Many clinicians and educators still identify ADHD as the janitor described. As a result, many with ADHD, especially girls, are overlooked.
Joseph Biederman (2002) studied the role of gender in diagnosis of
ADHD. He found that although girls and boys with ADHD have similar
patterns of severity with the problem, ten boys are referred to clinics for
treatment of ADHD for every one girl referred. Community samples show
a different gender ratio: three boys have ADHD for every one girl who has
the disorder.

In contrast, during adulthood the rates of referral for ADHD are more
balanced between women and men. Biederman (2004) suggested a reason: adults usually self-refer for ADHD evaluation because of problems
they recognize in themselves, whereas children and adolescents are usually referred for evaluation by parents or teachers—adults who are more
likely to identify those with obvious behavior problems.

Though their problems may not be so obvious, girls with ADHD can
suffer significant problems. Stephen Hinshaw (2002a, 2002b) compared
a large group of girls with ADHD to other girls of the same age and social
status. He found that girls with ADHD had much more trouble according
to several measures: cognitive tasks, academic performance, getting along
with peers, and ratings of emotional problems, social isolation, and behavior problems. Biederman (1999) studied a large group of girls six to
eighteen years old with ADHD and compared them to boys with ADHD.

He found that the girls with ADHD had problems in home and school that were just as serious as those of boys with the disorder. The primary difference between the two groups was how much trouble they made for other people. Serious behavior problems, such as oppositional defiant disorder and conduct disorder (explained in detail in Chapter 8), were twice as common among boys with ADHD. This 50 percent lower rate of disruptive behavioral problems in the girls with ADHD is probably the most important reason that girls are less often recognized as having this disorder.

But it is not only girls whose impairments are often overlooked. Many boys and men have ADD symptoms that go unrecognized because they are not boisterous troublemakers. This problem of delayed recognition or total failure to recognize ADHD in individuals who are not disruptive continues because many clinicians, educators, and persons in the general public still assume that attentional problems of ADHD are significant only when linked with hyperactivity.

This continuing mistaken assumption is not surprising, given that the very name of the disorder continues to hold the two terms together. The official *DSM-IV* label for the disorder is "attention-deficit/hyperactivity disorder," followed by a comma and the name of the subtype. For those whose ADHD impairments do not include significant problems with hyperactivity, this system results in a diagnostic label that says essentially "attention-deficit hyperactivity disorder, without significant hyperactivity," a rather clumsy and confusing label that perpetuates the overemphasis on behavioral problems.

Behavior Problems Are Not Necessarily a Part of ADHD

Some researchers continue to claim that the primary problems in ADHD are impairments in the control of behavior. In 1997 Russell Barkley introduced a new theory of ADHD that in many ways is similar to my model of ADD syndrome. He noted that problems in ADHD lie not simply in the individual's ability to pay attention or in excessive hyperactivity, but rather in the executive functions of the brain. Functions included in his model of executive functions are virtually identical to those in the model of executive functions described in Chapter 2, albeit with different labels and organization.

Yet Barkley's model differs from my model in two important ways. First, Barkley claims that his model applies only to the combined type of ADHD, not to the predominantly inattentive subtype. He has argued that the predominantly inattentive subtype of ADHD may be a disorder entirely distinct from the combined type of ADHD (Barkley 1997; Barkley 2001b). In contrast, my model of ADD syndrome is intended to describe all subtypes of ADHD, not just the combined or predominantly inattentive.

It is difficult to see how combined and inattentive subtypes of ADHD could be completely separate disorders. In most children with combined subtype, hyperactivity and impulsivity symptoms gradually attenuate during later childhood while their inattention symptoms persist; their ADHD usually develops into predominantly inattentive type by mid-adolescence. Moreover, the two subtypes appear not to be inherited separately. In a large genetic study of twins, Susan Smalley and colleagues (2000) found virtually complete genetic overlap for the two sets of ADHD symptoms. A parent with ADHD might have two children, one with ADHD who is extremely hyper and another with ADHD who is a couch potato; the strong inheritance component of this disorder does not predict which subtype will develop.

The second way in which Barkley's (1997) model of ADHD differs from mine is that he elevates behavioral inhibition as *the* primary executive function. Barkley specifies that behavioral inhibition "is critical to the proficient performance of the executive functions. It permits them, supports their occurrence, and protects them from interference." He describes the other executive functions as "dependent on behavioral inhibition" (p. 154).

In contrast to Barkley's approach, my model includes behavioral inhibition as just one among six clusters of executive functions, here called "monitoring and self-regulating behavior," without the other executive functions being especially dependent on that one function. I believe that inhibition, the ability to put on the brakes, is just one aspect of executive functions. Equally important are the brain's systems for ignition, transmission, and steering. All must interact to operate the car.

The difference between these two models is not simply academic. It has practical importance for how the difference between ADHD and normal variations of inattention is to be determined. If Barkley's model were used as a basis for diagnosis, only cases that include significant hyperactive and impulsive symptoms would qualify for the diagnosis of ADHD. My model is consistent with the *DSM-IV* criteria, which stipulate that a diagnosis of ADHD can legitimately be made for individuals with few or no symptoms of hyperactivity or impulsivity, provided that they are sufficiently impaired by the stipulated inattention symptoms. Problems of inhibition and inadequate behavioral control that result in hyperactivity or impulsivity symptoms may be present, but they are not required for an ADHD diagnosis.

ADHD Symptoms Are Not Always Obvious during Childhood

The criteria set out in *DSM-IV* stipulate that at least some of the impairing ADHD symptoms must have been present before age seven. But this requirement has no basis in empirical research; it was arbitrarily stipulated by the committee that wrote the diagnostic criteria for *DSM-IV*. Presumably the rationale was to establish that ADHD does not appear de novo later in life. Such a view makes no sense when ADHD is seen as a developmental impairment of executive functions, an impairment that in some persons may not become apparent until such functions are challenged by the demands of elementary or secondary school, or perhaps even later, when the individual experiences the trials of adulthood.

Russell Barkley and Joseph Biederman published an article in 1997 cautioning clinicians to avoid use of the age seven cutoff as a requirement for diagnosis of ADHD. They emphasized the lack of research to support it and argued that this age of onset requirement "deserves to be abandoned or very generously interpreted as occurring sometime in childhood, broadly construed." They noted that "to do otherwise would be simply arbitrary, surely discriminatory, and empirically indefensible" (p. 1209).

Increasing numbers of older adolescents and adults are now recognizing that they suffer from ADHD. Media coverage or prompting by friends or family leads them to realize that they have suffered for many years from ADHD impairments not recognized by their parents, their teachers, or themselves. Many have struggled throughout their schooling, frustrated by their inability to perform with any consistency to the level of their ability. Others were successful, perhaps very successful, in the early years of their education, then floundered in high school, college, or beyond. Chapters 5 and 6 provide examples of individuals whose impairments of ADD syndrome were not apparent until the tasks of adolescence or adulthood challenged their capacity to exercise executive functions. In my view, childhood ADHD should not be considered essential for diagnosis of ADHD in adults any more than childhood diabetes is required for the diagnosis of adult-onset diabetes.

People with ADHD May Also Have
Symptoms of Depression or Anxiety

Some individuals well past childhood have repeatedly sought help for their difficulties from psychologists, psychiatrists, or other mental health professionals who did not recognize their ADHD impairments. In years past, and even today, many professionals in these fields have received no adequate professional training to help them understand and recognize impairments of ADHD. They are, however, usually trained to recognize depression, anxiety, and personality disorders. Consequently, many doctors are quick to identify symptoms of these more familiar disorders in individuals seeking help. They may also assume that conventional psychotherapy or antidepressant medications will alleviate ADD impairments. Unfortunately, these misguided therapies have caused a large number of older adolescents and adults with ADHD to struggle unsuccessfully, and often for many years, to overcome their ADHD symptoms.

In 1992 John Ratey and others published a study that described sixty patients with ADHD who had sought and been given treatment in psychotherapy by experienced psychotherapists who had failed to recognize their symptoms of ADHD. In some cases these adults suffered from depression or anxiety as well as from ADHD, but received treatment aimed only at their symptoms of depression and anxiety. In other instances patients were given treatment for symptoms that were entirely misdiagnosed.

Because conventional treatments for depression, anxiety, and personality disorders are not effective in alleviating symptoms of ADHD, it is important that clinicians who treat adolescents and adults be provided adequate professional training to help them recognize and provide effective treatment for the disorder, which afflicts a large percentage of individuals who seek help from mental health professionals. Chapter 8 describes how ADHD often appears with one or several other disorders of learning, emotions, or behavior. Having symptoms of anxiety or depression does not rule out the possibility of ADHD; such symptoms may instead indicate a more complicated case in which two or more disorders are present.

Very Intelligent People with ADHD Are Often Overlooked

Sometimes persons with a higher overall IQ who suffer from ADHD are at greater risk of having their impairments overlooked. At Yale, Donald Quinlan and I studied adults who sought evaluation for chronic attentional problems, all of whom had a tested IQ in the superior range; in terms of intelligence, they were in the top 1 to 9 percent of the general population. Despite their very high IQ scores, 42 percent of these men and women had dropped out of their postsecondary schooling at least once, not because they were not smart enough to understand the work, but because they were not able to organize, focus, and sustain their efforts to deal with academic requirements. Some eventually returned to complete their education and achieved success in business or professions; others experienced continuing frustration and failure.

Virtually all of the very bright adults in this Yale study reported that they had suffered chronic and often severe impairments of ADD syndrome that were essentially ignored or denied by their parents, teachers, and themselves for many years. One thirty-eight-year-old woman described her experiences:

> I started reading sentences before I was in kindergarten and everyone in my family kept saying that I was so smart. When I was in elementary schools the teachers told my parents that I was almost a genius because I asked so many good questions and knew so much about so many things. In fifth grade they

tested my IQ and put me in a special group for "gifted" students. All that changed in middle school when I wasn't keeping up with my homework. I started high school in honors-level classes, but over a couple of years they dropped me out of all of them because I often wasn't prepared. I didn't read what we were supposed to read at home and I almost never did the papers that were assigned.

All that really interested me were the school plays and athletics. The guidance counselor and teachers kept telling my parents that I could do the work, if only I really wanted to; they thought I was lazy. My parents figured I was just bored. They thought the problem was poor teachers and that it would all get better when I went to college.

I got into a really good university because my SAT scores were really high and I had great references from my art and theater teachers. When I got there, I had a great time. There were so many interesting people to hang out with and learn from. But I couldn't get myself organized to get to classes enough and to get the reading done and to write the papers. Everything was always late or just not done. That got me put on probation and eventually they kicked me out in the middle of my second year because I was failing almost everything. For me it was all really interesting, but I just couldn't get organized and do enough of the work. Only after my daughter got diagnosed with ADD did I realize that there was something wrong with me other than laziness, a problem that could get fixed. Nobody including me thought that such a smart person could have any real problem in school.

Even today many educators and clinicians do not realize that those executive functions crucial to effective performance as a student can be severely impaired even in individuals who are very bright and talented. In many schools and families, bright but disorganized and poorly performing students with ADHD are still seen as stubbornly lazy, unmotivated, or defiant. Well-intentioned but uninformed teachers and parents often punish these bright, extremely inconsistent students for what appears to be a lack of motivation or a refusal to do what they need to do.

Perhaps worse than punishments meted out by frustrated teachers and parents is the self-criticism experienced by these extremely bright but floundering students. Often their ambitions and expectations for themselves have been inflated by accomplishments and recognition obtained in earlier years, when less focus and self-management was required. When confronted by the intensified academic challenges of some high school honors classes or university courses, many very bright individuals with ADD syndrome get so frustrated and demoralized that they give up on their education.

Adults with ADHD May Have Fewer Symptoms

According to the *DSM-IV*, a diagnosis of ADHD should be made only if an individual has at least six of the nine inattention symptoms or at least six of the nine symptoms of hyperactivity/impulsivity. And it is true that this disorder involves concurrent impairments in a wide variety of functions; it is a syndrome. But there is a big problem in this symptom count system when older adolescents or adults are being evaluated. The *DSM-IV* diagnostic criteria for ADHD are based on research data that included only children four to seventeen years old.

Kevin Murphy and Russell Barkley (1996) did a study to see how many adults in a community sample met *DSM-IV* diagnostic criteria for ADHD. They reported that although the "six of nine symptoms" rule from *DSM-IV* picks up the most severely impaired 7 percent of children with ADHD impairments, when used for diagnosis of adults, this rule picks up only the most impaired 1 percent of adults who should be eligible for diagnosis. Murphy and Barkley found that many adults who reported having only four or five of the *DSM-IV* symptoms suffered ADHD impairments severe enough to warrant treatment.

One might question why the cutoff point for symptoms differs so much from children to adults if the symptoms of ADHD do not disappear with age. One obvious answer is that the *DSM-IV* describes some ADHD symptoms in ways that do not apply to tasks of adulthood. Examples of difficulty in sustaining mental effort refer only to schoolwork and homework. Examples of losing things necessary for tasks and activities refer only to toys, school assignments, pencils, books, or tools. To find out whether an older adolescent or adult has ADD impairments, it is necessary to inquire with examples more appropriate to adult life. A good start on that task has been made by Lenard Adler, Ronald Kessler, and Thomas Spencer (2004), who created new, adult-focused examples for each of the eighteen *DSM-IV* criteria. The adult self-report scale they developed is available on the World Health Organization web site and at www.med.nyu.edu/Psych/training/adhd.html.

Another reason that the *DSM-IV* symptom cut-off system is not sufficient for adults is that even just a few ADHD symptoms may severely impair adults. For example, an adult who has significant, chronic difficulty sustaining attention while driving a car can cause very serious damage. Adults may create significant problems for themselves and others if they repeatedly forget to pick up their children at daycare or cannot remember to follow through on important tasks on their job. Later in this chapter I discuss the importance of weighting symptoms by their severity and significance, not just counting them, when assessing impairment.

The Limits of Neuropsychological Tests of Executive Functions

Some neuropsychological tests traditionally have been labeled as "tests of executive function" (EF tests). These include the Wisconsin Card Sorting Test, the Stroop Color-Word Test, the Tower of London, the Rey-Osterrieth Complex Figure Test, the California Verbal Learning Test, and various computerized continuous-performance tests. Most of these tests were originally developed to assess patients with schizophrenia or those who had suffered damage to the frontal lobes of the brain. At first glance, such tests might appear to be appropriate measures to assess ADHD. In fact, they are not.

When given to children diagnosed with ADHD, such tests give variable results. Alysa Doyle and colleagues (2000) administered a battery of seven "EF tests" to a group of children diagnosed with ADHD. They found that no single EF test accurately differentiated children with ADHD from children without the disorder. Using all seven tests combined, they found that about 18 percent of the boys with ADHD appeared significantly impaired on at least four tests, while about 5 percent of the boys who did not have ADHD showed similar impairment. They concluded that "neuropsychological tests of attention and executive functioning underidentify cases that meet these [DSM-IV] criteria." Stephen Hinshaw and others (2002c) obtained comparable results from a neuropsychological evaluation of girls with ADHD.

Neuropsychological tests of executive-function impairments in adults are no better. Aaron Hervey and colleagues (2004) reviewed thirty-three published studies that used neuropsychological EF tests to evaluate adults with ADHD. He found that current neuropsychological measures are not sensitive enough to pick up ADHD symptoms.

Any who seek to identify executive function impairments of ADHD primarily by means of scores for these EF tests are likely to be frustrated because of the "lamppost problem." "Lamppost" here refers to the old story of the drunken man whose friends came along on a dark night and found him on his hands and knees crawling around under a streetlamp. When they asked what he was doing he explained, "I lost the keys to my car and I'm looking for them so I can drive home." They asked, "Where do you think you lost them?" "Somewhere over there in the dark across the street where my car is parked," he responded. "Then why are you looking here?" they asked. He answered, "It's easier to look here because the light's so much better!"

Executive-function tests might appear to be a convenient way to assess impairments associated with ADHD, but they don't shed enough light on the areas that need to be examined. Patrick Rabbitt (1997) explained why methods traditionally used by experimental psychology cannot validly be applied to executive functions. The usual scientific approach in research is to isolate and try to measure one variable that reflects one specific process and not others. He argued that

> this venerable strategy is entirely inappropriate for analyzing executive function because an essential property of all "executive

function" is that, by its very nature, it involves the simultaneous management of a variety of different functional processes. (p. 14)

The usual "isolate the variable and test it" approach simply cannot encompass and measure the complex interactive nature of executive functions. Put another way, in seeking a new conductor for a symphony orchestra, one could not adequately evaluate candidates simply by having them rhythmically wave their arms or hum bars of a specific instrument's part in a section of a particular symphony. The ability to integrate and guide a large group of musicians through the performance of diverse musical pieces simply cannot be assessed with any isolated musical task. One would instead need to evaluate the candidate's ability to interact dynamically with the whole group of musicians as they play a variety of complex and challenging pieces.

Paul Burgess (1997) elaborated this same argument against trying to assess executive functions with simple tasks:

> Goethe's famous comment that dissecting a fly and studying its parts will not tell you how it flies could almost have been intended for the neuropsychology of executive function . . . executive processing is called into play only when the activities of multiple components of the cognitive architecture must be coordinated. . . . Thus if a methodology is used where a task is broken down into its component parts, no deficit will be discovered in dysexecutive patients. (pp. 99–102)

A person's ability to perform the complex, self-managed tasks of everyday life provides a much better measure of his or her executive functioning than can neuropsychological tests. Tim Shallice and Paul Burgess (1991) demonstrated this fact in a study where patients with frontal lobe damage were unable to perform adequately everyday errands that require planning and multitasking, even though they achieved average or well-above-average scores on traditional neuropsychological tests of language, memory, perception, and "executive functions." Similar efforts to assess executive functions in more "real life" situations have been reported by

Nick Alderman and others (2003), who assessed adults doing tasks in a shopping mall, and by Vivienne Lawrence and colleagues (2002), who monitored children as they followed a series of directions during a trip to a zoo. These contrived situations are likely to be more useful than laboratory tests of executive functions, although they lack the flexibility and scope needed to assess adequately the wider range of executive-function impairments in real life.

What then is "the test" for differentiating ADD syndrome from normal inattention? There is no one test that can determine whether a given individual meets *DSM-IV* diagnostic criteria for ADHD. It is not like a fracture where a physician can look at an X-ray and definitively see that the bone is or is not broken. This is a diagnosis that depends on the judgment of a skilled clinician who knows what ADHD looks like and can differentiate it from other possible causes of impairment.

The Clinical Interview: The Most Sensitive Assessment Tool

The most sensitive instrument for making a diagnosis of ADHD is a well-conducted interview in which a skilled clinician asks about the history and nature of the patient's current functioning and life situation as well as the patient's earlier life experiences, noting the presence or absence of patterns of impairment in school, work, family life, and social relationships.

Usually such an interview requires at least two hours, during which time the interviewer and patient will discuss the patient's (1) adaptive strengths and weaknesses, how the person does their work, what they do for fun, and what they struggle with daily; (2) strengths and stressors in the family background as well as any blood relatives with related problems; (3) health history, focusing on any medical or developmental problems that may be relevant; (4) history of school achievement and struggles with particular types of academic work; (5) relationships with peers, family, teachers, employers, and friends; (6) eating and sleeping habits; (7) current mood patterns and any significant difficulties with anxiety, temper, or behavior; and (8) history of previous evaluations or treatment.

For adolescents and adults, I make additional inquires about their strengths and problems in significant relationships, their history of vocational aspirations and work experiences, and their past and present use or abuse of alcohol and other drugs. Detailed formats to help clinicians in structuring clinical interviews for evaluation of ADHD in children and adults have been published by Barkley and Murphy (1998) and by me (1996a, 1996b, 1996c, 2001a, 2001b, 2001c).

Throughout an evaluation interview, I try to be alert to strengths and problems of the patient in utilizing executive functions in an age-appropriate way. I listen carefully to information given, asking for details and examples that will help to clarify the patient's abilities in a variety of relevant life situations.

Interviewing Children

In the evaluation of children, parents play a crucial role in providing relevant information, but the child's input is also essential. Since many executive functions impaired in ADHD involve cognitive processes not noticed by others, it is crucial that I interview the patient. Even young children can provide important information about their experience to a clinician skilled at asking relevant questions and listening carefully to responses.

For children whose schooling is mostly in a classroom with one teacher, information from that teacher may be very helpful. Such teachers usually can describe the child's responses to different types of tasks, and can compare the child's performance to that of many other children of the same age. Often elementary schoolteachers can also furnish valuable information about how the child gets along with classmates and how the child interacts with teachers and other adults on the school staff. Yet teachers alone cannot and should not make or deny a diagnosis of ADHD. In some children symptoms of ADHD are less obvious in school than elsewhere.

Observations from teachers are usually less valuable for the evaluation of junior high or high school students, who rotate among six or seven teachers each day. Unless the teacher is also an advisor, coach, or mentor of some kind to the student, he or she will usually see the child only for one period each day, perhaps less, and typically will have five different groups of perhaps twenty-five to thirty-five students daily—so is often not able to report about any one student in sufficient detail.

ADHD Rating Scales

Regardless of the age of the patient being evaluated, detailed ADHD symptom rating scales should be used. These scales are typically listings of cognitive, emotional, and behavioral problems often experienced by individuals with ADHD. Standardized scales have been administered to selected samples of individuals within a particular age group who have been carefully diagnosed with ADHD and to a sample of individuals matched for age and socioeconomic variables who are in the general population, not identified as having ADHD. Scores of a person being evaluated can then be compared with those in the general population to ascertain whether the levels of impairment are consistent with an ADHD diagnosis.

Keith Conners (1997), Conners and colleagues (1999) and I (1996c, 2001c) have published ADHD rating scales standardized for all ages from early childhood to adulthood. The Conners' Rating Scales-Revised (long form) and the Brown ADD Scales both include multiple items that assess symptoms of ADHD as identified by *DSM-IV.* They also include items that probe other symptoms often associated with ADD impairments not included in the current version of the *DSM.* The use of such rating scales generally provides cursory but more systematic coverage of symptoms, some of which may not be mentioned spontaneously by the patient or others in a clinical interview. Scores from these rating scales provide useful information about how much difficulty the patient seems to be having with symptoms related to ADHD and how these impairments compare with those experienced by the general population. Scores on these or any other rating scales, however, should not solely determine a diagnosis of ADHD.

The Conners and Brown scales have many similar items, although each also has some different emphases and a somewhat different style. Each is published in formats suited for children (in several age groups), adolescents, and adults. Both sets of scales have versions designed to be completed by teachers of children through elementary school. My scales also have self-report forms for children aged eight and older; the Conners' scales have self-report forms for adolescents. The Brown ADD scales for adolescents and for adults include scoring for both the patient and a parent, spouse, or friend; the Conners' Adult ADD Rating Scales have separate forms for self-report and for report by a collateral observer. A review of these and other rating scales for ADHD was published by Brent Collett and others (2003).

Interviewing Adolescents and Adults

When I assess an older adolescent or adult, I invite them to have a parent, spouse, or close friend join in at least a portion of their clinical interview. This is not essential, but it may provide helpful information and an additional perspective. Of course, it may not be possible or desirable to involve a parent in the evaluation. The parent may be unavailable due to long distance, ill health, or death. For adults, a parent may have little relevant information about the patient's current and recent abilities. In this situation the patient may choose to invite a close friend or relative.

Sometimes clinicians become too cautious about making a diagnosis of ADHD in adults because the data are essentially self-reported. They feel that some "hard evidence" must be provided, such as old report cards with some teacher comments about learning or behavior problems, or direct testimony from a parent or childhood friend. They feel that self-reporting is "too subjective." It is certainly possible for the self-report to be biased or deceptive, but most skilled clinicians are able to sort this out in a comprehensive clinical interview. Diagnostic decisions in many other fields of medicine are made based primarily on self-reporting. For example, there is no laboratory test or diagnostic instrument that can measure pain, so self-reported information about the location, intensity, and timing of pain may be crucial for diagnostic decision-making in medicine, especially when there are few other clues on which to base a diagnostic or treatment decision.

Indeed, self-reported information about mental processes and cognitive functioning should play a central role in assessment of symptoms of ADHD, particularly for adults. Patricia Murphy and Russell Schachar (2000) reported studies showing that adults can give a true account of their childhood and current symptoms of ADHD. And it makes sense that assessment for this disorder should not be an adversarial process in which patients are required to prove that they meet diagnostic requirements while the clinician functions as a "devil's advocate," arguing that they do not. I believe that an evaluation for ADHD should be collaborative, with the patient being encouraged to describe the problems that have caused him to seek treatment, and the clinician inquiring for examples and additional information to understand the context in which these difficulties exist and the factors that may be causing them.

In evaluating for ADHD, I always consider and carefully weigh alternative diagnostic hypotheses for the patient's problems. Not everyone who thinks they have ADHD does, in fact, have it. But usually people who seek evaluation and treatment, especially those who self-refer as older adolescents or adults, come because they are suffering from some significant difficulties for which they need help. The evaluator should be a sensitive and compassionate listener who uses clinical skills to elicit relevant information from the patient and then uses diagnostic abilities to identify underlying causes, to provide a plan for effective treatment, and to guide the implementation, monitoring, and refinement of that treatment plan.

Helpful Standardized Measures

Although self-reporting is a central component of evaluation for ADHD, and though there is no single test that is definitive for making an ADHD diagnosis, I have found that some standardized measures can provide useful information. One of these is a test of short-term auditory memory. Donald Quinlan and I (2003) reported a study in which we administered short-term verbal memory tests to adults diagnosed with ADHD by *DSM-IV* criteria. We used two stories, each twenty-five word units long, from the Wechsler Memory Scale.

We asked patients to listen carefully to two brief stories. After each story was read aloud, we asked the patient to repeat it back, using as many of the same words as possible. Detailed scoring criteria and published norms make it possible to determine how a given individual performs this task in comparison with others of the same age group. We then compared the patient's score on story recall with his overall verbal ability to see if there was a significant discrepancy.

We found that 66 percent of the adults with ADHD in our sample had a large discrepancy (one standard deviation or more) between their verbal IQ and their story memory; in the general public only 16 percent of adults show such a wide difference. Children with ADHD show a similar problem with listening and remembering. In 2001c I reported on use of a similar story-memory test administered to several age groups of children. Among those with ADHD, 57 to 73 percent showed significant impairment on story recall, while only 25 to 33 percent of children in the general population had such difficulties.

Taken together, these results suggest that across wide age spans, these tests of story recall offer a brief and effective way to test impairments of verbal working memory in individuals being assessed for ADHD. These simple tests take only about ten minutes to administer. The task allows the clinician to check the effectiveness of a patient's working memory on a task similar to many situations in daily life where one is given information orally and is able to hear it only once. It should be noted, however, that in each age group some persons with ADHD were not impaired on the story-recall task, while some who did not have ADHD were impaired. For this reason, results of such a test cannot be used alone to determine the presence or absence of ADHD. Multiple measures are needed.

A person's level of general intelligence has nothing to do with whether they have ADHD. Russell Barkley observed that "ADHD children are likely to represent the entire spectrum of intellectual development, with some being gifted while others are normal, slow learners, or even mildly intellectually retarded" (1998, p. 98). An individual's verbal IQ, performance IQ, or full-scale IQ score can tell nothing about whether they do or do not suffer from ADHD. Yet some IQ tests, for example, the Wechsler Intelligence Scales for Children, fourth edition (WISC-IV), introduced in 2003, and the Wechsler Adult Intelligence Scales, third edition (WAIS-III), available since 1997, have some subtests that are fairly sensitive to impairments in executive functions. Comparing a person's performance on these subtests can offer information useful for the assessment of ADHD.

In 2001c I considered the performance of ADHD-diagnosed children ages eight to twelve with the overall group of same-age test-takers on four index scores on the WISC-III. Two of the indexes—the Verbal Comprehension Index (VCI) and the Perceptual Organization Index (POI)—summarize subtests less sensitive to executive-function impairments; instead these identify one's general verbal ability and general perceptual organization abilities. Indexes more sensitive to executive-function impairments are the Freedom from Distractibility [Working Memory] Index (WMI) and the Processing Speed Index (PSI); these characterize one's working memory and speed on simple clerical tasks.

In my sample, over 61 percent of the children with ADHD showed a large (at least 15 points) discrepancy between their VCI or POI (whichever was higher) and their WMI or PSI (whichever was lower). Fewer than 25 percent of the children on which the test was standardized showed such a discrepancy (2001c). In my earlier samples of adolescents and adults, the differences for this measure were equally substantial (1996c).

These data show that comparisons of an individual's WISC or WAIS index scores may offer helpful information about the degree of weakness of that person's executive functions. Just as with scores for the verbal memory tests discussed earlier, however, such discrepancies are not shown by all individuals with ADHD and similar discrepancies are shown by as many as 25 percent of individuals not diagnosed with ADHD. This means that such index score comparisons should be only one part of an evaluation for ADHD.

Additional Disorders That May Cause or Complicate ADHD

There are many reasons that a child or adolescent may be unsuccessful at school or in social relationships, just as there are many reasons that adults may be unsuccessful in education, work, social relationships, or family life. ADHD is one possible reason, but not the only one. For this reason, any evaluation for possible ADHD should include screening for environmental problems and for other learning or psychiatric disorders that may be causing or complicating the symptoms presented as possible ADHD. The Brown ADD Diagnostic Form in versions for children, adolescents, and adults all include guidelines to assist clinicians in checking for possible additional disorders. The implications of these additional disorders for understanding ADHD are discussed in Chapter 8.

Educating the Patient

Once I have completed the clinical interview, scored the ADD rating scales, administered standardized measures, and screened for additional disorders, I ask the patient what information they have about ADHD. Some who come seeking evaluation for themselves or their children are very sophisticated in their understanding of ADHD. They have learned much about the diagnosis and treatment of this disorder from reading, taking courses, or talking with others who are well informed. Others come to the initial evaluation with very limited information about ADHD, and with many misconceptions. Once I ascertain what is already known, I try to provide information about ADHD at an appropriate level. I believe that teaching the patient and family about ADHD is a very important part of the initial evaluation.

I provide a concise description of the primary symptoms of ADHD impairment using clear examples to illustrate each one. Usually I do this in a format something like the description of symptom clusters in Chapter 2. After each symptom cluster has been described, I pause and ask the patient and family members present to indicate the degree to which the described symptom cluster fits or does not fit the patient's experience. I use follow-up questions to probe for relevant details or examples from the patient's daily experience. This process can enrich the patient's understanding of the disorder as well as yield additional information valuable for determining the diagnosis.

Critical Questions of the Evaluation

Once all elements of the evaluation are completed, a process that usually requires at least two hours, sometimes considerably more, I weigh the available data and make a determination: Does this patient meet the diagnostic criteria for ADHD? I find the answer not by simply adding up scores on rating scales or counting symptoms that the patient or family say are present. To make an adequate diagnosis, I need to use informed judgment to answer two critical questions: (1) Does this patient currently suffer from symptoms of ADHD in ways that impair his or her functioning in daily life to a degree that treatment may be warranted? and (2) Are these symptoms substantially caused by developmental impairments of ADHD rather than by other circumstances or disorders for which ADHD treatment would be inappropriate?

Resolving Conflicting Views

In some cases these questions can be answered, yes or no, with little hesitation or ambiguity. Other cases are much more complicated, making one or both questions considerably more difficult to answer. Sometimes there are striking contradictions in the information provided by various informants about the patient's symptoms. One parent may describe a child as having significant problems with organizing and completing homework, retaining learned information, and utilizing short-term memory. The other parent of the same child may emphatically deny that such problems exist. Either one could be correct, or each may be correct about only certain aspects of the child's functioning.

Sometimes a teacher feels strongly that a child has ADHD impairments while neither parent sees such problems. Or parents may see ADHD impairments in their child's efforts to do homework, household routines, and social relationships while the child's teacher reports no evidence of any such difficulties at school. Studies comparing data from parents and teachers usually find low rates of agreement in their assessments of any given child. Victor Mota and Russell Schachar (2000) compared ADHD symptom ratings of children by their parents and teachers. Their methods allowed them to identify which of the *DSM-IV* symptoms of ADHD were most important to parents and which were most important to teachers when a child's performance was being assessed for evidence of ADHD.

Mota and Schachar found that although parents and teachers disagreed considerably on the number of *DSM-IV* symptoms a child had, they more often agreed about whether the child was impaired relative to others. Using a sample of children ages seven to twelve referred for possible ADHD, they obtained ratings from parents and a teacher for each child. Using a sophisticated statistical analysis, they created a subset of symptoms most important to teachers and a separate subset of symptoms most important to parents. In addition, they found that not all *DSM-IV* symptoms predicted impairment equally well. Using their revised, separate, and shorter symptom lists, they increased the agreement between parents and teachers from very poor to extremely good.

Differences in such judgments between parents and teachers may be due to the child's performing very differently in the two settings, each of which has very different task demands. Or the variation could be due to the parents having unrealistic expectations of what a child of a particular age can do—whereas the teacher can compare each child with many others of the same age. Alternatively, the teacher may be inexperienced in assessing shortcomings in the child's learning and behavior, perhaps blaming either herself or the child too much for any problems noticed. Sometimes, too, the teacher may be caught up in a personality conflict with the child, or be ideologically opposed to recognizing any child as having impairments of ADHD.

In situations of conflicting reports I need to elicit examples from each parent, interview the child directly, and seek out additional information from teacher reports and standardized testing. Usually reviewing examples clarifies the causes for differences of opinion about a child's symptoms.

Are the Symptoms Truly Caused by ADHD?

In other situations, there may be little question about the presence of the symptoms, but considerable uncertainty about their causes. The parents, child, and the child's teachers may all agree that the child has some symptoms of ADHD, yet factors other than ADHD are likely to blame. For example, the family may be suffering from severe financial hardship with both parents unemployed. One parent may be seriously addicted to alcohol, causing disruption or abuse at home. An older sibling may be severely defiant toward the parents and intimidating to the patient. A beloved grandparent may be dying of cancer. Or a child's favorite teacher may have left on maternity leave for several months, replaced by a series of ineffective substitutes.

Such stressors, especially when more than one is present, may be the primary cause of the child's apparent ADHD impairments, or they may simply be exacerbating ADHD impairments that have been present since birth. The incidence of unemployment, marital conflict, substance abuse, and frequent changes of residence is elevated among individuals with ADHD. The presence of environmental stressors, even if they are many and severe, does not rule out a diagnosis of ADHD any more than such stressors would rule out a diagnosis of asthma.

Impairment by What Measure?

One important factor in determining impairment is the basis for comparison. To whom should an individual be compared in order to make a diagnosis of ADHD? The *DSM-IV* (2001) states that the ADHD symptoms must be "maladaptive and inconsistent with developmental level" (p. 92). For children, "developmental level" might be taken as referring simply to age groups. One could argue that a five-year-old is not impaired in her ability to pay attention if she can pay attention as well as most other five-year-olds. The *DSM-IV* does not, however, spell out the full range of meanings for "developmental level," which could also be taken to refer to level of intelligence. At the lower boundary, this reinterpretation would mean that one would not make the diagnosis of ADHD for an eight-year-old developmentally disabled child with an IQ of 60 by comparing his ability to sustain attention with that of other eight-year-olds with normal IQ. This is generally accepted.

What is more controversial is the assessment of impairment at the upper boundary of ability—that is, for the very bright individual whose overall cognitive competence as measured by standardized tests of intelligence is in, say, the top 5 to 10 percent of the age group. Should this individual be considered impaired if he is chronically unable to organize and sustain effort for his work, to remember what he has just read, or to perform other cognitive tasks as compared to a same-age student with cognitive abilities scored in a similar range?

If the superior-range student can perform most other cognitive tasks as well as other students in the top 5 to 10 percent of his age group, it would seem that symptoms of ADD syndrome that chronically and significantly depress his capacity to use his abilities should be counted as clinically significant impairment. Assessment of impairment ought to take into account the overall level of cognitive abilities in the individual being assessed—otherwise, only those whose impairments are most global and most severe will likely be eligible for treatment. A high school student who demonstrates superior ability on a standardized IQ test but consistently gets very low grades is certainly working below his ability. This failure might be due to depression, to substance abuse, to deliberate defiance of parental expectations, or to many other factors; one possible cause could be ADD syndrome.

Using Integrated Information for Diagnosis

This chapter asks how one can recognize those children, adolescents, and adults whose problems with executive functions warrant diagnosis and treatment for ADHD. My answer is that a comprehensive clinical evaluation is the most adequate way to differentiate those individuals who meet diagnostic criteria for ADHD from those who do not. As described earlier, this evaluation should include a careful clinical interview that focuses on the patient's past and present functioning and, if possible, includes information from others who know the patient well. The evaluation should also include use of a standardized, age-appropriate ADD rating scale such as the Conners or Brown scales and some standardized measures like the verbal memory test described earlier. For students of any age, a comparison of IQ index scores from the WISC or WAIS IQ tests may also be helpful. Yet when all of these data are gathered, a question remains: How severe does impairment from ADD symptoms have to be in order to be recognized as ADHD?

The Severity of ADHD Symptoms and Accurate Diagnosis

Some have attempted to answer this question by arbitrarily selecting for diagnosis a certain proportion of the population studied. For example, the

DSM-IV field study selected cutoff scores that included the 7 percent who were most impaired by ADHD symptoms, thus establishing that the remaining 93 percent of children would not be considered impaired enough to warrant diagnosis. But why should that be the cutoff for diagnosis rather than 3 percent, 10 percent, or 15 percent?

One way to address this question is to determine the percentage of individuals in the general population who typically meet diagnostic criteria for ADHD as defined by *DSM-IV*. The prevalence rate cited for ADHD in *DSM-IV-TR* is 3 to 7 percent of school-aged children. But this estimate has not been well documented in epidemiological studies. In 2001, Andrew Rowland and colleagues reported an epidemiological study that used parent and teacher reports about a population-based sample of children in North Carolina. This study found that 16 percent of the children in their sample were significantly impaired by ADHD symptoms, an incidence rate much higher than the estimate in *DSM-IV*. Some other studies have reported an even higher incidence of ADHD, while other researchers have found lower rates in the general population.

Whatever the incidence rate of *DSM-IV*-defined ADHD, how impaired are those who meet *DSM-IV* diagnostic criteria for ADHD in comparison to those who are just slightly below that cutoff? Lawrence Scahill and others (1999) reported a study that addressed this question. The group used a combination of parent and teacher reports to assign a large sample of children aged six to twelve years into three groups: those who fully met *DSM-III-R* diagnostic criteria for ADHD; a "subthreshold ADHD" group who had many symptoms, but fewer than what is usually required for diagnosis; and a non-ADHD group.

The Scahill study found that children in their subthreshold sample had less psychosocial stress—for example, less family dysfunction and less poverty and a lighter load of additional psychiatric disorders—than those who fully met diagnostic criteria for ADHD. Yet this subthreshold ADHD group still carried a burden of ADHD symptoms and, for many, additional psychiatric impairments relative to those in the non-ADHD group. Scahill concluded his report by noting that the subthreshold ADHD children, who had many ADHD symptoms but not enough to meet full diagnostic criteria, appeared to be at high risk of developing full ADHD; one-third of them already had another psychiatric disorder. I believe that such high-risk individuals, especially children, should be evaluated carefully and, if appropriate, considered for possible treatment.

A parallel might be drawn to a variety of medical problems. Individuals whose blood pressure is only slightly below the accepted cutoff for diagnosis of hypertension, or those whose blood glucose levels are just slightly below the accepted cutoff for diabetes, are generally recognized as "at risk" for problems that can easily become serious threats to health and functioning. In good medical practice, these at-risk individuals are generally provided interventions that may range from recommendations for a change of lifestyle to daily use of medication to reduce their risk to less dangerous levels.

Likewise, prescriptions for eyeglasses or contact lenses are not limited to children and adults whose vision is so impaired that they are virtually in need of a white cane. Rather, good practice usually provides corrective lenses for all those whose chronic impairments of vision interfere in any significant way with their performing the tasks of daily life. If medical practitioners employed the same pragmatic principles to guide interventions for ADHD as those used for patients with poor vision or borderline risk of hypertension or diabetes, it is likely that the number of those considered eligible for intervention would be much higher than the 3 to 7 percent estimated by the *DSM-IV-TR*. Yet there is still need for some threshold at or around which a clinician should be more inclined to offer diagnosis and treatment.

In its emphasis on the need for recognizing children whose ADHD impairments place them at risk of ADHD, the Scahill report called attention to the importance of early identification and intervention. As I explain in Chapter 4, some children show clear evidence of ADHD impairments from their earliest years. Parents and preschool teachers are able to recognize that this particular child is dramatically more impaired than most others of the same age in meeting the developmental challenges of his age group. In such cases, prompt evaluation is important, particularly if the child is extremely impulsive, hyperactive, or aggressive.

Severe ADHD impairments in preschool children may cause them to be at great risk of accidental injuries, rejection, and scapegoating by other children. They may also be vulnerable to emotional or physical abuse from siblings, parents, or other caretakers who are chronically frustrated by the untreated ADHD preschooler's relentless and exhausting demands. Even when a child's behavior does not cause such severe suffering, untreated ADHD in a young child can significantly hamper development of the basic skills and attitudes needed for success in the early years of school. The time for careful assessment and consideration of possible ADHD treatment of a child is that point when the impairments of ADHD are significantly interfering with that child's ability to meet age appropriate developmental challenges.

For those individuals whose ADHD impairments do not become apparent until later childhood, adolescence, or adulthood, evaluation for possible ADHD diagnosis and treatment may begin much later, but it can still lead to very important, life-transforming interventions.

I believe that the threshold for ADHD diagnosis should be one that identifies those children, adolescents, and adults who suffer from chronic developmental impairments of executive functions that significantly interfere with the tasks of daily life—and so are likely to be helped and not harmed by clinical interventions for ADHD. It is unlikely that these individuals can be adequately identified solely on the basis of counting the number of *DSM-IV* symptoms of ADHD that the person "often" manifests, because "often" is a subjective measure. It is also unclear what constitutes "clinically significant impairment."

How Much Do the Symptoms Interfere with Daily Life?

To assess an individual's difficulties only by counting symptoms would be like assessing a route for a cross-country hike using a map that offers no indication of the type of terrain to be traversed. To know the challenges to be faced by a hiker, one needs to know not only the mileage to be covered, but also the climate and characteristics of the ground that will be traveled; is it a single flat plain or rolling hills? Are there high mountains to be climbed or deep rivers to be crossed? Is the hike to be made over an open road or through a dense jungle with walls of vegetation?

To evaluate someone for ADHD, I need to gain a realistic appreciation of how much difficulty the various symptoms are causing for that person in meeting the challenges of their current life situation. This requires knowing something about the individual's tasks of daily life and the circumstances under which those tasks must be performed. It also requires an appreciation of how much trouble any given symptom of ADHD is consistently causing this particular individual relative to most others of the comparison group. Sometimes one or two symptoms may be severely impairing, comparable to a deep valley and a high mountain on the hiking path. In other persons the weight of ADHD impairment may be significant not from any one or two severely impairing symptoms, but from difficulties caused by an overwhelming combination of many less severe symptoms, none of which might be considered so problematic in isolation.

Making the Decision

The often unacknowledged truth is that there is no clear-cut, objectively measurable boundary between those persons whom we consider to be suffering from ADHD and those whose impairments of executive functions are slightly less severe. ADHD is a complex, multidimensional disorder for which a diagnosis must rest on the clinical judgment of a clinician who, hopefully, is adequately trained to use appropriate information from the patient and other relevant sources in a sensitive and reasonable way. Although many would wish for some more objective mode of determination, the judgment of an experienced clinician is the primary determinant of diagnostic decision making in many complex situations not only in psychiatry, but also in most other fields of medicine.

Discussing the Diagnosis with the Patient

Once I have arrived at a careful diagnosis, I try to explain the diagnostic formulation to the patient and family in a realistic and understandable manner. When the patient and those close to him have a clear picture of

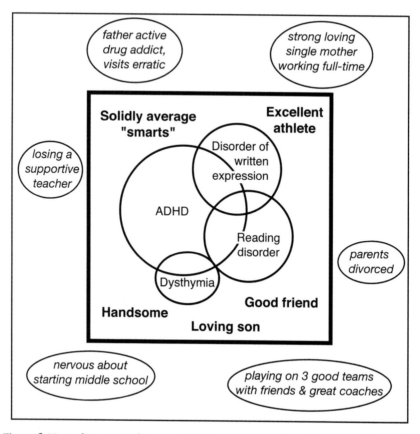

Figure 6 Venn diagnostic diagram. The inner square shows key strengths and impairments of an eleven-year-old boy evaluated as he was preparing for transition into middle school. Venn circles within that square identify overlapping diagnostic categories that currently apply, and the outer square highlights important supports and stressors in his immediate environment.

my understanding of the nature and causes of the patient's difficulties, they are usually more willing to collaborate in the development and monitoring of recommended treatments. They may also be able to correct aspects of my formulation that may be incomplete or mistaken.

I usually present the diagnosis with a simple drawing of two squares and overlapping circles. In a conversation with the patient (if the patient is old enough to understand and participate in such a discussion) and with key family members, I draw a moderately large square on a paper to represent the patient as a person. Within this square I note several important strengths of the patient, such as "very bright," "musically talented," "good at fixing things," "hard working," and "very supportive of family."

Within this "patient square," I then draw one or several overlapping circles to represent each appropriate diagnosis, which perhaps includes ADHD, explaining in understandable terms what each diagnostic term represents. These circles can be drawn as in the Venn diagram in Figure 6, each sized to represent the current importance of the problem to the patient, and overlapping to represent interacting effects.

After the patient square and overlapping circles are drawn and discussed, I draw a larger square around the first square, this one to represent the environment in which the patient lives and works. On this square important environmental strengths or stressors can be noted. These might include "a very understanding teacher," "Dad's expert help with math," "adjusting to a new job," "recently divorced," "being taught by an inexperienced teacher at school," "worrisome financial pressures," and so on.

The purpose of the overlapping circles in squares is to provide a clear and manageable description of the nature of the patient's current difficulties in the context of important personal strengths and environmental stressors. As part of this collaborative process, it is essential also to consider a wide range of other disorders that often occur with ADHD.

Chapter 8   Disorders That May Accompany
ADD Syndrome

MYTH: Someone can't have ADD and also have depression, anxiety, or other psychiatric problems.

FACT: A person with ADD is six times more likely to have another psychiatric or learning disorder than most other people. ADD usually overlaps with other disorders.

ADD syndrome is complicated. It includes chronic impairments in multiple cognitive functions. In addition, those with this syndrome often have difficulties with other aspects of their learning, emotional regulation, social functioning, or behavior.

The medical term for a person having more than one disorder is "comorbidity." Sometimes researchers use the term to describe situations where both disorders are present at the same time—for example, within a six- or twelve-month period. Others take "comorbidity" in a more inclusive way to refer to any disorder that occurs within the lifetime of an individual who has a specific disorder.

ADHD has extraordinarily high rates of comorbidity with virtually every other psychiatric disorder listed in the *DSM-IV,* both in the cross-sectional and lifetime analyses. For example, studies have found that about 5 to 10 percent of children in the general population suffer from anxiety disorders (Tannock 2000). Among children with ADHD, the rate of anxiety disorders is three to six times greater.

In the large Multimodal Treatment Study of Children with Attention Deficit Hyperactivity Disorder (MTA Cooperative Group 1999), of children ages seven to nine years diagnosed with ADHD, 70 percent were found to have met *DSM-IV* diagnostic criteria for at least one other psychiatric disorder within the preceding year. These included:

Oppositional-defiant disorder	40%
Anxiety disorder	34%
Conduct disorder	14%
Tic disorder	11%
Affective disorder (depression)	4%
Mania, hypomania	2%

The MTA sample included only young children; 80 percent were boys and most were in first, second, or third grade during the initial evaluation. Only children with combined-type ADHD were assessed; no children without significant hyperactive-impulsive symptoms of ADHD were included. The profile of psychiatric and learning problems characteristic of older children, adolescents, and adults with ADHD, especially women and those with predominantly inattentive-type ADHD, is likely to be different.

A study of somewhat older children in Puerto Rico yielded results different from the MTA. Among an equal mix of boys and girls ages nine to sixteen years from the general community, Hector Bird and colleagues (1993) found 48 percent who suffered from depressive symptoms, far more than the 4 percent of young children similarly identified in the MTA sample. Some disorders like depression tend to emerge later in life than others.

Studies of adults with ADHD show an even higher incidence of additional disorders accompanying ADHD. Rachel Millstein and others (1997) compared adults whose ADHD symptoms were predominantly inattentive (37 percent) with those who had the combined type (56 percent). Rates for some comorbid disorders were similar between these two subtypes of ADHD; others were different:

Diagnosis	Combined Type	Inattentive Type
Substance Abuse/		
Dependence	69%	43%
Major Depression	63%	63%

Oppositional Disorder	40%	16%
Multiple Anxiety Disorders	35%	23%
Conduct Disorder	30%	20%
Social Phobia	24%	31%

It should be emphasized that the percentages in this table are lifetime rates. For example, a forty-seven-year-old businessman with combined-type ADHD who had smoked marijuana heavily for a year during college and then had abstained from any marijuana use for the following quarter-century would be included in the 69 percent with a history of substance abuse or dependence.

To grasp the significance of comorbidity in adults with ADHD, a comparison with baseline rates in the general population is needed. The 2004 replication of the National Comorbidity Survey sampled the entire U.S. population in the fifteen- to forty-four-year age range. From this study Ronald Kessler (2004) reported that 88 percent of adults with ADHD had at least one additional psychiatric disorder sometime in their lifetime. This was sixfold the prevalence in the general population of adults. Here are the findings for the U.S. sample:

Disorder	ADHD adult sample	Odds ratio
Any mood disorder	45%	3.0
Any anxiety disorder	59%	3.2
Any substance use disorder	35%	2.8
Any impulse disorder	69%	5.9
Any psychiatric disorder	88%	6.3

The numbers listed under odds ratio show how much the ADHD sample exceeded the general population sample. An odds ratio of 1.0 means that the ADHD sample had the same percentage as was found in the larger population, whereas an odds ratio of 3.0 indicates that the disorder occurred three times as often in the ADHD population. These estimates do not include any learning or language disorders, but they do highlight the markedly elevated incidence of psychiatric disorders reported by adults with ADHD.

Epidemiological and clinical samples each give different information about the frequency with which various psychiatric disorders occur. Epidemiological studies yield information about how many individuals in a sample of the general population report sufficient symptoms to be diagnosed with a particular disorder. Typically investigators approach individuals at random and try to solicit their cooperation in answering multiple questions about psychiatric symptoms. Such inquiries may yield useful estimates of how many individuals in a population experience a particular problem, but such data have an important limitation: It is highly unlikely that most individuals will fully disclose their personal difficulties to an investigator whom they do not know and when there is no significant benefit to them that might offset the potential worry and embarrassment of such disclosures. For this reason, epidemiological studies are likely to underestimate the prevalence of psychiatric disorders.

Yet clinical samples, groups of people who have sought out help for themselves in psychiatric clinics, are likely to overestimate the incidence of comorbid disorders in the larger population. Clinical evaluations are likely to probe more fully and get more candid responses than can epidemiological studies. Patients are likely to disclose their multiple difficulties more fully to the doctor whose help they have sought. Their hope for relief from suffering may offset the embarrassment and shame that otherwise would cause them to avoid discussion of their private suffering. Yet those who seek treatment in clinics or hospitals are a selected population, likely to be characterized by more severe and complicated illness than are those in the general population who may suffer similar problems, but stay away from clinics or hospitals. Some with mild impairments and more financial resources may get treatment from private practitioners in the community whose records are not generally included in clinical studies; others may cope with a less intense form of the same problem without any treatment at all. As a result, reports describing comorbidity rates for clinical populations are likely to yield helpful information about the dramatic cases that appear in clinics, but may well overlook a broader range of individuals with similar problems not sufficiently severe or complicated to cause them to seek treatment in a clinic or hospital.

Whether gathered in an epidemiological study or reported from clinical samples, psychiatric diagnoses are simply a set of categories, conceptual pigeonholes, for classifying complicated aspects of impaired human functioning. Currently the *DSM-IV* lists over two hundred separate diagnostic categories, each described as though it were a discrete entity. These categories divide up impairments of human cognitive, emotional, and behavioral functioning somewhat like the boundaries of nation-states divide up peoples of the world. Both are the product of committees subject to complex political pressures and shaped by the historical setting in which they were developed.

Boundaries of some nations like North and South Korea arbitrarily separate groups with closely shared connections of culture and history, whereas boundaries of other nations like Iraq clump together disparate groups with conflicting history and cultures, creating an entity that is far from unified. Similarly, current diagnostic categories for cognitive, emotional, and behavioral problems divide some clusters of functions that have common causes and similar responses to treatment, while lumping together other clusters that might better be dealt with as separate entities. Once established, these boundaries become very difficult to change. Proposals for changes in either diagnostic or political boundaries can ignite earnest and intense conflicts.

Bruce Pennington (2002) has highlighted the need to reconsider existing boundaries for conceptualizing psychiatric disorders. He suggested a new framework to integrate emerging neuroscientific understandings of psychiatric disorders, one that includes three clusters of syndromes: disorders of motivation, disorders of action regulation, and disorders of language and cognitive development. In the following pages I have borrowed and adapted Pennington's categories to describe some of the complicated ways in which ADD syndrome overlaps other categories of psychiatric disorders. My model is shown in Figure 7.

Diagnostic Clusters

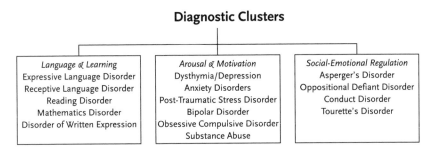

Language & Learning	*Arousal & Motivation*	*Social-Emotional Regulation*
Expressive Language Disorder	Dysthymia/Depression	Asperger's Disorder
Receptive Language Disorder	Anxiety Disorders	Oppositional Defiant Disorder
Reading Disorder	Post-Traumatic Stress Disorder	Conduct Disorder
Mathematics Disorder	Bipolar Disorder	Tourette's Disorder
Disorder of Written Expression	Obsessive Compulsive Disorder	
	Substance Abuse	

Figure 7 Executive-function impairments characterize most diagnoses. These three groupings, clustered according to important common elements, include a variety of learning and psychiatric disorders that often occur with ADHD. All of these disorders involve impairments in executive functions as well as other malfunctions specific to that disorder.

Disorders of Learning and Language

Dennis Cantwell and Lorian Baker (1991) studied the overlap between language disorders and ADHD in preschoolers referred to a clinic for speech or language problems. Almost all had serious problems relative to others of their age in being able to understand what was said to them or in being able to use verbal language to express themselves. Nineteen percent of these children with speech or language impairments also met diagnostic criteria for ADD, almost fourfold the baseline incidence of ADD reported at that time in the general population.

Joseph Beitchman and others (1996) did a longer-term study of preschool children with language disorders. In that sample, too, ADHD was found to be the most common psychiatric disorder, occurring in 30 percent of the preschoolers who had speech or language disorders. Findings from Beitchman's long-term study showed that children with impaired language function at age five were much more likely than others to have a psychiatric disorder at age twelve. Children with severe difficulty in using language and in understanding what others say to them are more likely to have significant behavioral problems; they are also likely to have poorer social skills. Communication difficulties may thus contribute eventually to failure in school or employment.

Because psychologists and psychiatrists generally have little training in speech and language impairments, the important role of these functions in academic, social, and vocational difficulties may often be overlooked. Many mental health workers assume that interpersonal problems are always caused by unrecognized emotional conflicts. For some individuals, however, interpersonal difficulties are more fundamentally rooted in an inability clearly to say what one is thinking or to understand correctly what others are trying to say.

Most physicians and mental health clinicians are similarly not educated to understand specific learning disorders (LD) that often overlap with ADHD. There are three major types of learning disorders: reading disorder, mathematics disorder, and disorder of written expression.

Reading Disorder

At age twelve, George was in fifth grade. He was a well-behaved boy who wanted very much to do well in school. His grades in math were always high, but he generally did poorly in reading and in any other classwork that involved reading. He was bright. On IQ tests he scored in the high average range. He had a strong vocabulary for listening and for speaking, but his reading vocabulary was very small. He could not read many words that were familiar when spoken to him. He could memorize a short list of words for weekly spelling tests, but he could not remember to spell those words correctly after the test and he was generally a very poor speller.

When called on to read aloud, George often mispronounced easy words and was tediously slow and halting. Despite getting extra help for reading since first grade, George could not sound out unfamiliar words. His mind seemed unable to retain what he had been taught about what sounds are associated with specific combinations of letters. He could not grasp the basics of phonics and had an intense dislike for reading because he found it so tedious and embarrassing.

Sally Shaywitz (2003) has described how most children, unlike George, learn to "break the code" in order to learn to read.

> The very first discovery a child makes on his way to reading is the realization that spoken words have parts. Suddenly a child appreciates that the word he hears comes apart into smaller pieces of sound; he has developed *phonemic awareness* . . . the ability to notice, identify and manipulate the individual sounds—phonemes—in spoken words. (p. 51)

Shaywitz noted that 70 to 80 percent of American children learn how to translate the code of written letters into spoken sounds without much difficulty. The remaining 20 to 30 percent have varying levels of persisting difficulty in learning to convert combinations of letters into spoken words. It is this impairment in learning to process phonemes, not the tendency to reverse letters and numbers, that is the major ingredient in dyslexia, another name for reading disorder.

There is strong evidence to suggest that dyslexia is associated with specific impairments in brain function. Sally Shaywitz and Bennett Shaywitz (2002) used functional MRI imaging to study the brains of dyslexic children compared to nonimpaired readers. In the brains of the dyslexic boys and girls, they found evidence of disrupted functioning in specific left hemisphere circuits that have been shown to be crucial for reading.

Mathematics Disorder

Twelve-year-old Lois is a sixth-grade student whose grades are all A's except in math. Since first grade she has always had great difficulty doing math problems. She is an excellent reader and has developed an exceptional vocabulary, but despite much effort she has not yet been able to learn her multiplication tables. She still uses her fingers to count and makes many errors when she attempts to do simple adding and subtraction. She seems to grasp the idea of multiplying, but is not yet able to multiply two numbers by two numbers. She finds simple division problems very confusing and still makes many mistakes in counting money or in reading the time from a clock. She has a digital watch because she has not yet mastered telling time from a conventional clock face.

Thus far there has been relatively little research to explore the underlying impairments in mathematics disorder. David Geary (1994) has described two distinct types of impairment in children with mathematics disability:

> The first involves difficulties in representing arithmetic facts in, or retrieving facts from, long term memory . . . many MD [mathematics disorder] children have problems remembering basic arithmetic facts such as $5 + 9 = 14$, even with extensive drilling. . . . The second involves difficulties in executing arithmetic procedures, such as carrying or trading in complex addition, or in executing counting procedures to solve simple addition problems. (pp. 155–156)

Much remains to be learned about the specifics of such impairments in the cognitive skills required for mathematics. There is some evidence that impairments in this domain, like those of dyslexia, are heritable, but the brain mechanisms involved are not yet known.

Disorder of Written Expression

Leo is an eleventh-grade boy who loves to read and gets excellent grades in all his courses in high school except those that involve extensive writing. Since early childhood he has shared with his father an intense interest in the Civil War. With his family he has visited every major Civil War battlefield. He has many books and videos about that war, and collecting Civil War memorabilia is his hobby. A history course that Leo took during the first semester of his junior year began with a unit on the Civil War. During class discussions Leo often contributed information and anecdotes that interested his classmates and impressed his teacher.

Yet Leo failed the first test of the semester, an essay exam requiring paragraphs to explain aspects of the Civil War that had been covered in the textbook and discussed in class. The teacher was annoyed by his overly terse answers and the lack of elaboration to support his responses. He felt that Leo knew the answers better than anyone else in class. He assumed that Leo had not taken the test seriously. Immediately after class the teacher met with Leo and required him to respond orally to each of the questions on the test. Leo's answers were all top-notch. When the teacher asked Leo why he had written such a poor test paper when he knew all the answers so well, Leo answered, "That happens to me all the time. I can know about something and can talk about it with no problem, but I just can't get the ideas written out on the page. All the teachers tell me that my answers are way too short and that I don't elaborate enough. I'm just a really poor writer."

Chapter 4 explains why written expression is much more demanding of executive functions than are talking or reading. The point here is that, like Leo, some children, adolescents, and adults experience extraordinary difficulty in expressing in writing, particularly expository writing, what they think, feel, and know.

After reviewing relevant research, Rosemary Tannock and I (2000) reported that all three of the basic learning disorders occur at rates two to three times higher among children with ADHD than among children in the general population. One of the few studies that looked for all three basic learning disorders in children with ADHD was reported by Susan Mayes and colleagues (2000). In a sample of children referred to a clinic, they found that 27 percent met diagnostic criteria for reading disorder, 31 percent for mathematics disorder, and 65 percent met diagnostic criteria for disorder of written expression. In sum, 70 percent of those children diagnosed with ADHD fully met the diagnostic criteria for at least one of these three learning disorders. Why are individuals with ADHD impaired by these learning disorders at such high rates?

For decades, ADHD and learning disabilities have been seen as completely separate disorders. ADHD was seen essentially as a disruptive behavior disorder that could be diagnosed by observation and treated with stimulant medications. In contrast, specific learning disorders of reading, mathematics, or written expression have generally been perceived as problems "hardwired" into the brain, problems that could be remediated only by employing special education techniques. Currently the boundary between these two categories of impairment is being reassessed.

In 2000 I argued that impairment of working memory plays a critical role both in ADD syndrome and in the cognitive functions that are disrupted in learning disorders related to reading, math, and written expression.

Reading involves holding in mind and integrating initial portions of a word, phrase, sentence, paragraph, chapter, and so forth long enough to connect these with subsequent portions so that connections can be made and various levels of meaning can be comprehended. Connections must be made between letter shapes and phonemes; diverse associations from elements of long-term memory must be quickly sorted out to select what is appropriate to context and to discard what is not. Smooth execution of these multiple linkages clearly involves not only the learning of phonemes and vocabulary, but also ongoing exercise of short-term working memory.

Likewise, most mathematical operations, from the borrowing and carrying of the simplest arithmetic to the intricacies of the most complex calculations for theoretical problem solving, are highly dependent on working memory. Multiple steps must be prioritized and sequenced, and information must be carried from one operation into another. To do arithmetic and mathematics one needs not only knowledge of specific procedures but also effective working memory. The problem solver's ability to transiently hold "on-line" these various numerical facts and relationships while analyzing problems and invoking appropriate learned procedure is another example of the exercise of working memory.

Similarly, working memory plays an essential role in written expression as one selects and weaves together words and verbal images to convey multiple levels of meaning. In writing, one must hold in mind an overall intention for what is to be communicated in the whole of the phrase, sentence, paragraph, essay, report, chapter, book, and so forth, while simultaneously generating the micro units of words and phrases that will eventually constitute the written work being produced. Complex and rapidly shifting interplay of micro and macro intentions is the essence of creating and self-editing that allows one gradually to shift from the glimmer of an idea, through crude approximations of rough draft, to the greater specificity and polish of a final product. . . . In addition to many more specific skills, the whole process of written expression involves ongoing and often intensive use of working memory. (pp. 38–39)

H. Lee Swanson and Leilani Sáez (2003) also emphasized the central importance of working memory and executive functions in learning disabilities (LD). They reported that "children and adults with LD are inferior to their counterparts on measures of short-term memory in which familiar items such as letters, words, and numbers, and unfamiliar shapes were recalled" (p. 189). They found

evidence . . . indicating both the phonological loop [of working memory] and the executive system as sources of deficit for participants with LD. Either one or both of these components play a significant role in predicting complex cognitive activities such as reading comprehension, arithmetic problem solving, and writing, as well as some basic skills (e.g. arithmetic computation). (p. 194)

Taken together, available data suggest that ADHD, language impairments, and specific learning disorders may not be so separate as has been generally assumed. The common element of impaired executive functions may account for a significant amount of the overlap between ADHD and specific learning disorders and between ADHD and some aspects of language impairment, particularly the pragmatic language impairments described in Chapter 4.

Yet specific learning disorders, speech and language disorders, and ADHD are not aspects of one problem. In speech/language disorders and in specific learning disorders, especially reading disorder, there is evidence that some brain functions are impaired in ways that are not found in individuals who have ADHD alone.

In Chapter 1, I suggested that if the brain is imagined as a symphony orchestra, executive functions impaired in ADD syndrome should be compared not to impaired players of the instruments, but to impairments in the conductor. In the overlap of ADD syndrome with impairments of language and learning, it would seem that this comorbidity reflects dysfunction in some of the players of instruments, as well as in the orchestra's conductor.

Disorders of Arousal and Motivation

Pennington (2002) proposed a category called "disorders of motivation," which includes (1) depression and dysthymia, (2) anxiety disorders, (3) post-traumatic stress disorder, and (4) bipolar illness. Each of these involves disruptions in the arousal/motivation system of the brain. To this category I have added obsessive-compulsive disorder as well as substance abuse and dependence. These two additional disorders are also essentially disruptions in the brain's normal regulation of arousal and motivation. Each of the six disorders in this expanded list occurs more frequently among persons with ADHD.

Depression and Dysthymia

Charles is a fifteen-year-old boy in ninth grade who was diagnosed with ADHD, predominantly inattentive type, when he was in fifth grade. Since that time he has been treated consistently with stimulant medication three times daily. Teachers, parents, and Charles himself report that this medication significantly improves his ability to stay focused on his schoolwork, to complete assignments, to organize his work, and to remember what he has read. His grades were honors level in junior high, but over the past year his academic performance has been in a slow decline.

Over the past two years Charles has become increasingly lethargic and withdrawn from social and athletic activities in which he had been very involved for several years. When not in school he now spends most of his time isolated in his room, usually playing video games or sleeping. His parents report that when friends call he avoids talking with them. He has declined their invitations to join in various activities so often that he now receives few calls. He rarely smiles, often makes self-deprecating comments, and appears chronically sad, though he denies that he is depressed.

Charles was not depressed in the sense of being immobilized by profound sadness or by a severe lack of energy. He was able to get out of bed and attend school regularly. He had no insomnia and his appetite was usually adequate, though he showed little interest in food. He gave no evidence of suicidal thoughts or actions and was not using drugs or alcohol, but all who had known him over time were struck by his persistent and increasing unhappiness, lethargy, and seeming inability to enjoy life.

The chronic, low-grade depressive symptoms shown by Charles are characteristic of dysthymia, a less dramatic but significantly impairing form of depression that has been described by Hagop Akiskal (1997). Charles was able to do most of what he was required to do, but found virtually no pleasure or satisfaction in most of life.

According to Thomas Spencer and others (2000) depression and/or dysthymia occurs in 15 to 75 percent of children or adolescents with ADHD. Since both ADHD and depression can be severely debilitating, any individual, like Charles, who suffers from both of these disorders should receive effective treatment for both. And some suffer not only from ADHD and depression, but also from anxiety disorders.

Anxiety Disorders

There are many types of anxiety disorders.

Separation anxiety is where a child experiences extremely excessive anxiety when separated or anticipating separation from home or persons to whom they have become attached. The child becomes terrified at the prospect of being away from primary caregivers and has extreme difficulty accepting a substitute caretaker even for short intervals. When required to stay with a babysitter, spend time in day care, or to attend school, the child may become extremely agitated and panicked.

Specific phobias involve an individual's being very fearful when faced with some specific situation—for example, encountering a dog, snake, or spider; sleeping alone in a dark room; entering an elevator; or flying in an airplane—though they may experience no extraordinary fear otherwise.

Social phobia, also known as social anxiety disorder, is an intense and persistently exaggerated fear of embarrassing oneself in interacting with or performing for other people. Usually this intense fear causes the individual to avoid the dreaded situations whenever possible, for example, by staying away from restaurants, parties, or other social gatherings. When the frightening situation cannot reasonably be avoided, such as when one is called on by a teacher to recite in class, one painfully endures the situation, getting it over as quickly as possible. Anticipation of such events often causes extreme stress, with nausea, tremors, stomachache, diarrhea, and so forth.

Panic disorder is characterized by recurrent panic attacks—brief but terrifying episodes of very intense fear that come on suddenly when there is no real danger and no anticipation of danger. Unlike phobic responses, the panic attack comes "out of the blue." The attack often includes shortness of breath, profuse sweating, chest pain, nausea, lightheadedness, and other sensations that may feel like one is having a heart attack and is about to die. Although such episodes usually peak within ten minutes, they are often followed by persistent fears of recurrence. Sometimes a panic attack is followed by strong fears of leaving one's home unless accompanied by a trusted companion: this is called panic disorder with agoraphobia.

Generalized anxiety disorder is a broader and more persistent pattern of chronic worry and fearful expectation that something bad is going to happen. Often individuals with this disorder spend long periods each day in uncontrollable, anxious anticipation of possible troubles or dangers. Additional symptoms such as chronic muscle tension, restlessness, excessive fatigue, or difficulty sleeping are often present. The focus of worry may vary considerably from one situation to another. Routine tasks and situations of daily life may become the focus of one's ruminating in gruesome detail about how badly events could turn out.

Although these various types of anxiety disorder are described as separate entities, they overlap with some aspects of normal development and often overlap with one another in afflicted individuals. To what extent are these various disorders perhaps variants of one larger problem?

Douglas Mennin and colleagues (2000) addressed the overlap among anxiety disorders in children with ADHD and in normal controls. His group found that being diagnosed with two or more specific anxiety disorders identified most children who were "significantly impaired by anxiety." This does not mean that an individual diagnosed with just one anxiety disorder does not warrant treatment. Mennin's measure simply identifies individuals for whom anxiety symptoms are especially impairing. According to this standard, 17 percent of the children with ADHD were severely impaired by anxiety.

Most of the children in the Mennin study had begun experiencing their anxiety disorders before the age of twelve. Several studies have shown that most individuals impaired by depression usually have a history of excessive anxiety antecedent to their hopeless feelings. Often these two streams, anxiety and depression, converge and continue to flow together over a person's lifetime.

The overlap and complexity of these various forms of anxiety is illustrated in the following case:

> Doug, a twelve-year-old boy in seventh grade, was diagnosed as having ADHD while he was in fourth grade, but received no medication treatment because his parents were apprehensive about possible adverse effects. He was brought for consultation during seventh grade because of longstanding problems with anxiety. Since early childhood Doug had been very fearful about being away from his family. When he started kindergarten he had great difficulty separating from his mother each day. Since that time he has generally been able to attend school regularly,

but has had episodic series of excessive absences because of vague complaints of headache, stomachache, or nausea.

Doug has a long history of difficulty falling asleep. He cannot get to sleep unless he is in a room with his brother or a parent. Even then he often is unable to get to sleep until sixty to ninety minutes after he gets into bed. Once in bed he will not leave his bed to go the bathroom unless a parent or his brother accompanies him.

He is very fearful of being alone, even in daylight. When taking a shower he often calls out to be sure that a parent is in earshot. He will not go outside his house to play unless accompanied by someone he trusts or by the family dog. He is easily embarrassed and extremely shy. Doug refuses any extracurricular activities, sports, or birthday parties unless one of his parents stays with him. Despite all this, he maintained a B+ average in school.

Doug met *DSM-IV* diagnostic criteria for several different anxiety disorders: separation anxiety, specific phobia (dark), social phobia, and generalized anxiety disorder. He also met criteria for ADHD, predominantly inattentive type. Although this laundry list of multiple diagnostic categories may sound like a variety of different problems, it would seem reasonable to think of Doug as simply a boy who has ADHD and is chronically extremely anxious in different ways in a variety of settings.

One way to consider Doug's situation is to compare him with a homeowner who has an overly sensitive smoke detector that screeches loudly and persistently any time bread is overcooked a bit in the toaster. In response to the slightest whiff of smoke, the detector sounds a protracted alarm as though the entire house is about to go up in flames. In the case of chronic anxiety, however, the "smoke detector" cannot easily be repaired or replaced.

Doug reported that he felt ashamed of his chronic fearfulness:

I know I'm scared of lots of things that are no problem to most other kids my age. I try to fight it and say to myself, "It's OK, just go ahead and do it. It's not really dangerous. Even my little brother can do it, no problem." Sometimes that works, but usually it doesn't. It's stupid, but if I try to walk around alone in the dark at night, even in our own house, or if I go outside alone, I get this terrible feeling inside, like something really, really bad is going to happen and I won't be able to stop it. I just can't make that feeling go away unless someone else is there with me. I get scared like I would be if I were standing in front of a truck speeding right at me or hanging off the edge of a cliff and losing my grip.

Such reactions involve intimate interactions among a very sensitive body chemistry, a set of recurrent thoughts and mental images and, presumably, some defect in the brain mechanisms that assess and respond to potentially threatening stimuli. Some of these elements may be inherited, some may be developed in response to frightening experiences, and some may emerge as a result of living with family members who themselves are much more alert to potential threats and dangers in the world than are most others. These variants of anxiety occur more often in individuals with ADHD, sometimes separately, sometimes in various combinations.

Obsessive-Compulsive Disorder

Joanne, a thirty-four-year-old divorced mother of an eight-year-old son and a ten-year-old daughter, supported her children by working an eight-hour shift each day as a registered nurse. Each morning she awakened early to dress, feed, and deliver her children to the day care center near their school. She then went to work her shift in the intensive care unit at the hospital, after which she picked up her son and daughter at day care, took them home, prepared supper, helped the children with their homework, bathed them, read them stories, and got them to bed. She then cleaned up the dinner dishes and did laundry or other household chores. After all this, every night she spent over an hour washing and stripping the wax off the floor of her kitchen and adjoining family room, letting it dry, and then re-waxing the floor and replacing the furniture.

Joanne explained, "I know it doesn't make sense for me to wash and rewax those floors every night. Most people don't do it even every month. But I have been doing it this way for years. I have to do it. If I try to let it go for a night, I just can't get to sleep. I get this feeling that my house is dirty and not good for the kids and me to live in, so I just have to get it done. I know it doesn't make any sense, but that's what I have to do."

Joanne recognized that her daily washing and rewaxing of her floors made no rational sense, but she felt compelled to do it. When she tried to end the day and go to sleep without completing this compulsive chore, she became so anxious that she was unable to relax and go to sleep. When she completed the task successfully, her anxiety was reduced enough so she was able to live her daily life without much difficulty. Her drive to complete this burdensome daily chore, despite her recognizing that it was not rationally necessary, is one example of the wide variety of compulsions that may be seen in obsessive compulsive disorder (OCD).

Compulsions are not always cleaning chores; problems with compulsions can become apparent in any of a wide variety of behaviors. One college student felt compelled to keep his large CD collection in perfect alphabetical order by name of musician; any time this order was disrupted, accidentally or deliberately, he felt compelled immediately to rearrange them, regardless of whether doing so meant missing a class or delaying required work. A girl in junior high felt compelled to count the number of steps on any stairway she walked on at home, school, or elsewhere and had to touch each side of a doorway once with each hand before she could walk through it. If she forgot, she felt she had to enter through the doorway again or go back to the foot of the stairs and walk up again, carefully counting. An eleven-year-old boy felt it necessary to confess to his teacher or parent anytime he looked at any girl's buttocks, repeatedly asking, "I did it again, is that OK?" Such inquiries were sometimes made many times an hour in school, despite the inevitable teasing from his classmates and the annoyance of his teacher and parents.

In another example, a forty-year-old teacher compulsively saved every daily newspaper for over ten years, neatly stacking them throughout her house until there was virtually no room to move around. When friends offered to help her move them out so she would have adequate living space, she responded, "I just can't bring myself to get rid of them. I keep thinking I may need to refer to them someday, even though I know it would be much easier to look anything up in the public library microfilms. I know it's stupid, but I just have this strong feeling that I have to store them in my own home."

These examples of cleaning, counting, arranging, checking, and hoarding are just a few of the enormous variety of tasks that people with OCD may feel compelled to perform every day. Usually a person's compulsions tend rather consistently to be of one type or another, though intensity of the symptoms may wax and wane. Some persons with OCD do not feel compelled to perform compulsive actions, but they repeatedly get stuck thinking about specific worries. Sometimes their worries are directly connected to compulsive behaviors that seem intended to relieve the worry. For example, the nurse who had to wash and wax her floors daily had a persisting worry about whether her house might be dangerously dirty. Others have concerns that are troubling in that they seem to require persistent preoccupation, but they are not accompanied by compulsive behaviors.

Examples of obsessional worries without accompanying compulsions include a nine-year-old girl who reported chronic preoccupation with fears that her five-year-old sister might suddenly die and a fifteen-year-old boy who reported daily preoccupation with worries that he had contracted AIDS, despite his awareness that he had had no experiences that would realistically put him at risk of such an infection. Although neither of these individuals engaged in compulsive behaviors, each reported successive months when such thoughts persisted in their thinking for two hours or more each day, despite their efforts to think about other things instead.

As I have described elsewhere (2000), most children, adolescents, and adults experience occasional preoccupations with disturbing thoughts and many engage in compulsive behaviors that do not make rational sense. To qualify for diagnosis as OCD, obsessions or compulsions must significantly disrupt the individual's daily functioning, usually consuming at least an hour each day. It is this daily impairment that distinguishes the obsessions and compulsions of OCD from the repetitive worrying or superstitious behaviors that may occur from time to time with most people.

In a group of children diagnosed with ADHD, Daniel Geller and others (2002) found that over half also had some form of OCD. Previously, in 1996, these researchers had found that one-third of children diagnosed with OCD also met full diagnostic criteria for ADHD; usually the ADHD occurred much earlier, more than two years before the OCD symptoms developed. Children who had both ADHD and OCD tended to have significantly worse daily functioning than those who had either disorder without the other.

Post-Traumatic Stress Disorder

Another anxiety disorder seen more commonly among individuals with ADHD is post-traumatic stress disorder (PTSD). Primary symptoms of PTSD have to do with an individual's persistent disturbing reactions to an event or series of events in which they had reason to believe that his or her life was in danger. This disorder was first recognized in soldiers who returned from combat, where they had been exposed to acute risk of severe injury or imminent death, and where they had seen their comrades suffer agonizing pain after being felled by bullets or bomb fragments.

For weeks, months, and years after exposure to such trauma, some soldiers repeatedly re-experienced the terrifying events as though a video of the situation were suddenly being replayed in their memory. In those moments of flashback, sometimes occasional, sometimes many times a day, they recalled the situations in painful detail as though they had suddenly been returned to the original experience. Each time they felt the same intensity of anxiety and other emotions that had accompanied the initial experience, a situation that seriously disrupted their sleep and daily life.

Study of Vietnam veterans suffering from PTSD yielded evidence that these terrifying experiences had been etched into memory in a unique way that the brain apparently reserves for situations of acute danger. For some veterans, PTSD symptoms diminish gradually over time; they have been able to heal from their trauma with some success. For others, the terror repeats over many years, and, for some, for the rest of their lives. Research suggests that the severity and duration of PTSD symptoms are not directly linked to the severity or duration of war trauma experienced; instead, some individuals are more vulnerable to such reactions than others.

Gradually clinicians recognized that some victims of trauma other than combat show similar persistent symptoms of flashbacks, sleep disturbances, and so forth. These occur in some individuals traumatized by rape, a severe motor vehicle accident, being trapped in a burning building, or some similar situation where, for terrifying moments or more, it appeared to the victims that they were about to die a terrible and unexpected death or where they witnessed such a fate in others. PTSD symptoms also occur in some people who experience life-threatening dangers in natural disasters such as earthquakes or floods.

Similar etching of painful events into memory occurs in some who have been subjected to physical and/or sexual abuse as children. PTSD also has been found in adults who have experienced relationships in which they were repeatedly battered physically and emotionally by parents or partners. Apparently there is a broad array of situations after which an individual may experience this recurrent misfiring of the brain's mechanism for acute alarm.

Among individuals with ADHD there is an elevated incidence of certain kinds of PTSD. Sally Merry and Leah Andrews (1994) studied sexually abused children and found that while 44 percent met the diagnostic criteria for PTSD, 25 percent also met those for ADHD; this is more than threefold the incidence of ADHD in the general population. This finding does not necessarily indicate that those with ADHD are more vulnerable to all types of PTSD. It may be that those with ADHD are more likely to be in situations where certain reactive or interactive types of acute danger to life or safety—such as accidents, or physical or sexual abuse— may be experienced.

Combined type ADHD may increase the risk of PTSD resulting from child abuse. Often those toddlers and young children have chronic difficulty in getting to sleep at night and are often defiant and unwilling to follow directions from their caretakers. As suggested in Chapter 4, parents or other caretakers forced to cope with the stress of managing such a child, especially late at night when they are likely to be overtired themselves, may be more likely to lose control of their anger and violently punish that child.

As they get older, individuals with ADHD, particularly those with combined type, may be quicker than most to seek out risk and adventure. They may be less likely to avoid risks that can be anticipated or may push the envelope by driving faster, climbing higher, or getting closer to the edge of the cliff, sometimes with terrifying or disastrous results.

In addition to not behaving carefully, many with ADHD often have excessive difficulty in regulating their emotions and in sizing up social interactions with others. This may lead some to get into interactions or relationships where they encounter or provoke excessive threats, danger, or violence, which in turn may cause PTSD. In some cases, then, the elevated incidence of PTSD among individuals with ADHD may be due more to their impulsively getting themselves into situations of increased physical or interpersonal danger than to a constitutional vulnerability to anxiety, though these are not mutually exclusive possibilities.

Bipolar Disorder

Bipolar disorder (BPD) is also among diagnoses classified by Pennington as "disorders of motivation and arousal." Formerly known as manic-depressive disorder, this syndrome is characterized by episodes during which the individual manifests an intense increase in elation, grandiosity, and rapid or racing thoughts, usually with decreased need for sleep and often with hypersexuality or increased frequency of other activities that may be pleasurable, but are likely to create serious difficulties for the individual. Such episodes alternate in longer or shorter intervals with episodes of major depression. Switches between the manic and depressive moods may occur with no clear cause. Individuals with BPD also have elevated risk for substance abuse and suicide.

For decades BPD was thought to occur only in late adolescence or adulthood. In 1995, however, Janet Wozniak and Joseph Biederman reported an elevated incidence of BPD (16 percent) among children and younger adolescents diagnosed with ADHD in their clinic; they suggested that mania might be far more common among psychiatrically referred children, particularly those with ADHD, than previously thought. Because some symptoms of ADHD overlap with those of BPD, these reports led to controversy among child psychiatrists as to whether the children being described simply had severe ADHD or did, in fact, suffer from childhood-onset bipolar disorder.

A team headed by Barbara Geller (2002a, 2002b) reported that children and younger adolescents with genuine BPD had four specific symptoms—elated mood, grandiosity, flight of ideas or racing thoughts, and decreased need for sleep—that occurred in them far more than in those with ADHD or in community controls.

Geller and colleagues (2002b) pointed out that some other symptoms characteristic of BPD also occur in many children with ADHD or other disorders. They found chronic irritability in 98 percent of the children with BPD, 72 percent of those with ADHD, and just 3 percent of those in the community control group. However, Eric Mick and others (2005) recently showed a critical difference in the irritability of bipolar children: their irritability tends to be much more extreme and explosive than in children with ADHD. Irritability in bipolar children tends to be severe, often physically aggressive, destructive, and dangerous. The difference between ADHD irritability and bipolar irritability might be compared to the difference between the pressure of a garden hose and that of a powerful fire hose.

It is not only the severity of irritability that differentiates these two disorders. Geller found that suicidal tendencies occurred in 25 percent of the BPD children; psychosis was seen in 60 percent; and mixed mania, a combination of manic and depressive symptoms, occurred in 55 percent of the BPD children. None of these are characteristic of those with just ADHD.

Although there is some overlap between symptoms of BPD and those of ADHD, and a wide range of severity in both disorders, there are important differences. Most of those with BPD meet diagnostic criteria for

ADHD, but are also characterized by a number of other seriously impairing symptoms that are not part of ADD syndrome.

Substance Use Disorders

Substance use disorders, which are characterized by abuse of or dependence on alcohol, marijuana, heroin, cocaine, methamphetamine, or a variety of other drugs, significantly disrupt one's motivation to pursue education or work, interact with others, and maintain one's self and household. Often the long-term goals and more immediate intentions of these individuals are seriously interrupted as they crave, seek, use, and react to substances of abuse. Persons given this diagnosis often suffer from excessive arousal, being excessively "hyped-up" in certain phases of drug use while being excessively slowed down or somnolent in other phases of abuse or dependence. These disruptions of motivation and arousal appear to be closely connected to anticipated, immediate, and delayed effects of the abused substances on the brain.

Among individuals diagnosed with ADHD, there is a markedly elevated incidence and severity of abuse and dependence on alcohol and other drugs over the lifetime. This difference does not become clear in group data until after mid-adolescence, however, when many of those with ADHD tend to become caught up in escalating problems with substance abuse. Joseph Biederman and Timothy Wilens (1997) published data comparing ADHD boys' and normal controls' use of drugs and alcohol at baseline and four years later. They found no difference between the ADHD adolescents and controls in rates of substance use disorders up to age fifteen years. Yet an earlier study of adults indicated that 52 percent of those diagnosed with ADHD had qualified for diagnosis of substance abuse or dependence at some point in their lives, while only half that percentage (27 percent) of adults without ADHD met the diagnostic criteria for substance use disorder.

According to data presented by Wilens and others (1998, 2000) having ADHD (1) heightens the risk of developing a drug use disorder, (2) accelerates twofold the transition from less severe drug or alcohol abuse to more severe dependence, and (3) more than doubles the duration of substance use before remission. Apparently those with ADHD tend to become more involved in seriously impairing substance abuse during late adolescence and early adulthood when most of their peers are reducing their abuse of such substances. This raises the question of why such a difference should occur at that particular point.

One indirect answer to that question might be derived from the 2003 review by Wilens and colleagues of six studies involving more than a thousand adolescents with ADHD, some of whom had been treated with stimulant medications during childhood and adolescence and some of whom had not. Their goal was to assess the effects of stimulant treatment for ADHD on the rate of substance abuse. Results showed an almost twofold reduction for risk of substance use disorders in individuals with ADHD who had been treated with stimulants, compared to individuals with ADHD who had not. In fact, those treated consistently during childhood and adolescence with stimulant medications had a rate of substance abuse and dependence not significantly different from the baseline rate in the population. Apparently there is something about living with untreated ADHD that increases the likelihood of abuse or dependence on drugs or alcohol. Multiple factors may be at work. For instance, impairments of the brain's reward system, described in Chapter 3 as an aspect of ADHD, a system managed primarily by dopamine networks, may cause affected persons to seek out and repeatedly use addictive substances that tend to stimulate that section of brain. Medication treatment for ADHD may reduce that vulnerability while it alleviates symptoms of ADHD.

Untreated ADHD may also cause an individual to be more frustrated and less successful in school. The lower-achieving student is more likely to be placed in lower-track classes with less able and less motivated classmates, a peer group where extensive and frequent use of drugs is more common. In such a situation the student may self-medicate with illicit substances to alleviate frustration, worry, and shame over poor achievement. In a study of adolescents in treatment for substance abuse, two-thirds reported to Beverly Horner and Karl Scheibe (1997) that they had continued use of illicit drugs not primarily for pleasure, but to improve their mood. A combination of interacting biochemical and psychosocial factors is likely to be behind the elevated rates of many disorders of motivation and arousal among those with ADHD.

Similarities among Disorders of Motivation and Arousal

Among the various disorders of motivation and arousal discussed in this section there are obvious differences, but also underlying similarities. Dysthymia and depression both involve a significant reduction in motivation and arousal associated with chronic feelings of hopelessness, as though an unsatisfying outcome to one's efforts were already determined. Anxiety disorders are characterized by an intensification of arousal often combined with avoidance of what is assumed to be an inevitably dangerous outcome. Bipolar disorder, in the manic phase, is marked by intense exaggeration of arousal and an often pathological intensity of certain motivations; the depressive aspect, whether phasic or mixed, falls to the opposite extreme.

Comparison of these comorbid disorders with the characteristics of ADD syndrome shows considerable overlap as well as differences. Management of arousal, ability to activate for tasks, ability to sustain effort for tasks, management of emotions, ability to effectively utilize working memory, ability to size up and regulate actions in social situations—these interacting executive functions tend to be impaired in each of these comorbid disorders. Yet each of the comorbid disorders of arousal and motivation is also characterized by more extreme intensity or absence of arousal, and/or by motivation that is more extreme in its variability or fixity, than is usually found in ADD syndrome itself. These extremes of arousal and motivation, combined with specific related impairments of these various disorders, occur among persons with ADHD more often than in most others without ADHD. The high rates of comorbidity between ADHD and these various disorders of motivation and arousal may be seen as another example of concurrent impairments in the conductor of the orchestra and in specific components of the orchestra itself.

Disorders of Social-Emotional Regulation

In my reformulation of Pennington's categories, I have grouped together the following disorders, all of which are characterized by various types and degrees of disruption in social-emotional regulation of action: Asperger's disorder, oppositional defiant disorder, conduct disorder, and Tourette's syndrome.

Asperger's Disorder

Chapter 2 describes how individuals with ADD syndrome often are impaired in their ability to manage frustration and modulate emotions, as well as in their ability to monitor and self-regulate actions. These and other facets of ADD syndrome often cause children, adolescents, and adults to have difficulty in their social relationships. But among those individuals with ADD syndrome are some whose impairments in social interactions are much more severe. Some of those meet diagnostic criteria for Asperger's disorder, which is considered by some experts to be a variant of autism.

Fred Volkmar and Ami Klin (2000) have described differences between autism and Asperger's syndrome (AS) this way:

> In contrast with individuals with autism, individuals with AS experience social isolation, but are not withdrawn or devoid of social interest; in fact, they often approach others, but in eccentric ways. Their interest in having friends, girlfriends/boyfriends, and social contact may in fact be quite striking. (p. 59)

This longing for social interaction combined with impairments of Asperger's disorder is illustrated in the following description by the mother of a thirteen-year-old girl in seventh grade:

> My daughter has ADHD, but she also has a lot of social problems that most kids with ADHD just don't have. She has never been able to catch on to how kids get along with other people, especially with other kids. Stuff that most kids just pick up by listening and watching other people, she doesn't absorb even when we try to explain it to her. She just doesn't get it! That's why all the other kids pick on her and call her weird. They won't have anything to do with her. It's been this way since about sec-

ond grade, but it has gotten a lot worse now that she is in middle school.

Sometimes she will beg another girl to come over to our house and even offer to pay her to play with her. If the girl says she might come over "sometime," my daughter will get on the phone and call her eight to ten times on the same day to try to get her to come over right away. If the girl says she's busy, my daughter keeps asking her why she can't come a little later that day. She can't tell when someone is lying or teasing or just trying to put her off. She takes everything literally. She's not stupid. Her grades are mostly C's and B's; sometimes she gets an A. She can understand a lot about computers and science, but she never seems to get how other people feel or why they get mad at her or laugh at her.

This girl's impairment in understanding and managing social interactions is qualitatively different from that of most other children with ADHD. Her problems affect the various executive functions that comprise ADD syndrome, but she is also impaired in more fundamental ways that have to do with the ability to read and understand emotions communicated by others in implicit, nonverbal ways. She has Asperger's disorder as well as ADHD.

Patients with Asperger's also tend to have a lot of trouble shifting focus flexibly between details and context. Martha Denckla (2000) described this problem as it appears in adults with nonverbal learning disabilities affecting not only their social relationships, but also other aspects of their thinking.

Having an overly local . . . cognitive style, such adults manifest "forest for trees disease"—that is, they miss the "big picture" and get stuck on detail. Despite good verbal skills, they write poorly because they do not summarize or relate pieces of information. Asked for the main idea, the overarching concept, or the hierarchy (rather than the sequence) of priorities inher-

ent in academic or vocational material, the adult . . . will be
baffled. (p. 313)

Psychologist Byron Rourke (2000) has shown that many individuals
with Asperger's have essentially the same profile on psychological tests
as do those identified with nonverbal learning disorders (as described by
Denckla). He notes that this may be a basis on which those with Asperger's
and individuals with high functioning autism might be differentiated.

Consequences of these more fundamental problems of individuals
with Asperger's are shown in a description by Simon Baron-Cohen (2003)
of individuals with Asperger's disorder seen in his clinic:

> Most did best at factual subjects such as math, science and his-
> tory . . . [but] were weakest at literature, where the task was to
> *interpret* a fictional text . . . or enter into a character's emotional
> life . . . they found it difficult to make friends; males with AS
> found it particularly difficult to establish a girlfriend relation-
> ship. . . . Most . . . had said things that had hurt others' feel-
> ings . . . yet they could not understand why the other person
> took offence if their statement was true . . .
>
> Many adults with AS have held a series of jobs, and have ex-
> perienced social difficulties leading to clashes with colleagues
> and employers . . . their work is often considered technically
> accomplished and thorough, but they may never get promoted
> because their people skills are so limited. . . . Some have had a
> series of short-term sexual relationships. Such relationships
> usually flounder, in part, because their partner feels they are
> being over-controlled or used, or because the person with AS
> is not emotionally supportive or communicative . . . their few
> friends are usually somewhat odd themselves. Typically, their
> friendships fall away because they do not maintain them. . . .
> A significant proportion of adults with AS experience clinical
> levels of depression and some even feel suicidal because they
> feel they are a social failure and do not belong. (pp. 144–145)

No specific medication treatment has been found to alleviate the complex impairments of Asperger's disorder, but when patients who have it manifest symptoms of ADD syndrome, they often benefit from treatment with stimulant medications, as do those with pervasive developmental disorder as described by Jean Frazier and others (2000).

Oppositional Defiant Disorder

My oldest daughter has always had a mind of her own, ever since she was a toddler. It's like she never got over the "terrible twos" where they say "No!" to everything you ask them. Now she is twelve and wants to think that she is all grown up and doesn't need to listen to anybody, regardless of who they are. I know a lot of teenagers are that way, but she's really extreme, even for a teenager.

At school they have always told me about how she's very smart, even though she has ADHD, but most of the teachers get fed up with her attitude. She is always arguing with whatever they say. They say white and she'll argue, "No, it can't be that way. It's really black." They call her "the lawyer" because she's always going on and on with her arguments. Sometimes she can be funny, but she doesn't know when to stop. The principal has suspended her three times this year for being disrespectful to teachers. They say this isn't part of her ADHD.

She seems to get along all right with other kids. She's one of the ringleaders of a group of girls at school. They play sports together. She's actually pretty good at soccer, and swimming and lacrosse. Coaches get frustrated though because anytime she makes a mistake, she always blames somebody else. She won't take responsibility for what is her own fault. She does the same thing at home. It's always somebody else who didn't do what they were supposed to. Nothing is ever her fault.

When her father and I set limits and won't let her go someplace she wants or won't buy her something she has decided she needs, she has a tantrum that can go on for a couple of hours,

with lots of swearing and throwing things and repeated slam-
ming of doors. We just don't know what to do with her! She's
not a bad kid. She gets herself to school and practice every day
and usually gets pretty good grades, but she's got a big-time attitude problem that we haven't found any way to improve much
over the past ten years.

This girl's chronic negativistic and oppositional attitude extend beyond impairments usually associated with ADHD. According to her mother's report she has a long history of being defiant toward not only parents, but also teachers and other adults. She is not delinquent, but she
reportedly maintains a very oppositional and defiant attitude in her interactions with most adults. This is an example of oppositional defiant disorder (ODD).

Overlap between ODD and ADHD is usually reported as very high,
particularly when only the combined type of ADHD is considered. Usual
estimates are that about 40 percent of children with ADHD also meet diagnostic criteria for ODD. Characteristics of ODD are mostly variants of
excessively negative emotional reactions and their behavioral manifestations. These include frequent angry outbursts, arguing with or defying
adults, annoyance with or blaming of others, touchiness, resentfulness,
spitefulness, and vindictiveness. Most children who meet criteria for ODD
do not have the more severe problems of conduct disorder (CD), a chronic
pattern of more delinquent behavior that is discussed later.

I explained in Chapter 2 that problems in managing frustration and
regulating emotion are one aspect of ADD syndrome. This is consistent
with my earlier work (1996, 2001) as well as reports of other researchers
such as Russell Barkley (1997), Keith Conners (1997), Conners and colleagues (1999), and Paul Wender (1995); all of us have reported problems
in regulating emotion as an important aspect of the impairments of individuals with ADHD. But current diagnostic criteria for ADHD include no
mention of problems with regulation of emotion. The very high incidence
of the ODD cluster of negative emotional reactions among children with
ADHD raises the question of whether chronic problems in managing

emotions, especially frustration, may be an aspect of ADHD that was mistakenly excluded from the *DSM-IV* description of the disorder.

Ross Greene and others (2002) reported on large samples of boys and girls, average age about ten years, who met diagnostic criteria for ODD alone or ODD with conduct disorder. He compared these children with others who had other psychiatric problems, but not ODD or CD. Comparisons showed that socioeconomic status was significantly lower for families of children with ODD alone, and for ODD with conduct disorder, than for families of children with other psychiatric disorders not including ODD or CD. These findings suggest that children with ODD and/or CD are more likely to come from relatively disadvantaged families.

Greene found that schoolchildren with ODD and/or CD had higher rates of placement in special education classes, though his three groups did not differ in rates of repeated grades or need for tutorial assistance. This suggests that children with ODD or CD were seen as needing more intensive supervision in school. But problems of children with ODD were not limited to school settings. Social impairments of those with ODD, with or without CD, cut across all domains of social functioning, including relationships with parents, siblings, and peers. Individuals with this combination of executive function impairments (from ADHD) and chronic problems in managing negative attitudes and emotions (which characterize ODD) tend to make significant difficulties for themselves and others in virtually every social setting.

Greene and colleagues (2002), as well as others, have reported that families of children diagnosed with ODD, with or without CD, tend to show significantly poorer family cohesion and significantly higher levels of family conflict. One possibility is that ADHD impairments with ODD symptoms of the child tend to create more conflict with parents. Another is that parents of these children may be more harsh and more likely to provoke the child, thus establishing a pattern of intensified reciprocal anger and chronic conflict that the child carries to other situations. It is likely that socioeconomic disadvantage also contributes substantially to chronic stress in many of these families.

Conduct Disorder

Mike is a sixteen-year-old boy whose ADHD diagnosis describes only a small portion of his chronic difficulties. He has been getting failing grades in most of his high school courses for the past two years since he moved into a new foster home placement. Often he cuts classes or just doesn't show up for school. Mike has been in foster care since he was seven years old; he is currently in his fourth placement. Each of his previous placements has ended because of serious behavior problems, for example, bullying younger children in the household, torturing pet cats in the neighborhood, and repeatedly stealing money from the foster parents.

Mike was arrested and put under juvenile court supervision when he was twelve. At that time he had started a fire in the garage of a neighbor; the garage and its contents were destroyed. He has been arrested three additional times for shoplifting. Mike is usually not overtly hostile; he tends to appear apathetic and sullen, as though he just doesn't care. Foster parents note that he can be pleasant at times, but can't be trusted to tell the truth, to keep his commitments, or to respect others' property. He smokes cigarettes openly and is suspected of drinking alcohol and smoking marijuana, though the evidence on this is not clear.

Mike is the youngest of five children. His father is an alcoholic who was physically abusive to his wife and children when drunk. He served time in jail for auto theft and assaulting a police officer. Mike's mother, also an alcoholic, had Mike placed in foster care because she was afraid of his repeatedly playing with matches in their home. She feared that he might set their house on fire when she was asleep.

The *DSM-IV* characterizes conduct disorder (CD) as having symptoms arranged in four clusters: (1) aggression toward people or animals, (2) destruction of property—for example, deliberate fire setting, (3) deceitfulness or theft, and (4) serious violations of rules, such as truancy or

running away from home before age thirteen. Only three of the fifteen behavioral symptoms listed are required for diagnosis of CD; consequently,
there are a wide variety of subtypes, one of which is characterized by various types of overt physical aggression and another in which behavior is
more covert and nonaggressive, though still delinquent.

Stephen Hinshaw and Carolyn Anderson (1996) noted that while individuals diagnosed with CD almost always have already met the criteria
for ODD, fewer than 25 percent of individuals with ODD eventually develop the more severe problems of CD. Hinshaw and Anderson also emphasized that there are many reasons that children become delinquent,
only a small percentage of which are directly related to the CD diagnosis.
The *DSM-IV* recognizes this distinction by stipulating that the CD diagnosis should be made only when the symptoms appear to be due to internal dysfunction.

Bruce Pennington (2002) summarized genetic studies showing that
children with ADHD and those who have conduct disorder tend to share
very similar genetic profiles. This led him to suggest that environmental
factors may play an important role in determining the CD outcome: "With
optimal parenting, a child with this genetic profile will develop ADHD
only. With harsh parenting, the same child will also develop comorbid
ODD or CD" (p. 183). These observations are consistent with family studies showing that harsh, abusive, and/or extremely inconsistent parenting
practices tend to set into motion a vicious cycle of aggressive behavior
from a child, which then elicits more harsh and punitive behavior from
parents. Pennington also notes that peer-group and other neighborhood
influences may cause some adolescents to engage transiently in the antisocial behaviors that characterize conduct disorder.

Usually the CD diagnosis is applied to individuals who engage in serious and persistent antisocial behaviors, some of which may be described
as psychopathic. Donal MacCoon, John Wallace, and Joseph Newman
(2004) have described how psychopathic individuals often are severely
impaired in being able to use awareness of others' emotions to restrain
themselves from taking aggressive actions. What causes most individuals

to care about and respect other persons, to treat others with respect for their rights and feelings, and to cope with frustrations without harming those who appear to be causing (or not alleviating) that frustration? Why do some individuals persistently ignore or show disdain for the pain and suffering that they may cause to others?

Daniel Siegel (1999) has described how children with "disorganized" attachments to their caregivers tend to develop hostile and aggressive patterns of interactions with others. From this point of view it appears that developing or maintaining positive emotional attachments to parents or other caretakers may increase the likelihood that the child will perceive others as persons to be respected. This is consistent with James Blair (1995), who suggested that a deficit in the ability to respond to distress cues in others (a failure of empathy), produces a failure to inhibit aggressive behavior.

This emphasis on the role of positive emotional attachments in controlling aggression toward others does not rule out the influence of biological factors. Pennington (2002) noted that low levels of serotonin correlate with antisocial behavior and excessive aggression. Low resting heart rate also has been shown to be characteristic of many individuals who demonstrate excessive aggression or antisocial behavior. Jame Ortiz and Adrian Raine (2004) reviewed studies involving more than 5,800 children or teenagers manifesting antisocial behavior. Their results strongly demonstrated that antisocial children tend to have a lower resting heart rate, especially when stressed, in comparison to both normal and psychiatric controls; they showed less of the usual fear response.

Direct links between biological factors and the diverse symptoms of CD have not been adequately established. One can only suspect a reduced biological vulnerability to fear, which might result in a relative lack of responsiveness to social cues, less fearfulness about incurring disapproval from others, or other characteristics. In any case, it seems likely that the destructive and self-damaging impairments of CD are shaped by some combination of inherited biological factors and the environmental influences of family and neighborhood.

Tourette's Syndrome

Tourette's syndrome (TS) is a disorder characterized most noticeably by chronic vocal and motor tics that occur many times virtually every day for at least a year. These motor tics may include repetitive eye squinting, nose twitching, facial grimacing, mouth opening, or shoulder shrugging. Sometimes more complex movements such a lifting an elbow and rotating a wrist may occur, but the simple tics are more common. Vocal tics may include throat clearing, sniffing, snorting, or other repetitive noises. Many patients with TS report that patterns of their tics tend to shift from one movement or noise to another over time, and that they can suppress them under certain conditions, but usually the tics tend to reemerge after suppression, sometimes in a more intense way.

Elkhonen Goldberg (2001) described two other characteristics often seen in patients with TS: an excessive urge to explore by touching, looking at, or smelling incidental objects that catch their interest, and "verbal incontinence," by which he means not only coprolalia, the tendency to make obscene or profane comments in socially inappropriate situations, but also a broader pattern of making critical or derisive comments in social settings where they are likely to hurt others' feelings or provoke anger or rejection.

This "verbal incontinence" includes impulsively uttering observations or reactions to others that many non-TS individuals might think, but never say aloud. As Goldberg explains: "What is on his mind may immediately be on his lips. It may be unflattering epithets, slurs of various kinds, obnoxious editorial comments—anything forbidden" (p. 183). Many TS patients describe themselves as having chronic difficulty in suppressing the impulse to say or do what is forbidden, once that possibility enters their mind. Goldberg observed that "in Tourette's the urge to release internal tension may be ever present and unquenchable" (p. 183). He quotes one of his TS patients who described irrepressible urges to touch or smell: "It is a heightened sensory curiosity and lack of inhibition. I become focused on a body part or an object. Once I focus on it, the urge becomes uncontrollable" (p. 185).

The chronic difficulty of many TS patients in resisting the impulse to say or do the socially inappropriate, the forbidden, suggests that they suffer from a particular failure of the brain to control emotional reactions such as frustration, curiosity, or anger. They seem unable to employ an awareness of others' emotions to hold back the comment or gesture that may be hurtful or embarrassing to that person or themselves. The resulting outbursts cause some TS patients to experience frequent rejection and sometimes dangerous punitive reactions.

Although tics can become embarrassing and problematic for those who suffer with TS, they are not usually the most troubling symptoms for those with this disorder. As David Comings (1988) and others have pointed out, most patients diagnosed with TS also suffer from ADHD and often also from OCD as well. Often it is symptoms of these other disorders, especially the ADHD, that cause most of the impairment suffered by those with TS.

Thomas Spencer and colleagues (1998) studied children with Tourette's syndrome and found that the vast majority, 81 percent, also fully met diagnostic criteria for ADHD. Spencer concluded: "Little doubt remains that ADHD is highly prevalent in patients with Tourette's syndrome and often represents the main clinical concern and the principal source of dysfunction and disability" (p. 1041). The group also found that OCD was much more prevalent in the children with TS (21 to 28 percent) than in the normal controls (2 percent). These findings suggest that TS may essentially be an especially severe variant of ADHD complicated by tics and often also by OCD and other disorders. For those with these complex impairments, a combination of treatment strategies is likely to be needed.

Similarities among Disorders of Social-Emotional Regulation

Among the various disorders of social-emotional regulation discussed in this section, there are many differences, but also some underlying similarities. Asperger's disorder involves extreme forms of impairment in the ability to recognize and respond to emotion in other persons. In a somewhat different way, ODD and CD involve extreme disruptions in the ability to recognize and respond appropriately to emotions of others; persons with these disorders tend to be strikingly insensitive to the feelings and needs of others and have a lot of trouble holding back verbal or, in some cases, physical expressions of aggression toward others, seeming to lack sensitivity to the others' pain. In TS there is rarely the deliberate verbal aggression of ODD or criminal behavior that may be seen in CD, yet TS too reflects significant impairment in the ability to modulate the expression of emotion by anticipating the emotional reactions of others. Thus all disorders in this group involve problems with using empathy to regulate one's actions.

As indicated, sizable percentages of persons with ADD syndrome tend to meet diagnostic criteria for the disorders of social-emotional regulation, but in each case, the impairments extend well beyond the symptoms of ADD syndrome alone. Persons with ADD syndrome and any of these disorders of social-emotional regulation tend to suffer not only from a chronically impaired conductor of the brain's "orchestra," but also from impairment in additional brain functions—from the inability of a section of players in the orchestra to interpret and follow the conductor's lead.

Why Does ADD Syndrome Often Overlap with Other Disorders?

Having described three clusters of learning and psychiatric disorders that very often overlap with ADD syndrome, we now return to the question I raised earlier in this chapter. Why is it that having ADD substantially increases the likelihood of having another disorder? Why is it that a child with ADHD, if untreated, has twice the risk of developing a substance use disorder at some time in his or her life? Why do children with ADHD have double or triple the risk of having reading disorder, math disorder, or disorder of written expression? Why do adults with ADHD have additional psychiatric disorders at six times the rate reported for the general U.S. population? Many researchers and clinicians point to genetics, as though one afflicted with ADHD is just unfortunate in being much more likely to be burdened with the inheritance of additional disorders of learning, emotions, or behavior. But there is another way to look at the high incidence of overlap between ADD syndrome and other learning and psychiatric disorders. Rather than considering ADD as just one separate disorder among others, this syndrome might be seen as a cluster of impairments that cuts across other diagnostic categories. To return to our oft-used metaphor, we could say that while a very weak brass section might impair the orchestra's playing of scores strongly reliant on brass, this weakness would not affect the orchestra's work as much as would having a conductor who had chronic difficulty in organizing and directing the musicians. A poor conductor can handicap the entire orchestra, especially when sections of the orchestra are required to play together. Many psychiatric disorders involve such high levels of coordination.

Put another way, executive functions are basic and essential to the integrated operation of many diverse activities of the mind; consequently, individuals with weaknesses in the development of their executive functions are likely to be more vulnerable to many other types of psychiatric impairment, just as anyone with weak bones is more vulnerable to fractures and one with a weak immune system is more vulnerable to a wide variety of infections.

Indeed, impairments of the ADD syndrome described in this book are not *specific* to ADHD; they occur in many other disorders as well. In 2002 Joseph Sergeant and colleagues published an article asking "How Specific Is a Deficit of Executive Functioning for Attention Deficit/Hyperactivity Disorder?" They noted that whereas children, adolescents, and adults with ADHD have been shown in many studies to have performance deficiencies on some executive-function tasks and tests, similar impairments had been shown in individuals with other disorders—for example, oppositional defiant disorder, conduct disorder, Tourette's syndrome, learning disorders, and high-functioning autism. The article concluded: "EF specificity for ADHD remains to be established" (p. 24).

I would argue that impairments of executive function are not likely ever to be established as specific to ADHD, because most other psychiatric disorders involve both executive-function impairments and additional dysfunctions of more specific cognitive systems. Thus an individual with reading disorder has impairments of executive functions such as working memory as well as specific problems in aspects of the brain involved in decoding and understanding words. A person with Asperger's disorder not only has impairments of executive functions involved in shifting focus, managing emotions, and monitoring action, but also has more specific disruptions in aspects of the brain that are essential for noticing and monitoring emotional communications of others.

In fact, it does not make much sense to think of such combinations of impairments, some of which involve executive functions, as chance occurrences of separate disorders. The situation is not like having a sprained ankle and influenza at the same time. Rather, impairments of executive function might be compared to disruptions of the operating system of a computer that interferes in various ways with running a wide range of software.

Executive Functions Can Be Impaired in Ways Other Than Just ADHD

Although impairments of executive functions that I call ADD syndrome seem usually to be inherited and to occur relatively early in life, they can also result from traumatic brain injury, the hormonal changes of menopause, and brain changes common in later stages of old age. In these ways, symptoms very similar to ADD syndrome may occur in some persons who have shown no evidence of ADHD earlier in life.

Traumatic Brain Injury

Joan Gerring and colleagues (1998) studied boys and girls aged four to nineteen years diagnosed with severe to moderate closed head injuries (CHI). Most had been injured as pedestrians or as drivers or passengers in a motor vehicle; many had been in a coma for about ten days. Gerring found that 20 percent of the children with CHI had ADHD prior to their head injury. This elevated incidence is consistent with the expectation that children with ADHD are more likely to behave in impulsive or careless ways that put them at risk of such injuries.

During the year following their CHI, an additional 19 percent of children and adolescents in this sample developed sufficient ADHD symptoms to warrant diagnosis. This development suggests that impairments of ADHD may be acquired by certain kinds of physical damage to the brain. Similar results were obtained in studies by Jeffrey Max and others (1998).

Menopausal Cognitive Impairments

Many middle-aged women report that during menopause, whether naturally occurring or surgically induced, they experience for the first time a constellation of persisting symptoms that closely resembles ADD syndrome. They note significant declines in short-term memory, in the ability to screen distractions and to sustain attention, in the organization and prioritizing of tasks, and so on. Some of these women are very competent, well-educated professionals and business executives who until menopause have never experienced significant impairments of ADD syndrome. In addition, women who have been diagnosed before menopause with ADD often report that their ADD symptoms tend to worsen for several days each month at about the time their estrogen level is probably lowest. As they enter menopause, many of these women also report significant exacerbation of their long-standing ADD symptoms.

Basic neuroscience research by Bruce McEwen (1991) suggests that estrogen plays an important role in the release and reloading of dopamine within the brain, particularly in brain areas associated with executive functions. If this is so, significant inconsistency or persisting reduction of estrogen levels in a woman's body may exacerbate ADD symptoms in women who suffer from ADD syndrome. Declines in estrogen related to menopause may also produce symptoms of ADD syndrome in some women who have never had them before.

Barbara Sherwin (1998) has reported that administrating estrogen to postmenopausal women enhances verbal memory and maintains the ability to learn new material. Sally Shaywitz and colleagues (1999) demonstrated in an MRI study that administration of estrogen to postmenopausal women increased activation in specific brain regions during verbal and nonverbal working memory tasks. None of these researchers was looking at the full range of ADD syndrome impairments described in this book. Yet their reports, combined with neuroscientific evidence about the role of estrogen in modulating dopamine release in the brain, suggest that further investigation of menopausal cognitive impairments similar to ADD syndrome is warranted. At present there is no evidence about the role of hormonal changes on the cognitive functioning of males.

Cognitive Impairments of Normal Aging

Many men and women complain of increasing problems with attention, working memory, and other executive functions as they reach late middle age and beyond. Denise Park and Trey Hedden (2001) evaluated men and women aged twenty-nine to ninety to determine how performance on tests of perceptual speed and working memory changes across age groups. They found that the rate of decline on measures of processing speed, working memory, and long-term memory was consistent across the lifespan.

> The loss of processing function that occurs from ages 20–29 is approximately the same as the loss that occurs from 60–69. The only difference is that the proportionate loss for the 69 year old is greater than for the 29 year old, given that a 20 year old has more processing resource than a 60 year old.
>
> As an analogy, if you start a bank account with a thousand dollars that doesn't accrue interest and withdraw $100. each decade beginning at age 20, you would decrease your financial resources by 10 percent on your 20th birthday and have $900. remaining. On your 70th birthday, you would have $500. left and your $100. withdrawal would at that point represent a 20 percent loss of your now meager financial resources, leaving you with only $400.
>
> As this analogy illustrates, the absolute decline in working memory function may be equivalent across decades, but the proportion of processing resources lost is greater as one gets older. (p. 154)

Park and Hedden concluded that this disproportionate loss of cognitive resources, combined with the fact that there is some threshold where declining resources significantly interfere with daily life, explains why older adults tend to complain about a drop in cognitive function as they get older, while younger adults usually do not.

Park and Hedden also showed, consistent with the work of Timothy Salthouse described in Chapter 3, that cognitive processing speed was the primary determinant of how individuals performed on most of the cognitive tasks. The slower cognitive-processing characteristic of older individuals can affect performance in two ways. First, it may leave an individual with insufficient time to complete all aspects of a task. Second, when working slowly there is an increased risk that one will forget earlier aspects of a problem before the problem is solved.

But the process of cognitive decline is not the same for everyone of a particular age. Donald Stuss and Malcolm Binns (2001) reported that whereas frontal or executive functions of the brain tend to deteriorate earlier than many other cognitive functions, they do not all decline at the same rate. Moreover, as Scott Johnson and John Rybash (1993) observed, age differences in information processing depend not only on the quantity of information to be processed, but also on what is required for specific tasks.

Individual differences also play a role in the persistence or decline of executive functions as one ages. The late Fergus Craik (1987) and colleagues compared three groups of elderly persons on performance of cognitive tasks. They found that the healthier, more engaged, higher-income adults performed most like young adults. Their group of lower income but actively engaged adults was intermediate in their cognitive performance, and the group of adults who had both low income and low activity levels tended to show the worst performance of the three groups.

Multiple Routes to Impaired Executive Functions

These studies show that many impairments of executive function seen in ADD syndrome can occur in persons who did not have ADHD in their earlier years. For some, head injuries, the hormonal changes of menopause, or cognitive changes of old age create a cluster of impairments that looks very much like ADD without the lifespan history of symptoms. It seems likely that severe chronic substance abuse and a variety of other psychiatric or medical disorders may have similar damaging effects on executive functions. It also seems likely that external challenges like these would cause some individuals who have a lifelong history of ADD syndrome to experience a worsening of their ADD symptoms.

Moreover, now we know that the brain's circuits responsible for integrating and managing its various components develop very slowly, gradually becoming capable of managing progressively more complex tasks. In some cases these management circuits simply do not develop adequately. In others, they develop well and then subsequently are damaged by trauma or compromised by disease or processes of aging. Given these facts, it is very difficult to continue to think of psychiatric impairments as discrete disorders with clear boundaries and relatively discrete causes.

Much remains to be learned about ADD syndrome and how it changes across the lifespan in different ways for various persons. Likewise, the subtle complexities in overlap of executive functions and other disorders are still barely understood. What does seem clear is that these various disorders are complex, overlapping and often interacting. This overlap of ADD syndrome with other disorders might be seen as an extension of Pennington's (2002) view that what differentiates various psychiatric disorders is not that each has a unique set of causes, but rather that each disrupts, in various levels of severity, different factors common to many disorders. Further, the kind of disorder that evolves depends in part on the variety of environmental challenges and supports encountered at various points of development.

I am suggesting that impairments of executive functions are a larger aspect of many psychiatric and learning disorders than has thus far been recognized. If accurate, this interpretation may have important implications for treatment of persons with other disorders. Perhaps some treatments demonstrated useful for ADHD might also be helpful as adjunctive treatments for some cases of other disorders such as depression or traumatic brain injury. Such treatments may also have some benefit for certain developmental conditions in which ADD syndrome may have a later developmental onset—for example, cognitive impairments that may come with menopause or old age. Research is needed to address these questions.

Questions about treatment also involve questions about the severity of impairment. Just as there are no clear lines between one psychiatric disorder and others, so to there is not a sharp boundary between what is psychopathology and the wide range of what is to be considered normal. As Pennington (2002) suggested, psychological disorders may be simply extreme points on various ranges of normal. This does not mean that such disorders do not require treatment. Hypertension, for example, is defined as the extreme end of the normal distribution of blood pressure, but it is also known that persons with chronic hypertension are at serious risk of stroke and a variety of other damaging or life-threatening problems.

Applying this idea to ADD syndrome means that we can recognize the impairments of those diagnosed with ADD syndrome as relatively extreme manifestations of difficulties experienced by everyone in some degree. This continuity does not mean, however, that the symptoms of ADD syndrome do not warrant treatment. Persons with significant impairment from symptoms of ADD syndrome are likely to suffer sustained and potentially very damaging effects if their symptoms are not recognized and effectively treated. As indicated in this chapter, such impairments of ADD syndrome are often further complicated by one or more additional disorders. Regardless of whether other disorders are present, it is important that appropriate treatment be provided.

Chapter 9 Medications and Other Treatments

MYTH: Medications for ADD are likely to cause longer-term problems with substance abuse or other health concerns, especially when used by children.

FACT: The risks of using appropriate medications to treat ADD are minimal, whereas the risks of not using medication to treat ADD are significant. The medications used for ADD are among the best researched for any disorder.

The most important aspect of treatment for ADD syndrome is education of the patient and family about the nature of the disorder and how it can be treated. Education does not change the chemical problems underlying executive function impairments, but if the patient and the patient's family do not adequately understand the uses and limitations of medications and other treatment options, they may jump into use of interventions that are not safe or helpful. They may develop wildly unrealistic expectations for the benefits to be gained from medications, or they may be too quick to stop treatments that would have been effective if only they had been adequately adjusted to the individual.

Education is also essential for helping each patient and family to recognize problematic feelings and mistaken assumptions they have developed about ADD syndrome and themselves. From their early years, individuals impaired with ADD syndrome tend to develop strong feelings of self-blame and inadequacy based on the "willpower" theory of ADD. Learning some of the science behind ADD syndrome can help individuals and their families to reduce excessive self-blame while avoiding use of the ADD diagnosis as an excuse for all personal shortcomings.

246

Yet although education about ADD syndrome is the foundation for effective treatment, it does not change the core problems in executive functions. Throughout this book ADD syndrome has been described as a cluster of cognitive impairments that, in most cases, results from chemical problems in the brain, specifically malfunctions in the dopaminergic and noradrenergic systems that regulate most executive functions. Because ADD syndrome is essentially a chemical problem in the brain, it makes sense that, in the vast majority of cases, the most effective way to alleviate its impairments is to change relevant aspects of the brain's chemistry. Additional treatments may be quite useful, but the most effective treatment for ADD syndrome is almost always well-managed medication.

Medication Offers Relief, Not a Cure

At present, there is no cure for ADD syndrome, but there are medication treatments that have been demonstrated safe and effective in alleviating symptoms of ADD syndrome in 80 to 90 percent of children, adolescents, and adults who have the disorder. Just as eyeglasses do not repair the patient's eyes and cure impaired vision, so medications that alleviate ADD syndrome do not cure problems of brain chemistry that cause these impairments: the improvements last only as long as the medication is active in the body. Yet, when carefully and appropriately utilized, these medications can facilitate substantial improvement in the daily functioning of most persons impaired by ADD syndrome, although not with equal effectiveness for all. For some patients, medication for ADD brings improvements that are dramatic and pervasive; for others, effects are significant, but not huge; for others, results are more modest; and for 10 to 20 percent of those affected with ADD syndrome, current medication treatments are not effective at all.

For the most fortunate of those who suffer from ADD syndrome, well-managed medication alleviates their impairments to the extent that not much further treatment is needed. These individuals have a good understanding of what they ought to do in most situations; they are just unable consistently to do it unless adequately treated. Unmedicated, they are too often unable to activate themselves at the right times, or to sustain the necessary focus and effort, or to engage their working memory and monitor their actions enough to do what they know they need to do. But when appropriate medication is in place to correct the chronic chemical problems that have impaired their executive functions, they generally function well.

Medication Alone May Not Be Enough

For others with ADD syndrome, medication helps, but does not sufficiently improve their functioning in school, employment, social relationships, and/or family relationships. Pills do not teach skills that some with ADD syndrome need and have not acquired. For these individuals, an important effect of the medication is to make them more ready to learn. Previously teachers, parents, supervisors, and friends may have struggled to coach them to develop important understandings and skills, only to find that, despite good intentions on both sides, the learning simply did not "stick," or carry over from one situation to another. With the help of adequately managed medications to alleviate their ADD symptoms, these individuals may become better able to remember and use their learning in ways that were never possible for them while their ADD symptoms were untreated.

For those whose ADD impairments are complicated by symptoms of depression, anxiety, dyslexia, substance abuse, or other disorders, treatment with medications effective for ADD symptoms may be helpful, but not helpful enough. Treatment in these situations often requires very skilled diagnosis and multiple treatment interventions, possibly including careful trials of two or more different medications used in combination. Psychosocial or educational interventions may also play a crucially important role.

For reasons that often are complicated (some of these are discussed in Chapter 10), many individuals think of medication as a treatment of last resort for impairments of ADD syndrome. They argue that psychosocial, behavioral treatments are preferable to medication and should always be tried first. This approach might have made sense long ago when ADD was seen as essentially a behavioral problem of young children; in fact, there is research evidence supporting the idea that a structured program of consistent behavior modification can be effective in getting most young children, including many with ADHD, to refrain from being disruptive in classrooms and at home. But it is difficult to see how even the best behavioral treatment program can modify an individual's impairments of ADD syndrome as they affect working memory or hamper one's ability to sustain attention enough to understand what one is reading, to write an essay, or to drive a car. And it is very difficult to imagine how such approaches could be used effectively for adolescents or adults with ADD syndrome who struggle to function as students in high school or university, or as working adults, or parents—situations where no one is available to monitor their complex behaviors or manage their reinforcements.

How Can Medications Help?

In assessing effectiveness of treatments for ADD syndrome, it is important to ask: What is the desired outcome? Some studies answer this question by analyzing how stimulant medications affect a patient's performance not on combined *DSM-IV* symptoms of ADHD, but on specific tasks orchestrated by executive functions. Seven of these studies are briefly described here.

Often persons with ADD work too quickly and don't recognize when they need to slow down to do a good job. Deborah Krusch and others (1996) studied the accuracy and processing speed of children with ADD. On the medication the children showed improvement on several executive functions: focus, self-monitoring of action, and processing speed.

Virginia Douglas (1999) demonstrated an even broader effect of methylphenidate (MPH) on self-regulation in children with ADHD. When provided MPH, boys with ADHD appropriately speeded up for more automatic, faster-paced tasks and slowed down as needed for complicated tasks that required more concentration and effort.

Persons with ADHD often complain of being too easily distracted. Caryn Carlson and colleagues (1991) found that while on medication boys with ADHD were better able to ignore distractions and to sustain focus and maintain speed and accuracy on their primary task.

Some parents and teachers believe that tangible rewards will motivate children with ADHD to work better on tasks that do not interest them.

Mary Solanto and others (1997) studied whether medicine or rewards would work better to get children with ADHD to keep working on a long, boring computer task. Their results showed that both the money-earning and the medication improved accuracy overall, but the MPH was significantly more potent; MPH also improved the ability of the children to sustain their attention and effort on the task, while the monetary rewards did not.

John Chelonis (2002) tested whether MPH significantly improves working memory in children with ADHD. In a series of trials, children with ADHD were significantly more accurate and efficient in remembering shapes correctly when on the MPH than when off it; on medication, their performance became as efficient as that of normal children of the same age range. The medication normalized their impaired working memory.

Individuals with ADHD are often too quick to give up when frustrated. Richard Milich and colleagues (1991) asked boys with ADHD to solve a series of puzzles, some of which were unsolvable. They tested whether while taking MPH these boys, after experiencing frustration from failing to solve some unsolvable puzzles, would keep trying to solve other puzzles longer than they did when taking a placebo. They found that

> the boys did significantly better on medication than on placebo
> following exposure to unsolvable puzzles . . . in fact, the boys'
> best performance occurred in the medication/insolvable condi-
> tion. . . . ADHD boys on placebo tend to get discouraged and
> exert less effort after failure experiences. . . . In contrast, on
> medication they adopt a more adaptive strategy of trying even
> harder after experiencing problems they could not solve. (p. 530)

Often children and adults with ADD syndrome are too impulsive; that is, not able to hesitate long enough to make a sensible response. Anne-Claude Bedard and others (2003) used a computer task to test children with ADHD on their ability to hold back a response until a signal was given. On medication, the children stopped themselves more quickly from making incorrect responses and were quicker and more consistent in making accurate responses. The researchers suggested that

> MPH may influence global cognitive processes, such as atten-
> tional capacity or working memory, that are deficient in children
> with ADHD and result in improvements in aspects of response
> inhibition, as well as response execution. (p. 325)

Taken together, these various studies demonstrate that stimulant medications improve a variety of functions impaired in ADD syndrome. These
include sustaining alertness, focus, motivation, and effort for tasks that
are not intrinsically interesting; shifting attention as needed; utilizing
working memory; adjusting processing speed to the demands of the task;
sustaining processing speed for efficient performance; managing emotions to persist despite frustration and failure; and monitoring and self-
regulating actions. These laboratory measures stand with a large body of
research over the past half-century that powerfully demonstrates the effectiveness of stimulant medications for alleviating a wide variety of impairments associated with ADD syndrome.

Thousands of Medication Studies

In the decades since stimulant medications were first introduced, several
thousand scientific studies have assessed the effectiveness of these medications for alleviating ADHD symptoms. C. Keith Conners (2002) published a comprehensive review of research that covered hundreds of studies involving over ten thousand individuals. He reported that evidence
from many hundreds of researchers, who assessed many thousands of
children with ADHD in a wide range of diverse settings, powerfully demonstrates that stimulant medications significantly improve symptoms of
ADHD for most of those who are treated.

Stimulant Medications for Adults with ADHD

For many decades, most of the studies of stimulant medications for ADHD
assessed only children. More recently, studies have also tested the effectiveness of medications for treating ADHD in adults. Stephen Faraone
and colleagues (2004) published a meta-analysis of the efficacy of MPH
for treatment of ADHD in adults. Across studies he found strong evidence

that this medication is as effective in alleviating ADHD in adults as it is in helping children and adolescents with the disorder.

Brain Imaging Studies Show Stimulants in Action

Although the positive results of medication treatment for ADHD symptoms have been widely recognized for many years, it is only in the past four or five years that newly developed imaging techniques have made it possible for researchers to begin to understand the mechanisms by which these medications benefit patients. Nora Volkow and colleagues (2002) developed a technology for using positron emission tomography (PET) to observe directly the effects of stimulant medications in the brain.

Volkow has shown that MPH reaches peak concentration in the brain about sixty to ninety minutes after ingestion and that therapeutic doses of oral MPH block more than 50 percent of the dopamine transporters in the brain. This blocking slows the normal reuptake process so that a larger amount of the dopamine is held a bit longer at countless synaptic junctions, thereby improving communication in those neural networks operating on dopamine. Her explanation is that this process enhances neuronal signaling for specific tasks and decreases "noise," or competing signals that might divert or disrupt the network.

Volkow also argued that dopamine modulates motivation. In 2004 she and others illustrated this with brain-imaging studies of healthy adults whose motivation for doing math problems increased significantly while given MPH. When on the medication, they were more "turned on" to the task. This was shown not only in their self-reports, but also in a visible increase of metabolic activity in brain scans of specific sectors of their brains.

In other words, increased dopamine in the synapse can act almost as a kind of "Viagra" to encourage the brain's response to the task. Thus MPH may counter the chronic problem with motivating oneself to do necessary, but not intrinsically interesting, tasks. In this way stimulant medication may help to alleviate the problems described in Chapter 1 as "impotence of the mind."

Volkow found, however, that MPH does not completely control the amount of dopamine in the synapses. Individuals vary in the rate and amount of dopamine released in various networks of their brain, so there is only so much dopamine that can be sustained by blocking the dopamine transporters at the synapse. If the quantity released is insufficient, slowing down its reuptake is not likely adequately to alleviate the problem. She notes that in persons who suffer chronically from insufficient release of dopamine, amphetamine (AMP) might be more helpful than MPH because amphetamine is not so dependent on cell firing to release dopamine into the synapse. Amphetamine not only slows reuptake; it also facilitates an increased release of dopamine from within the cells where it is stored.

Sometimes One Stimulant Works Better Than Another

This difference between the two primary stimulant medications may explain why some individuals with ADHD respond to one medication better than another. Eugene Arnold (2000) reviewed studies that compared patients with ADHD on consecutive trials of both MPH and AMP. Of these patients, more than 66 percent responded well to AMP and over 56 percent responded well to MPH; most responded equally well to both. The overall response rate to one or another of these stimulants was 85 percent.

There are biological reasons to expect that subtle differences will cause some persons with ADD syndrome to respond better to one stimulant medication than to another, but there is no way to tell at the outset which medicine will work best for which patient. As Arnold summarized:

> Although very similar in many ways, the two stimulants are in some ways complementary in patient responsiveness. The clearest lesson gained from the controlled studies is that . . . nonresponse or intolerable side effects with one stimulant do not preclude a good response to the other . . . "symptomatic improvement is unpredictable and can only be determined by an empirical trial on an individual basis." Each should be tried before stimulant treatment is abandoned. (p. 135)

Sometimes the first stimulant tried with a particular patient will work well with only minor adjustments. Yet often multiple adjustments in dosage are needed to elicit the optimal response. Further, sometimes the initial stimulant tried does not work at any dose or produces adverse effects that make it necessary to try an alternative. For some patients, too, none of the stimulants works well and other, nonstimulant medications are clearly preferable. Overall, a given individual with ADD syndrome is 80 percent likely to respond positively to treatment with one or another of the stimulant medications. But a careful "fine-tuning" of the dose and timing is essential to establish the optimal regimen.

Finding the Most Effective Dose

Some medications are prescribed best according to the patient's age, weight, or severity of symptoms. But stimulant medications do not reliably follow such guidelines. Nora Volkow and James Swanson (2003) described individual differences that affect one's response to stimulant medications. Mark Rapport and Colin Denney (2000) demonstrated that body mass fails to predict optimal dose for ADHD patients. Some very young and small children need quite large and frequent doses of stimulant to get a positive effect; whereas other children, adolescents, and adults may benefit from very small doses of stimulant and may have adverse effects to larger doses. In short, more medication is not always better. And since it is not possible to predict the optimal dose from age, weight, or symptom severity, the usual approach is to begin with a very small dose of one or another of the stimulant medications and then increase the dose gradually, allowing about three to seven days on a dose before trying a larger one.

For decades, stimulant medications were available only in preparations effective for just four to five hours; for some whose bodies metabolized these agents more quickly, the effectiveness was much shorter, sometimes just two to two-and-a-half hours. This meant that schoolchildren were required to go to their teacher or a school nurse once or twice during the day to receive additional doses, and that adults on this medication had to remember to take three to four doses each day during their employment and daily routines. Given that persons with ADD syndrome are often chronically forgetful—and that classmates, teachers, or coworkers who did not understand or respect the reasons for such medications often had negative reactions to those who took them—many with ADD used these shorter-acting stimulants inconsistently, if at all.

Many improved, longer-acting formulations of stimulant medications are now produced. In countries where they are available, these extended-release preparations have revolutionized stimulant medication treatments for ADHD. They make it possible for children to avoid taking medication at school, and they reduce the number of times each day that adults must remember to take their tablets.

The American Academy of Child and Adolescent Psychiatry (AACAP) has published approved guidelines for use of stimulant medications in the treatment of children, adolescents, and adults (2002). For immediate release (short-acting) methylphenidate (MPH; sold as brands Ritalin or Methylin, or as generic methylphenidate), its recommended starting dose is 5 mg administered twice daily, increasing as needed by 5 mg weekly up to a usual maximum of 20 mg per dose; a third daily dose may eventually be added at the clinician's discretion. For preschoolers the starting dose is usually lower. Laurence Greenhill and colleagues (2004) reported that initial doses of 1.25 mg of MPH with gradual increments of 1.25 mg as needed, up to 7.5 mg three times daily, worked well for 85 percent of three- to five-year-olds in a multisite study sponsored by the National Institute of Mental Health.

For all ages, each weekly increase is to be made only after monitoring the effectiveness of the drug, the patient's weight and vital signs, and any side effects. Increases are made only when the current dose is not producing an adequate response and is not causing significant adverse effects. If a given dose continues to produce significant side effects, the dose is to be reduced or the medication stopped with the option of trying another compound. Standard dosing of short-acting MPH is three times daily, given at times adjusted to fit the individual's schedule and activities. Some individuals may require more frequent dosing, whereas others may respond better to taking the medicine only twice each day.

An alternative form of short-acting methylphenidate is Focalin. This formulation is produced by removing from methylphenidate one of its two components that reportedly is more likely to cause adverse effects.

The resulting dexmethylphenidate is a more potent compound available in 2.5, 5, and 10 mg doses usually started at about half of the usually administered dose of conventional methylphenidate; increases are also made at half of the usual increments for regular MPH. The medication is effective for about five to six hours. Some patients find it easier to tolerate this formulation than conventional MPH.

For short-acting dextroamphetamine (DEX; sold as Dexedrine or Dextrostat) or mixed amphetamine salts (AMP; available as Adderall or generic mixed amphetamine salts), AACAP-recommended doses are smaller than those for MPH. This is because DEX and AMP compounds tend to pack a bit more "punch" per milligram. The recommended starting dose of these agents is 2.5 mg for children and 5 mg for older adolescents or adults given once or twice daily, with increases of 2.5 mg every week until a good response is obtained. Once an effective dose has been identified, it is usually administered two to three times daily, depending on the patient's individual needs.

Although a single dose of fast-acting MPH, DEX, or AMP is effective for about four hours, some individuals get a much longer or much shorter response. This is one reason that it is so important for stimulant medication to be carefully monitored and adjusted to each individual's needs.

Medication for More Than Just School or Work

For many years, physicians prescribed stimulant medications to children only for school days or for weekend days when homework needed to be done. In recent years, however, clinicians have come to recognize that non-academic tasks are also impaired with ADD syndrome. A child who has great difficulty in maintaining focus, sustaining effort, utilizing working memory, managing frustration, monitoring action, and so on in school is likely also to have similar difficulties when playing Little League baseball, attending religious services, or interacting with friends and family. Most adults with ADD syndrome who are excessively distracted and forgetful at work are likely to have similar difficulties while shopping, driving their car, managing their children, or interacting with colleagues and family.

Recognition of the pervasiveness of impairments from ADD syndrome has led many clinicians to prescribe stimulant medications to cover not only school or workdays, but every day of the week. In practice, the use of stimulant medications by persons with ADHD varies as does the use of eyeglasses. Just as some individuals wear their eyeglasses all day, every day, because the help they provide is needed for virtually everything they do, so do many with ADD syndrome maintain their stimulant medication coverage throughout virtually every day. Others, like those who need their eyeglasses only for reading or for watching TV, will plan with their physician to use their medication only when they need it for specific types of activities like schoolwork or employment.

AACAP has advised that the usual maximum daily dose of short-acting MPH be 60 mg while the maximum daily total dose for DEX and AMP is usually 40 mg, but their report noted that some patients may need larger doses to provide full relief or to accommodate a longer day of activities. In such situations the clinician is advised to document that the symptoms cannot be controlled at lower doses and that the higher doses are not producing adverse effects such as significant weight loss, an increase in blood pressure, or agitation.

Longer-Lasting Medicines

Currently there are several longer-acting stimulant preparations, some deliver methylphenidate in two or three doses within one capsule (Concerta, Metadate-CD [Equasym-XL in the UK] and Ritalin-LA). Focalin-XR delivers two doses of dexmethylphenidate in a single capsule, while others provide extended release versions of dextroamphetamine (Dexedrine Spansules) or mixed amphetamine salts (Adderall-XR). These preparations come in various sizes and differ considerably in their speed and intensity of onset, as well as in their duration. Just as for shorter-acting stimulant medications, careful tailoring of dose and timing is needed to provide optimal coverage for any given patient. One size or formulation does not fit all.

Methylphenidate is available in two formulations that provide a medium duration of coverage. Ritalin-LA, currently available in 10, 20, 30, or

40 mg sizes, releases about 50 percent of its dose within an hour of ingestion and the other 50 percent about three to four hours later. Metadate-CD (Equasym-XL) currently available in 10, 20, and 30 mg sizes, releases about 30 percent of its full dose within the first hour after ingestion and the remaining 70 percent in another pulse about three hours later. For most individuals these two medium-duration preparations provide about six to eight hours of coverage. Both Ritalin-LA and Metadate-CD are capsules containing tiny beads, some of which are designed to release their contents quickly, while others provide delayed release to extend the duration of coverage; for both of these formulations the capsules can be opened and sprinkled on a tablespoon of applesauce, pudding, or ice cream for a young child who is unable to swallow a pill.

A longer-acting preparation of methylphenidate is provided in Concerta, currently available in 18, 27, 36, and 54 mg sizes. Concerta releases about 30 percent of its dose via absorption of its coating, which activates within about an hour. The rest of the dose is released in two subsequent pulses over the ensuing six hours. For most individuals this provides a fairly smooth distribution of coverage over a total of about ten to twelve hours. Concerta capsules should be swallowed whole because cutting or breaking them destroys the time-release system.

Focalin-XR is available in 5, 10, and 20 mg capsules that release about 50 percent of the medication within about an hour after ingestion, and the remainder about 3 to 4 hours later. Focalin-XR capsules can be opened and sprinkled on food as described above. Dextroamphetamine is available in longer-acting spansules containing 5, 10, and 15 mg of medication. These release about one-third of the dose within about one hour after ingestion and the remaining two-thirds about three hours later. Dexedrine spansules usually are effective for about six to eight hours. Opening of Dexedrine capsules is not recommended. Mixed salts of amphetamine are available in Adderall-XR, a preparation currently available in 5, 10, 15, 20, 25, and 30 mg sizes. A two-phase release is provided by the mix of tiny beads inside this capsule, which can be opened and sprinkled on foods for children who cannot swallow the capsule itself. Adderall-XR provides about ten to twelve hours of coverage.

Startup Dosing for Longer-Acting Stimulants

The AACAP guidelines recommend that all patients prescribed stimulants be started on twice-daily dosing with a shorter-acting formulation and then switched to a longer-acting version once it is clear that they can tolerate the medication in its immediate-release form. This approach may be problematic for schoolchildren, however, who do not want to have to go to the teacher or nurse during the school day to receive a second dose. An alternative approach is to start with a very low dose of longer-acting stimulant and then gradually increase the dose at intervals of at least four to seven days until an adequate response is obtained. As with shorter-acting preparations, the dose should not be increased if the patient is experiencing significant adverse effects.

The maximum recommended dose of Ritalin-LA and Metadate-CD is 60 mg for the day. But research with Concerta has shown that for 37 percent of a sample of adolescents, the optimal effect was not obtained until the dose was increased to 72 mg administered at one time (Spencer and Greenhill 2003); in 2004 the FDA approved 72 mg as a maximum dose of Concerta for adolescents. The maximum recommended daily dose is 40 mg for Dexedrine Spansules, 30 mg for Adderall-XR, and 20 mg for Focalin-XR; many patients respond well to lower doses.

Published maximum dosage guidelines do not take into account that for many adolescents and adults, and for some children, once-daily administration of the longer-acting formulations is not sufficient; for many, these need to be supplemented by administration of shorter-acting stimulants to provide more adequate coverage of their full day of activities. Some experts have advised that the usual maximum recommended doses may not be sufficiently robust to meet the needs of some patients.

Virtually no studies have been done to test the combined use of longer-acting and shorter-acting stimulant formulations, or twice-daily dosing of longer acting stimulants, but many clinicians report that such combinations provide more adequate coverage for patients. Many older children and adolescents who take longer-acting stimulants just before leaving for school at 6:30 to 8:00 a.m. find that the medicine wears off long before they have completed their homework—particularly if they participate in sports or other activities that prevent them from starting their homework until after dinner. Many adolescents with ADHD also want coverage in late afternoon and into the evening to help them sustain attention when they are working a part-time job or driving a car. Adults, too, also often require longer coverage in order to alleviate their ADHD symptoms not only during their work day, but also in the evening when they interact with family, attend evening meetings, or do reading or paper-work at home.

To address such problems, some clinicians prescribe a "booster," a dose of shorter-acting stimulant to be taken in mid to late afternoon to ex-tend coverage into the early evening. For some patients who must take their morning dose of stimulant very early, or who metabolize stimulants very quickly and have shorter than usual duration of action, twice-daily dosing of the longer-acting stimulants might be prescribed. Careful mon-itoring is important: This extended coverage may cause the patient to have excessive difficulty in getting to sleep at night or may suppress appetite so much that the person loses too much weight or does not eat nutritiously enough. Such difficulties can usually be alleviated, but careful planning and further monitoring may be needed.

Alleviating Any Adverse Effects

Adverse effects of stimulants include some responses that are common and transient or easily adjusted for, such as slight stomachache, headache, and (especially for the first few days on longer-acting agents) extended delay in getting to sleep. Many patients taking stimulants also find that their appetite is diminished while the medication is most active; they may not feel very hungry until the medication has worn off, which is some-times not until almost bedtime.

Stomachaches and headaches, if experienced, are usually not severe and often go away within a few days, after the person's body has become more accustomed to the medication. Stomachache is less likely if the pa-tient can eat some food, even just a piece of toast or a glass of milk, before taking the medication. And diminished appetite is often simply delayed appetite. Many patients taking stimulants eat very little during the day

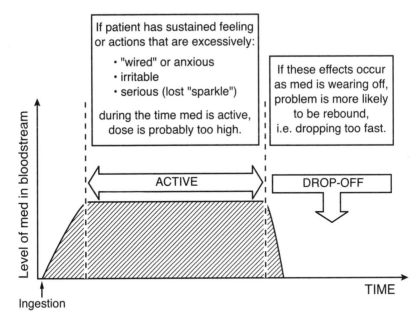

Figure 8 Stimulant time frames and "rebound." Unpleasant reactions may occur while the stimulant medication is at full strength or as it wears off. If the reaction is limited primarily to when the medication is active, the dose may be too high, whereas if the reaction occurs only later, as the medication is wearing off, the problem is more likely one of "rebound," an excessively quick drop-off of medication effect. Each of these problems requires a different intervention.

while the medication is most active, feel slightly hungry for dinner in early evening, and then become quite hungry later in the evening. If they are encouraged to eat when they feel hungry, possibly having a second dinner shortly before bedtime, appetite difficulties usually become less problematic. In fact, many patients report that their appetite returns to a more normal schedule after they have been on stimulant medications for at least a couple of months.

Recognizing Excessively High Doses and "Rebound"

If an individual is receiving a dose of stimulant that is too high for him or her, that person is likely to experience one or more of the following symptoms while the medication is active:

feeling excessively "edgy" or "wired" (as after drinking too much coffee),

feeling excessively irritable, or

feeling very tired, sad, or "blunted" emotionally, with loss of usual "sparkle"

When such uncomfortable, atypical emotions begin shortly after the stimulant medication kicks in and continue for hours, remitting only at about the time the medication is expected to wear off, the most likely explanation is that the dose of medication is too high for this person. An individual should be able to be their "regular self" when taking stimulant medications. If they become steadily tense, irritable, or "zombie like" while on a stimulant, the dose should be reduced. And if this does not alleviate the problem, a different medication should be tried instead.

If, however, these unpleasant emotional reactions arise in late afternoon or early evening when the medication would normally be expected to wear off, they are more likely part of a "rebound." Such reactions are not usually the result of an excessively high dose. If that were the problem, it would have become apparent while the medication was active and at peak levels. Usually rebound reactions result from the medication level dropping too fast as it wears off. Often such difficulties can easily be alleviated by administering a small dose of immediate-release stimulant shortly before the rebound usually begins. Hence, if a patient complains of feeling excessively wired, irritable, or serious while taking a stimulant, the physician will need to determine whether this reaction occurs when the medication is most active, or as it wears off, in order to find the appropriate remedy. Figure 8 illustrates the different time frames for each of these two problems.

Determining Effectiveness

Patients and families often wonder how they will be able to determine whether a given dose of medication for ADD is effective. If an individual is suffering from significant hyperactive or impulsive symptoms of ADD, an improvement due to medication may be noticed by others who observe the patient's shift to more calm, appropriate, and better-controlled behavior. Improvement of inattention symptoms of ADD may not be so obvious to others; however, it should be noticeable to the patient as soon as an effective dose is obtained. Changes noted might include reduced distractibility, improved attention to task, better short-term memory, more effective completion of work, and so on.

Sometimes an individual does not notice a difference in how he feels during the day but does notice an improvement in how he functions. For example, a college student said he felt nothing from the medication. Yet he said he could tell it was helping him because he noticed that he had been taking much more detailed and comprehensive notes during class and had been getting much more of his assigned reading done than prior to starting medication. The cause of this improvement was confirmed one day when he forgot to take his medication and found that he was feeling very sleepy and not taking many notes in class.

In assessing effectiveness it is very important to remember that improvements produced by these medications last only as long as the dose of medication is actively working. Once it wears off, symptoms are likely to return to their baseline levels.

Tic Problems

If an individual has a tendency toward tics (repetitive involuntary movements or noises), taking stimulant medication might make those tics worse (though sometimes medication helps alleviate tics). Even if tics occur, however, they may cause less difficulty than the ADD symptoms that the stimulant medications are helping, so the administration of medication may still be a good choice.

Growth Rate

In the past, some doctors felt that taking stimulants regularly might slow the growth of a child or teenager. This concern was based on findings that groups of children treated with stimulant medications tended to be, on average, about 1 centimeter shorter than children without ADHD. Longer-term studies showed that this average difference in height disappeared when the groups were compared later in adolescence. It was assumed that the delay in reaching full height was caused by the stimulant medication.

Thomas Spencer and colleagues (1996a) studied groups of children with ADHD treated with stimulants and compared them with groups of children diagnosed with ADHD who had not been treated with stimulants. Both groups showed the same delay in reaching their full height. This led him to conclude that most or all of the difference in height between the two groups was due not to the medication, but to having ADHD. Children with ADHD, with or without medication treatment, tend as a group to take a little longer into adolescence to reach their full height. The problem appears to be not the treatment, but the disorder itself.

It should be noted, however, that these are group data. Not all individuals with ADHD are smaller than most of their peers during childhood and early adolescence. Some are smaller and others are on the taller end of the range. The point here is simply that stimulant medication does not seem to have a very significant effect on growth rate for most who take it. If parents have specific concerns about the growth of their son or daughter, they should consult their pediatrician.

Nonstimulant Medications for ADHD

Although stimulant medications are effective in alleviating ADHD symptoms in most children, adolescents, and adults who suffer from the disorder, about 20 to 30 percent do not respond well to stimulants. For these individuals, nonstimulant medications may be effective. Even among those who do experience significant relief from their symptoms when taking stimulants, there are many who experience significant difficulties with mood, anxiety, tics, or other problems that may be exacerbated, or at least not helped much, by stimulants. For these individuals, too, treatment with nonstimulant medications may be preferable. This chapter does not provide an exhaustive review of all nonstimulant medications used for treatments of ADHD; only those prescribed most often are listed here.

Atomoxetine

At present only one nonstimulant medication, Atomoxetine (ATX), has been approved by the FDA specifically for treatment of ADHD. (Nonstimulant medications approved for other uses are often used for ADHD treatment; they are discussed later.) Approved in November 2003, ATX has already been subjected to extensive testing. In controlled scientific studies including over 1,600 individuals, ATX has been demonstrated to be safe and effective as a treatment for ADHD in children, adolescents, and adults.

Marketed under the brand name Strattera, ATX is not a stimulant. Unlike stimulants it is not classified as a "Schedule II" medication; that is, it has very low potential for abuse and is not subject to the strict rules enforced for stimulants, pain medications, and other compounds that, if misused, could cause addiction. This means that ATX can be obtained more conveniently by patients. Physicians can provide samples, can phone prescriptions to the pharmacy, and can provide refills without having to write a new prescription each time.

ATX takes a different approach than stimulants to alleviating the impairments of ADHD. While stimulants target primarily the dopamine system in the brain, ATX targets primarily the noradrenergic neurotransmitter system. ATX helpfully slows the reuptake of norepinephrine at noradrenergic synapses in the brain in much the same way that stimulants helpfully slow transmitter reuptake in synapses of the dopamine system. As described in Chapter 3 of this book, the noradrenergic and dopaminergic systems are the two neurotransmitter systems most involved in management of executive functions impaired in ADD syndrome. The relative influence of each of these two systems on specific aspects of ADHD impairments has not yet been determined.

Adequate "head-to-head" research has not yet tested whether ATX provides the same degree of improvement for inattention symptoms of ADHD as the stimulants usually do. But clinical trials have clearly shown in sizable groups of children, adolescents, and adults that, for many, this medication can significantly alleviate both inattention and hyperactive or impulsive symptoms of ADHD. In addition, ATX has the advantage of lasting longer than stimulants. Some parents report that while on ATX their ADHD children are easier to get along with throughout the day and evening, are able to fall asleep with less difficulty at bedtime, and are able to awaken the next morning with less irritability and oppositional behavior. There is also some evidence that ATX may help to alleviate the anxiety and depressive symptoms that often appear with ADHD and are less likely to be alleviated by stimulants.

One disadvantage of ATX is that it does not provide noticeable benefits until the patient has been taking it daily for three to five weeks. By comparison, stimulants are usually noticeably effective within an hour after the patient has ingested a dose that is of optimal strength for them. Common side effects of ATX may include stomachache (especially if taken on an empty stomach) and drowsiness; usually these gradually diminish after a few days or weeks on the regimen. Another disadvantage is that the capsules should be swallowed whole; but this is usually a problem only for very young children who are unable or unwilling to swallow a pill.

The dopaminergic and noradrenergic systems both contribute to the biological elements underlying ADD syndrome. And individuals with ADD syndrome vary considerably in which aspects of the ADD syndrome are most problematic for them. Given these factors, it is likely that some patients with ADD syndrome will respond better to ATX than to stimulants while others will respond better to treatment with a stimulant. Unfortunately, there is not yet a sufficient base of research and clinical experience for clinicians reliably to predict which of these medications will be most helpful to any particular patient. Clinical experience and research should eventually yield useful guidelines for such decisions.

While it is usually preferable to treat ADD syndrome with just one medication, there may be some circumstances where neither stimulants nor ATX alone provide adequate alleviation of an individual's impairment from ADD syndrome. In such cases, carefully combined use of these two medications might be considered. In 2004, I presented case reports on the successful use of ATX and stimulants in combination for some patients who did not respond adequately to either agent alone. Yet I cautioned that there is not yet research to guide such combined use, so very careful clinical monitoring is essential.

While ATX is the only nonstimulant medication thus far approved by the FDA specifically for treatment of ADHD, a number of other nonstimulant medications have been demonstrated helpful for treatment of the disorder. Guidelines from the American Academy of Pediatrics (2001) identified tricyclic antidepressants and buproprion as "second-line agents" for treatment of ADHD. Clinicians are advised to utilize second-line agents for ADHD only if an individual fails to respond adequately to adequate trials of at least two stimulants and ATX.

Tricyclic Antidepressants

Tricyclic antidepressants (TCAs) were introduced in the late 1950s as an effective treatment for major depression. Medications in this class include imipramine, desipramine, nortriptyline, and others; all act primarily on the noradrenergic system. TCAs remained the primary agents for treatment of depression until the advent of selective serotonin reuptake inhibitors in 1987. Most of the research on use of TCAs for treatment of ADHD has focused on desipramine and nortriptyline.

These medications have the advantage of lasting relatively long, so they do not require multiple daily doses and do not produce the "hills and valleys" or "rebound" effects sometimes found in treatment with stimulants. They tend to be quite effective in alleviating hyperactive and impulsive symptoms of ADHD, though they have not generally been found to improve the inattention symptoms of ADHD as much as do the stimulants. TCAs tend to be especially helpful for ADHD patients who suffer from comorbid depression, anxiety, oppositionality, or tics.

Timothy Wilens and colleagues (2002) recommended that dosing with TCAs should start with 25 mg daily with a gradual increase to a maximum of 5 mg per kg of patient weight per day, except for nortriptyline, whose dosing should be limited to a maximum of 2 mg per kg per day. Often responses to TCA treatment are not very noticeable until the regimen has been continued for three to five weeks. Adverse effects with TCAs may include sedation, weight gain, dry mouth, constipation, and sexual dysfunction. Usually nortriptyline produces fewer adverse effects than do the other TCAs.

The primary disadvantage of TCAs is their relatively narrow margin of safety. If these medications are taken in a significant overdose, accidental or deliberate, they can cause severe, even fatal, cardiovascular problems. This is an important risk factor, especially in households with young children or for individuals with depressive problems. Despite a substantial body of research showing the effectiveness of desipramine for treatment of ADHD, many physicians stopped prescribing it, at least for prepubescent children, after sudden deaths were reported in four children who had been taking appropriate, not excessive, doses of desipramine for ADHD. Joseph Biederman and others (1995a) have reported that the risk of sudden death when taking appropriate doses of desipramine is elevated only slightly above the normal risk for sudden, unexplained death in children. Nevertheless, caution is advised when considering this specific medication for prepubescent children. For ADHD most clinicians feel more comfortable prescribing nortriptyline because it tends to have fewer adverse effects than most other TCAs.

Nontricyclic Antidepressants

The other nonstimulant medication recommended by the American Academy of Pediatrics (2001) as a second-line treatment for ADHD is buproprion (BUP). Marketed under the brand names Wellbutrin and Zyban, buproprion is classified as an antidepressant, but its chemical structure is quite different from that of most other medications in this class. BUP acts on the noradrenergic system and indirectly on the dopaminergic system. Controlled studies have found BUP to be effective for treating ADHD in children (two trials) and adults (two trials). One open-label study found BUP useful for treating patients with ADHD and comorbid bipolar disorder. Wilens and colleagues (2002) suggested that treatment with BUP for ADHD patients should be initiated at 37.5 mg and increased every three or four days up to a maximum of 300 mg daily in younger children and 450 mg daily in older children or adults. Adverse effects may include excessive activation, irritability, insomnia, and (rarely) seizures.

Antihypertensives

Clonidine and guanfacine, marketed as Catapres and Tenex, respectively, were originally developed as medications to reduce high blood pressure. They have been found helpful for reducing excessive hyperactivity and impulsivity in children with ADHD, but there is currently no evidence that these agents improve the cognitive impairments of ADHD. The effects for clonidine usually persist for about six hours, while guanfacine usually lasts a bit longer. Usual daily doses reported by the group led by Wilens (2002) are 0.05 to 0.4 mg for clonidine and 0.5 mg to 3 mg for guanfacine. Many physicians using these medications do a baseline ECG and monitor the patient's vital signs during treatment. The most common side effect of these antihypertensives is drowsiness, although they can also cause depression or rebound hypertension as they wear off.

The sedating properties of clonidine have been exploited to help alleviate the chronic difficulties in falling asleep that are common in many children with ADHD. Jefferson Prince and colleagues (1996) reported that of sixty-two children and adolescents treated with clonidine about an hour before bedtime, 85 percent had significantly less difficulty falling asleep. Many of these children (68 percent) were being treated successfully with stimulant medications during the day and were given small doses of clonidine, typically either a half or full 0.1 mg tablet, about an hour before bedtime.

Combined Medications

Because many patients with ADHD suffer from one or more comorbid psychiatric disorders, one medication is often not sufficient to control their symptoms. For example, as described above, many patients whose ADHD symptoms respond well to treatment with stimulants throughout the day continue to have great difficulty falling asleep at night. A significant percentage of these patients experience much less insomnia when taking a small dose of clonidine about an hour before bedtime. Yet for most of these patients, clonidine is of little or no help in alleviating the cognitive impairments of ADD syndrome and also tends to be too sedating to take during the day. For such patients the combination of stimulant medication during the day and atomoxetine or clonidine at bedtime may provide much better alleviation of ADHD symptoms without significant adverse effects.

Similarly, as discussed in Chapter 8, many individuals suffer from severe episodes of depression, crippling anxiety, or very burdensome obsessive compulsive disorder in addition to persistent ADHD. For these patients, concurrent treatment with a stimulant and a selective serotonin reuptake inhibitor (SSRI)—for example, fluoxetine, sertraline, paroxetine, fluvoxamine, or citaprolam (marketed, respectively, as Prozac, Zoloft, Paxil, Luvox, and Celexa)—or another such agent may alleviate both sets of symptoms in ways that no one medication alone could. Davis Gammon and I (1993) reported a study in which fluoxetine was successfully administered with stimulants to children who had ADHD as well as depression and other symptoms. Recent findings about an increase in suicidal thoughts or behavior in a small percentage of children or adolescents taking SSRIs, however, has led the FDA to urge close monitoring of use of any antidepressant prescribed for any purpose to children and adolescents.

Treatment with combinations of medications for ADHD and various comorbid disorders is now relatively common and apparently is becoming more widespread. Daniel Safer, Julie Zito, and Susan dosReis (2003) reported that in the mid-1990s more than 20 percent of youths in outpatient psychiatric treatment and 40 percent of those receiving inpatient psychiatric care were given two or more concurrent psychiatric medications. Their findings indicate that the frequency of such combined treatment is becoming increasingly common, especially for youths being treated with stimulants for ADHD. This is not so different from other fields of medicine; combined medication treatments have been shown to be significantly more effective than single medication treatment for HIV, intractable seizures, congestive heart failure, and hypertension.

The problem of combined medication treatments in psychiatry, especially when used for the treatment of children, is that the effects of medicines given for psychiatric disorders are more difficult to measure than those used to treat many medical problems for which critical levels of antibodies, blood pressure, seizure activity, coronary output, and other vital readings can be easily ascertained. Another important problem is that very little research has been done to assess the risks and benefits of treatment with these various combinations of medications.

There are a few published examples of such research, however. In addition to the studies by Prince and others (1996) and Gammon and Brown

(1993) cited earlier, Gabrielle Carlson and colleagues (1992) have reported on the combined use of MPH and lithium for children with bipolar disorder and ADHD. More recently Russell Scheffer and others (2005) reported a controlled trial of mixed amphetamine salts in combination with a mood-stabilizing medication in bipolar children whose ADHD was impairing even after their mood problems had been stabilized. And Biederman and colleagues (2000) reviewed the use of mood-stabilizing medications, antidepressants, and stimulants. The Tourette's Syndrome Study Group (2002) and Hazell and Stuart (2003) reported positive results using clonidine and stimulants in combination. And Michael Aman and colleagues (2004) summarized two studies on the combined use of stimulants and risperidone for disruptive behavior disorders. Since some of these were chart reviews or relatively small, open-label studies, there are limitations to what conclusions can validly be drawn; such findings are more suggestive than definitive.

Some are quick to criticize clinicians who employ combined medication strategies for treatment of ADHD and various comorbid disorders since there is so little research evidence to guide such treatments. While there is good reason to prefer treating patients with just one medication in accordance with guidelines supported by extensive clinical trials, in some cases combining medications may relieve substantial suffering while incurring what seems to be a relatively small risk.

Is it preferable to treat a child only with a stimulant that improves his severe problems with inattention and impulsivity, but does not aid his chronic, severe insomnia? Should a clinician treat an adolescent with severe bipolar mood swings only with a mood stabilizer and leave untreated the student's ADD syndrome impairments, which make it impossible for him to do his schoolwork even minimally well? Faced with such dilemmas, many clinicians, in consultation with the patient and family, choose to prescribe combined medication treatments for ADHD and comorbid disorders, despite the lack of sufficient research to guide the process. In such situations the apparent risks of not providing the combined treatments may appear to outweigh considerably the uncertain risks of providing such treatment while monitoring carefully for possible adverse effects.

Behavioral Treatments for ADHD

Although there is a vast body of evidence that certain medications alleviate many symptoms of ADHD, medicine alone is not sufficient treatment for some with ADHD, especially those children and adolescents whose behavior is seriously disruptive in school, with peers, and/or at home with their families. Many of these children need systematic help to develop more adaptive patterns of behavior. Also, current medications are not effective for all individuals with ADHD; as mentioned earlier, 20 to 30 percent of all patients diagnosed have no significant response to medication. In these situations, behavioral treatments may be helpful.

Children and adolescents with disruptive behavioral problems are the ones who primarily benefit from behavioral treatments, which are of limited use for improving cognitive functions such as working memory, processing speed, and sustaining alertness. Behavioral strategies may also help to reduce the common tendency of parents, teachers, and others unwittingly to reinforce a child's disruptive behaviors. For an overview of the extensive body of research showing the effectiveness of these interventions for disruptive behavior orders, including ADHD, see William Pelham and Daniel Waschbusch (1999).

Principles of Behavioral Treatment

Although behavioral treatment for ADHD can be summarized in a few simple principles, for example, "You catch more flies with honey than you do with vinegar" and "Don't feed what you don't want to grow," the design and implementation of effective behavioral treatments for a particular child can require as much clinical skill and individualized tailoring as the design of an effective medication regimen. Some think of behavioral treatment as just putting a checklist on the refrigerator door and then pasting on stars when the child is "being good." It's not that simple.

The first element of behavioral treatment is a careful assessment of problematic behaviors to determine what encourages a child in various contexts and what specific changes might be helpful. Targets might include getting a child to stop hitting others when angry, to comply with parental directions without arguing, to sleep in one's own bed every night, or to follow established routines for getting up, dressed, and ready for school in time for the bus pickup. Often parents have a long list of changes they want to see in the behavior of their child with ADHD. A clinician may need to assist the parents (and child) in selecting the most important and then stating each goal in a clear and positive way. For example, "Show a positive attitude" is too general. "Use polite language without swearing" is more specific and less likely to lead to arguments about whether the behavior has been performed. In addition, it is usually helpful to target no more than five behaviors for change at one time.

The next step is to monitor compliance. Some target behaviors like "Make bed each morning before leaving on time for school" involve a simple "yes" or "no" for the day. Other behaviors, like "Speak politely to other family members without swearing," might be reinforced more effectively if the child is assessed four to five times each day. In this way, if the desired behavior is not shown during one time period, the child still has the opportunity to improve over the course of the day.

The third task is to identify consequences, positive and/or negative, that the parent will impose in response to how the child performs the target behaviors. Following the "more flies with honey than with vinegar" rule, a parent who wants a child to speak more politely is most likely to obtain the desired change by rewarding the child for every time period in which the child complies. "Reward" here may mean any of many different privileges or gifts; and it often does not need to have monetary value. Some children will work hard for verbal praise, hugs, smiles, or nods of approval from a parent. Other children will make the desired changes in behavior only if it means a privilege like extra reading time with a parent before bed or a chance to play with a special toy that is desirable, but not always available. Other children are more likely to change their behavior only to earn points that can eventually win them a specific amount of money or opportunity to rent a new video game.

Often behavior change requires not only rewards, but also some penalty for a specific misbehavior. For example, a child who hits younger siblings might be rewarded for each time period over the day when he keeps hands to himself. Yet the behavioral treatment plan may also specify that each time the child does hit a sibling, he or she is required to sit on a certain chair or go to a particular room for a time-out. The time-out period should be brief, perhaps just five minutes for a younger child or fifteen minutes for an older child. Its purpose is to interrupt the maladaptive behavior and then to get everyone back on the track, working toward the desired behavior.

The fourth element of behavioral treatment is monitoring the effectiveness of the intervention, evaluating what is working and what needs to be changed. This may sound simple, but success lies in a sensitive, detail-oriented implementation of the plan. For example, if a child is given a time-out for a temper tantrum, the time-out should be timed with a kitchen timer that will ring at the end of the set time. If the child gets up too early or persists in screaming and shouting, the timer should be restarted until the specified time is completed quietly in the right place. If the parent shouts to tell the child to keep quiet or to remind the child what the consequences will be, the system collapses; the child is then being encouraged to continue the tantrum rather than learning that compliance ends the punishment more quickly. If a parent gets intensely involved with a child, even to scold, in reaction to undesirable behavior, the child may be more likely to repeat that negative behavior. Don't feed it, if you don't want it to grow! For many children, both positive and negative attention from parents are reinforcing.

Training for Parenting Children with ADHD

Most parents need some help to learn how to design and effectively implement behavioral programs. Useful strategies for all children have been described by Thomas Phelan (2003) in his book *1-2-3 Magic*. Russell Barkley (2000), in his *Taking Charge of ADHD*, also offers ways for parents to deal with many behavioral problems associated with ADHD. And systematic training programs to help parents learn how to apply behavioral treatment strategies to children with ADHD have been described by Arthur Anastopoulos and colleagues (1998) and Charles Cunningham (1998).

Despite such training, some parents—especially those who themselves have ADD syndrome—have great difficulty making behavioral treatment programs work. For example, Edmund Sonuga-Barke and colleagues (2002) reported a study of preschool children with ADHD and their mothers in which the children of mothers who themselves had relatively high levels of ADHD symptoms showed the least improvement after their mothers had received parent training. This suggests that the benefits a child receives from behavioral treatment at home are strongly influenced by the ability of the parent to consistently implement the program plan, a task that may be very difficult for the 25 percent of parents of children with ADHD who themselves suffer substantial impairments from ADD syndrome.

Some Children Respond Poorly to Behavioral Treatment

Parental problems are not the only factor that may interfere with a child's benefiting from a behavioral treatment program. Some children suffer from emotional and behavioral problems that make standard behavioral treatment programs much less likely to succeed. Ross Greene wrote in *The Explosive Child* (1998) about children who have extraordinary difficulty managing frustration and tend to "melt down" into protracted tantrums and disorganization, which makes them unresponsive to the usual strategies of behavioral treatment.

Many might consider these children to be just exceptionally stubborn or unmotivated to comply with requests of parents and teachers. But Greene proposes that some of these children may be like a mediocre basketball player given the opportunity to play on a professional basketball team with a very high salary—as long as their performance is outstanding. Though they may be strongly motivated to perform well, they may lack the ability to do what is expected and required to get the reward. Their capacity to tolerate frustration and change their behavior may not be sufficiently developed, and unlike most other children, they seem unable to respond to anticipated rewards or even to harsh punishments.

For such children, Greene proposes that the guiding adults reprioritize their usual expectations. He suggests that parents and teachers prune their priorities and seek to enforce with the child only those rules that are so essential to safety that it is worth enduring the stress of a meltdown by the child. Greene proposes a process of then working with the child to com-

municate, negotiate, and compromise on an increasing range of other behaviors important for development (but not worth a major meltdown) as
the child develops the abilities needed to meet more age-appropriate expectations.

There certainly are children whose impairments with severe ADD syndrome prevent them from responding to the usual behavioral treatments
(particularly when comorbid Asperger's disorder or pervasive developmental disorders are involved), yet allow them to respond to the approach
described by Greene. Most children with disruptive behavioral disorders,
however, will respond to more conventional behavioral treatment programs at home and in school.

Behavioral Interventions at School

Behavioral strategies have also been developed to support and improve the
functioning of children with ADHD and related problems in school. Details about approaches for schools are not reviewed in this book, but are
readily available elsewhere. George DuPaul and Gary Stoner (2003), for example, have described in detail a variety of ways that children with ADHD
can be supported in school. And Sandra Rief (2005) has written a book
offering practical suggestions for teachers who want to adapt their classroom to maximize learning opportunities for their students with ADHD.

One behavioral treatment strategy that can be helpful for parents is
the daily report card. This is a simple device that allows a teacher quickly
to record each day how well a student has performed on several specific
target behaviors in the classroom. Parents can then recognize and reward
their child at home for specific good behaviors at school on the very day
they occur. Sometimes weekly report cards, too, can be very helpful and
less burdensome for a busy classroom teacher.

Behavioral strategies need to be adapted carefully to each context and
to the developmental level of each child. Some approaches that work well
at school for many younger children with ADHD do not work as effectively for older children or adolescents, who usually interact with five to
seven teachers daily. Getting accurate, up-to-date information about how
an adolescent is performing in school—whether their homework is being

completed adequately and handed in on time, whether they have been prepared for quizzes and tests, whether they are participating in class discussions, and when they are supposed to be working on longer-term assignments, for example—is much more difficult when a student has multiple teachers throughout the day.

Strategies for Parenting Adolescents with ADHD

Arthur Robin (1998) has written guiding principles for parenting adolescents with ADHD and has provided explanations and multiple examples of how these can be implemented:

> Facilitate appropriate independence seeking
>
> Maintain adequate structure and supervision
>
> Establish bottom-line rules for living in your home and enforce them consistently
>
> Negotiate all issues that are not bottom lines with your adolescent
>
> Use consequences wisely to influence your adolescent's behavior
>
> Maintain good communication
>
> Keep a disability perspective and practice forgiveness
>
> Focus on the positive. (p. 307)

These principles highlight developmental issues that emerge during adolescence, requiring changes that are often difficult for adolescents and parents alike. Robin's emphasis on encouraging appropriate independence-seeking reminds parents that their task during the adolescent years is to nurture their son or daughter's efforts to function with more self-management and less intensive dependence on parents and teachers. His mention of the need for forgiveness acknowledges the inevitability of adolescents sometimes behaving, sometimes deliberately, in ways that are disappointing or hurtful to their parents. Forgiveness can help to repair and put into perspective such mistakes so they do not unnecessarily disrupt the bond between parent and child that is so crucial to facilitating mutual growth.

Other books that may be helpful to parents of adolescents with ADHD include Marlene Snyder's 2001 book on problematic issues that often arise as adolescents with ADHD begin driving motor vehicles and Chris Dendy's practical guidebooks on parenting adolescents with ADHD (1995) and teaching adolescents with ADHD (2000).

Comparisons of Medications and Behavioral Treatments: The MTA Study

Sometimes parents and clinicians wonder which type of treatment, behavioral or medication, is more effective for treatment of ADHD. Until recently there was very little empirical data to address that question. This situation changed with completion of the Multimodal Treatment Study of Children with ADHD (MTA Cooperative Group 1999). This massive research project, sponsored jointly by the National Institute of Mental Health and the U.S. Department of Education, sought to answer three questions: (1) How do medication and behavioral treatments for ADHD compare with each other over the long term? (2) Are there additional benefits when the two modes of treatment are used together? and (3) What is the effectiveness of systematic, carefully delivered treatments versus the routine care usually delivered in most communities of the United States?

At six different sites in the United States and Canada, children were recruited to participate in the study. All were aged seven to 9.9 years when the study began, and all were found after comprehensive evaluation to meet the *DSM-IV* diagnostic criteria for ADHD, combined type; no children with predominantly inattentive type were included. After evaluation these children were randomly assigned to undergo fourteen months of treatment in one of four different groups:

1. *Medication monitoring only.* Patients were given carefully tailored medication treatment for ADHD, which was monitored each month and adjusted according to prearranged formulas to optimize response. These children and their families were provided no other treatment for ADHD.
2. *Behavioral treatment only.* Patient families were given a comprehensive behavioral treatment package: parent training, an intensive eight-week summer day camp for the child with trained specialist counselors; episodic expert consultations for the child's

classroom teacher; twelve weeks of trained aides working with the teacher in the child's school classroom, and a daily report card to maximize school-home communication. These students received no medication treatment for ADHD.

3. *Combined medication and behavioral treatment.* Patients received the full medication management treatment and the full behavioral treatment program.

4. *Community care only.* Participants received no direct treatment in the study. Those randomized to this group were evaluated and then asked to seek out treatment in their community; this could be from their pediatrician, a psychologist, social worker, or whatever other resource they chose. Treatment could include medication, behavioral treatment, counseling, and so on.

After fourteen months of treatment, children in all groups were reevaluated to compare relative levels of improvement in the four groups. Since all children had received the same comprehensive evaluation, met the same diagnostic criteria, and been randomly assigned to one of the four groups, the results could reasonably be taken to reflect the relative effectiveness of the four treatment options. Most of those who had heard about the study expected the combined treatment group, the one getting both carefully managed medication and the intensive behavioral treatment program, to do the best. They assumed that more treatment leads to better results.

Many were surprised by the results of this carefully controlled study. Children in each of the four groups showed significant reductions in their ADHD symptoms over the fourteen months, but there were notable differences in the degree of change. Medication management was superior to the behavioral treatment program and to routine community care, even though many in the community care were taking medication for ADHD. What was most surprising was that the combined treatment did not yield significantly better results for improvement of ADHD symptoms than did the medication treatment alone. Combined treatment was a bit better for some non-ADHD symptoms and for some measures of positive functioning, but the mean group scores for core ADHD symptoms in the combined treatment group were not significantly better than the mean group scores of the group that did not receive any treatment other than carefully managed medication for ADHD. These data clearly support the notion that the primary impairments in ADHD are chemical and can often be alleviated with appropriate medications alone.

It should be noted, however, that these results were group means, the averages, for improvement on various symptoms that had been selected in advance. When the data were reanalyzed to determine the percentage of individuals who had obtained excellent improvement from treatment, the advantages of the combined treatment were more apparent. James Swanson and colleagues (2001) reported the percentages of children who obtained "excellent," normalized responses from their treatment:

Community Care (with or without medication)	25%
Behavior Treatment only	34%
Medication Management only	56%
Combined Behavior Treatment and Medication Management	68%

These data show that the combined treatments yielded a 12 percent increase in the percentage of children obtaining an excellent response. They also show that some in each group obtained an excellent response while even the most effective treatment left fully 32 percent of children in that condition with a less than excellent response. Keep in mind that most of those not listed as having an excellent (that is, normalized) response to treatment still benefited in varying degrees from their treatment experiences. Follow-up studies will continue to monitor the results of this treatment study for at least ten years, even though some participants have discontinued or switched their treatments.

In assessing the results of the MTA study, it is important to keep in mind the age of the participants. All the subjects were young children with combined-type ADHD; the behavioral treatments that proved effective for many of the young children in the MTA study may have much more limited effectiveness for the ADHD impairments suffered by older children, adolescents, and adults, as well as for those who have predominantly inattentive-type ADHD.

The Role of Parents, Mentors, Coaches, and Therapists

Although ADD syndrome is fundamentally a problem in the chemistry of the brain, and though appropriately managed medication is usually the most effective treatment for ADD syndrome, medication alone is often not enough. Growing up with untreated ADD syndrome can expose an individual to daily frustrations and embarrassments that can take an enormous toll on self-confidence and personal hope. Battling every day with even well-intended criticism from frustrated parents, teachers, friends, and even oneself—"You should be able to do this; you know it's important, why don't you just do it?" causes many children with ADD syndrome to form "defensive images" of themselves and others.

> "Everybody is always picking on me, wanting too much."
> "I just can't do a lot of things they think I can do."
> "I'm just one of those people who's always a day late and a dollar short."
> "They think I'm really smart, but it's not true. Underneath it all, I'm stupid."
> "If I set my sights on accomplishing much, I'll just be disappointed."

With such recurrent thoughts, some learn to reduce their expectations of themselves and to avoid opportunities that may lead to higher grades, more friends, better jobs, and increased status. By this process some individuals with ADD syndrome learn early in life to see themselves as "losers," "victims," or both. Some react with sullen resentment; others with a demanding sense of entitlement. Some labor to win others with their quick wit or clown antics; others slide into quiet resignation or a quirky independence from conventional social expectations. In interactions with others, such attitudes and postures tend to create feedback loops in which the individual finds those around him acting and reacting in ways that confirm and reinforce his defensive images of himself. This can become an important aspect of the person's "representational model" of herself and others as described by John Bowlby and discussed in Chapter 6.

If an individual with ADD syndrome has developed such self-defeating assumptions about himself and others, medication treatment is unlikely to cause a lasting change. To counter the persisting effects of such self-defeating assumptions and attitudes, the patient will need help recognizing and revising them in the context of an emotionally engaged relationship.

This process of attitude change and revising assumptions is not a purely intellectual process that can be derived from listening to a lecture or reading a book. Such resources may be helpful, but real change will involve subtle and powerful emotions, not just an exchange of words and ideas. The interaction may occur in a series of intensive, closely spaced conversations, or it may happen over many months or years.

For some, the partner in this process is a parent who persists in recognizing the strengths of this son or daughter despite recurrent setbacks and disappointments. Some parents are amazingly adept at nurturing a positive and hopeful attitude in their children while also providing reasonable limits and honest feedback about shortcomings in the son's or daughter's plans or behavior. They cultivate recognition of the child's strengths and they provide generous and sustained reinforcement for constructive efforts. They encourage their child to pursue opportunities that can be reached with extra effort, yet they avoid supporting unrealistic expectations likely to lead only to frustration. In countless conversations at times when the child must make critical decisions or is responding to the delights of success or the pain of defeat, such parents can share the emotions of their child and nurture the child's developing strengths.

Yet despite the best efforts of their parents, some children and many adolescents and adults need more specialized help to recognize and overhaul self-defeating assumptions and attitudes developed in reaction to their ADD syndrome. The most fortunate encounter and connect with a wise and empathetic teacher, professor, or work supervisor who is willing to serve as a mentor, providing ongoing guidance and emotional support for their efforts to revise their ways of doing business with themselves and other people. For others it may be necessary to consult and employ a professional counselor, a psychotherapist, or an ADD "coach" to provide perspective and support for the process of self-change that may be needed, especially in the early stages of coming to terms with an ADD diagnosis.

Getting such support is not always easy. Many counselors and psychotherapists still do not understand ADHD. And persons who present themselves as ADD "coaches" vary widely in their educational background, level of training, and competence. Some have as their main qualification their desire to be helpful to persons with ADD and their willingness to maintain frequent contact by phone or face-to-face meetings. Others have professional training in social work or a related field and have specialized training to increase their understanding of ADD syndrome—training that has given them strategies to help patients and families clarify goals, organize tasks, and sustain the effort required to attain reasonable objectives. Development of a system for assessing qualifications and providing credentials for ADD coaches is still in its infancy. Patients who have worked with coaches have had reactions ranging from grateful and enthusiastic appreciation to frustrated disappointment.

At present, it cannot reasonably be assumed that every licensed counselor, psychotherapist, psychologist, or psychiatrist is familiar with ADD syndrome and can competently assist those who have it. Only a small percentage of professionals in the present generation have received even a minimal education about how to recognize and treat the various forms of this disorder. Increasing numbers are learning about the assessment of ADD and its treatment with medications. But relatively few, at present, have been trained to deal with assessment, medication adjustments, and the more subtle issues of identifying and treating the problematic assumptions and attitudes of patients with ADD syndrome. Organizations like Children and Adults with ADHD (CHADD) and Attention Deficit Disorder Association (ADDA), listed in the resources section of this book, may offer some information helpful for finding trained professionals.

Cognitive-Behavioral Treatment

One promising way to address problematic attitudes and behaviors that persist in some with ADD syndrome, along with medication, is to use cognitive behavioral therapy techniques. Steven McDermott (2000) and Russell Ramsay with Anthony Rostain (2004) have described strategies and case examples of this approach with adults. Arthur Anastopoulos and Lisa Gerrard (2003) have described similar processes with children and adolescents. Typically cognitive behavior strategies seek to identify the patient's self-sabotaging assumptions and strategies, undermine these with cognitive behavioral interventions, and encourage behaviors that will facilitate development of more positive and helpful approaches.

Marital and Family Treatments

Usually untreated ADD syndrome affects the entire household of the person experiencing the symptoms. Problems may emerge in couples even when there are no children. As I described in Chapter 6, adults with ADD syndrome often partner with someone who provides support that compensates for some of their own weaknesses. Without consciously realizing it, a person with untreated ADD syndrome may feel drawn to someone who is exceptionally tolerant or amused by their chronic tardiness, inattention, and disorganization, or to someone willing to take on the tasks of managing joint finances and scheduling medical appointments and social events. Some opt for partners more forceful and confrontational, who take on a parenting role toward the adult partner with ADD, perhaps even by continuing a nagging style that had been familiar, if not comfortable, in the family of origin.

As such relationships evolve, however, the ADD syndrome impairments of one partner may become less amusing, more annoying, and more burdensome to the other. Or the individual with ADD syndrome may gradually start to feel resentful about the nagging demands or condescension of the "helpful" partner. One or both may become chronically irritable or react with increasing distance and eventual emotional or physical abandonment. Such pressures can be even more problematic if the couple has a child—especially if, as often happens, the couple has a child with ADHD.

Indeed, children with ADD syndrome present a continuing series of worries, frustrations, and management problems to their parents. Although deeply loved, they can be very "high maintenance" relative to

most other children of the same age. And they may consume a disproportionate amount of time and attention from their parents, often leaving siblings frustrated and resentful over what may constitute genuine
unfairness.

Jeanne Safer (2002) grew up with an emotionally troubled older brother.
She described the complex, painful, and often unacknowledged feelings
that can affect brothers and sisters of children with chronic problems.

> No one with an abnormal sibling has a normal childhood. . . .
> Family gatherings and significant events become occasions for
> anxiety and suppressed shame. . . . [Healthy siblings] . . . feel
> tormented by the compulsion to compensate for their parents'
> disappointments by having no problems and making no de-
> mands. . . . Their success is always tainted by their sibling's fail-
> ure, their future clouded by an untoward sense of obligation and
> responsibility. . . . You are ashamed that you are related, guilty
> that you have a better life, envious that nothing is expected of
> him, relieved that you are not the misfit to be scorned or pitied.
> Because a sibling is your closest relative, you are eternally en-
> meshed with each other. (pp. xviii–xix)

Not every individual with a sibling who has ADHD suffers such intense burdens as Safer describes. Many enjoy and benefit from most of
their interactions with their brother or sister who has ADHD. Yet there are
certainly some children impaired by untreated ADHD, especially those
with severe comorbid problems, who daily disrupt family life over many
years. These children may drain so much parental time and attention that
the remaining siblings chronically get short shrift.

But it is also true that some brothers and sisters exploit their ADHD
siblings, setting them up to be unfairly punished for misdeeds they did
not commit, or gaining more favorable treatment for themselves by directing parental attention to otherwise unnoticed shortcomings of the
ADD child. Families with members who have ADD are subject to the full
range of sibling rivalries and complex emotional alliances often found in
other families.

Parental Polarization in Raising Children with ADHD

One common form of stress in families with a child suffering from inadequately treated ADD syndrome is the polarization of parents as they struggle to deal with daily challenges of parenting a chronically impaired child. Often one parent takes on the role of the "enforcer," emphasizing repeatedly that loving the child requires making reasonable but firm demands on him or her:

> We have to be firm and confront this kid. If we don't get on his case and punish him when he doesn't do what he's supposed to, he's never going to learn to do the right thing. He'll always be looking for some excuse. And he'll never learn how to do what he has to do to make it in the real world.

Meanwhile, the other parent, "the marshmallow," equally worried and equally loving the same child, is likely to argue:

> But this kid is in trouble all the time, every place he goes. Everybody is always on his case. Don't you think he needs some place where he can feel accepted as who he is, some place where he is not constantly being pushed, with some people who will keep loving him even when he's having a hard time doing what he's supposed to do? If he doesn't have support at home, where is he going to get it?

The dilemma, of course, is that both views are partly true. Unfortunately, this is often not recognized when parents polarize into extremes, each fighting, sometimes fiercely, with the other to press for their own view while rejecting the other. Extreme "enforcer" and "marshmallow" polarization can occur as parents battle over how to punish their children or adolescents for not doing homework, getting poor grades, harassing their siblings, being disrespectful to teachers or parents, getting drunk, stealing money, or wrecking the family car. But if they argue too vehemently, parents can become diverted from the difficult task of deciding together when to be tough and confrontational and when to be more flexible and supportive. And when such arguing becomes chronic, it can seriously undermine the quality of the relationship between the parents themselves.

When parents chronically disagree about how to deal with a problematic child, the entire family, even extended family members such as grandparents, may become involved in complex alliances. One parent may take on the role of defender of the ADHD child, spending a lot of time talking sympathetically with and about that child, often making excuses for wrongdoing or failures. The defending parent may even conspire with the ADHD child to keep secret from the other parent negative reports from the school or complaints from other siblings.

Meanwhile, the other parent may become so consumed with frustration and anger that he or she gives up trying interact with the spouse or the ADHD child, aligning instead with another son or daughter. Such alliances may be skewed by a parent's earlier life experiences with their own siblings, or by unrecognized wishes to be more firm or sympathetic, or less uptight or intrusive, than their own parents seemed to be.

Sometimes grandparents, uncles, aunts, and neighbors become directly involved in parental conflicts as they provide solicited support or intrude without being asked. Such conflicts can become intense, charged with strong emotions that can contaminate interactions of the entire family system and obscure the strengths and needs of family members over many years.

Not every family that has a member with ADD syndrome is as disrupted as these examples. Many families have one or several members with ADHD, including both parents and children, and function extraordinarily well. In cases where family interactions become very problematic, however, it may be wise to consult a skilled counselor who understands not only the dynamics of family life, but also ADHD and related problems. In such situations it is very important that the difficulties be conceptualized as a problem of the family system, involving multiple family members, and not just as fallout from the impairments of one person. Craig Everett and Sandra Everett (1999) have written about how theories and strategies of family therapy can be adapted to help couples and families affected by ADHD.

Accommodations at School or Work

Some individuals with ADHD continue to be quite impaired despite treatment. Moreover, some individuals are not able to acquire or sustain appropriate treatment for ADHD. In such situations, some changes, or "accommodations," in the requirements and procedures at school or work may provide a fairer chance for the individual with ADHD.

The most commonly requested accommodation is extended time for taking tests and examinations. Because of their slow cognitive processing speed and impairments of working memory, many children, adolescents, and adults with ADD syndrome have great difficulty completing tests and examinations within standard time allotments. To compensate for their ADD impairments, they often need to reread directions and test items multiple times and need repeatedly to recheck their answers. This may slow their work so much that they are unable even to attempt many items on the test. Thus they may get a low grade, not because they did not know the material and gave wrong answers, but because they were unable to complete the exam.

If such students are allowed extended time, usually 1.5 times the usual time allotment, their scores may improve significantly simply because they were able to answer more questions. Extended time may also alleviate the excessive anxiety that plagues such students when they take examinations. Knowing that they often are unable to finish the test within the usual time, these individuals often work even more slowly because they worry excessively: "Will I be able to answer all the questions before we have to hand in our papers? I have to hurry!" Such accommodations can be critically important for individuals taking "high stakes" examinations that determine their eligibility for more advanced or specialized levels of education or certification. Another accommodation for examinations might include allowing a test-taker the opportunity to take the examination in a setting where external distractions are minimized—that is, where there are fewer people moving around, tapping their feet or pencils, and so on in ways that may be excessively distracting for some individuals with ADD syndrome.

In school, some students with severe ADD syndrome impairments may be allowed a reduced amount of homework. This accommodation is generally considered appropriate, however, only when a student takes twice as long (or longer) to complete homework assignments. In such situations students are usually asked to work on every other math problem, spelling word, and so forth so they can try all the levels of difficulty included in the assignment.

Another accommodation helpful to younger students with ADD syndrome is more frequent reports from the teacher to parents about the child's academic performance and behavior. This allows parents to monitor the child's performance more closely and to provide extra encouragement. These reports may be very frequent, such as the daily "report card" mentioned earlier, or less frequent—for example, weekly progress reports. Such feedback can help the child to be more aware of the quality of their performance, good and bad, than they would be from quarterly report cards or bimonthly progress reports.

In the United States, federal regulations stipulate that children and adolescents with certain impairments, including ADHD and specific learning disabilities, must be allowed special accommodations in school in accordance with the results of a professional evaluation and extensive documentation about which accommodations are needed. Requirements for these processes in the United States have been summarized by George DuPaul and Thomas Power (2000). Many other nations have not yet set up such protections for impaired students.

For those U.S. patients beyond secondary school, some provisions of section 504 of the Rehabilitation Act of 1973 and the Americans with Disabilities Act of 1990 may provide certain similar accommodations and protections in colleges, universities, and workplaces for those who meet specific qualifications. Reviews of these laws and regulations, as well as a discussion of the problems involved in establishing eligibility, are included in a book by Lynda Katz and colleagues (2001) and in summaries of legal issues in accommodations by attorneys Peter Latham and Patricia Latham (1996, 1999, 2005).

More Specialized Treatments

As mentioned earlier, some persons with ADD syndrome also suffer from severe learning disorders such as reading disorder, math disorder, or disorder of written expression. During the school years, they are likely to need special education services in addition to treatment for ADD impairments. Others with ADD syndrome are actively caught up in abuse or dependence on alcohol, marijuana, or other drugs; for them, effective treatment of their substance abuse will be required before their ADD impairments can adequately be alleviated. Still others with ADD syndrome may have chronic and severe problems with panic attacks or OCD. And severe social impairments on the Asperger's/autistic spectrum or severe problems with mood regulation, depression, or bipolar disorder can also complicate the patient's struggles with ADD syndrome. Detailed information about treatment options for ADHD in combination with these various comorbid disorders is the primary focus of my edited textbook *Attention Deficit Disorders and Comorbidities in Children, Adolescents, and Adults* (2000).

Unproven Treatments

In addition to the well-researched treatments discussed thus far, there are many other treatment options claiming to alleviate impairments of ADHD more easily or without need for medication. Most of these alternative treatments lack credible scientific evidence that they are effective and, for some, there may be reason to question their safety. The primary problem with such unproven treatments, however, is that they may delay an individual's receiving treatment that has been proven safe and will likely be effective.

Elimination Diets and Diet Supplements

Elimination diets are based on an assumption that if an individual with ADHD refrains from consuming certain specific foods such as sugar, candy, dietary salicylates, and artificial food colorings, their symptoms will disappear. The best-known of these is the Feingold diet. Eugene Arnold (2002) reviewed the literature on elimination diets for ADHD and concluded that most research shows no credible evidence for the effectiveness of such diets in treating ADHD. He did note that such diets may be helpful for a small subset of children who have specific food allergies, but there is no evidence that children with ADHD have any greater incidence of such food allergies than children in the general population.

Diet supplements—typically herbal remedies, high-dose vitamins, or other consumable products sold over the counter in health food stores or supermarkets—are often touted as being able to, for example, "improve focus" or "strengthen memory." Because the FDA regulations that control advertising for prescription drugs do not apply to diet supplements, there is virtually no limit to the extravagance of claims that can be made for such products. Although a few compounds—for example, essential fatty acids—have shown some possible benefits for ADHD patients in pilot studies, most of these products have not been proven effective thus far. Some, such as megadose vitamins, may carry a mild risk of damage to the liver.

Some believe that any substance advertised as "natural" must be safer than a pharmaceutical product. In fact, many "natural" substances in the environment are quite toxic, sometimes even in small doses. Arsenic, for example, is a natural substance. The most widely publicized example of a "natural" diet supplement causing health problems was a series of cases in 1989 where onset of eosinophilia-myalgia was linked to use of tryptophan. Arnold (2002) noted that those cases may have been due more to impurities in the tryptophan than to the compound itself. This explanation highlights another problem with many diet supplements: their production is not regulated by the FDA to maintain high standards of quality and purity.

EEG Biofeedback or Neurofeedback Treatments

Practitioners of biofeedback (or "neurofeedback") often claim that their treatments can train a child, adolescent, or adult with ADHD to change their brain wave patterns and thereby alleviate their ADHD impairments. This treatment consists of electrodes being attached to a patient and then hooked up to a computerized monitor that displays the frequency rates of certain types of electrical activity that normally vary in the human brain.

The patient is given directions about how to relax himself or herself, much as might be done in hypnosis. On a monitor the patient is then able to see how successfully he can modify those brain waves. As Russell Barkley (2003) has pointed out, however, there is no active ingredient in the process that directly affects the brain waves. The equipment is simply a fancy monitor that provides immediate feedback about how successfully the patient can relax.

Although practitioners of neurofeedback claim that evidence of the success of their treatment techniques has been published, reviews by Sandra Loo (2003) and by Russell Barkley (2003) indicate that this published research does not meet basic scientific standards for evidence of effectiveness. Studies published thus far are deeply flawed by failure to randomize patients, failure to use a placebo control, failure to "blind" patients or evaluators, contamination of results by allowing intervening or concurrent interventions with other treatments, and various other problems. Indeed, Loo reports that the one and only published study of neurofeedback that came close to following accepted scientific standards provided no evidence that neurofeedback was effective. Given the understanding of ADD syndrome proposed in this book, and the physiological processes that support executive functions, it is difficult to imagine how conscious efforts to relax oneself, with or without an electronic monitor, could cause any lasting improvement in the complex cognitive processes that constitute executive functioning. Neurofeedback treatments appear to be rooted in a simplistic notion of ADHD as an individual's simply being too tense or revved up and needing to learn to relax.

Exercise Treatments

A program of individualized exercises purported to improve "cerebellar developmental delay" is currently being marketed as a new alternative treatment for alleviating dyslexia and attention deficit disorder. Claims have been made that prescribed programs of exercise done for five to ten minutes twice daily—for example, balancing on one foot while throwing a beanbag from one hand to the other, can produce dramatic improvement in reading ability and fully alleviate ADD symptoms without medication. Testimonials claim that these exercises have improved reading, writing, and comprehension difficulties, poor concentration and organizational skills, clumsiness, poor memory, low self-esteem, and difficulty controlling emotions in large numbers of children, adolescents, and adults.

While a consistent program of manageable exercise may contribute to overall health and self-esteem for anyone, there is no scientifically recognized evidence to support such wild claims for alleviating the complex impairments of ADD syndrome or learning disorders. Like neurofeedback, this alternative treatment is founded on an overly simplistic view of the nature and underlying physiology of ADD syndrome. Unfortunately, such alternative treatments are often marketed in ways that cause many families who lack a scientifically based understanding of ADD syndrome to waste money and valuable time on unproven treatments while avoiding treatments that are adequately researched and likely to be helpful.

Tailoring Treatments for Individuals and Families with ADHD

Some clinicians claim that every patient with ADHD should receive "multimodal treatment." This fancy phrase simply means that medication alone is often not enough to fully treat ADHD. Typically, behavioral treatments and education are added to the list of treatment modalities that "should be" provided for every patient. But although it is true that educating the patient and family about the nature of ADHD and its treatment is an essential component of any adequate treatment plan, it is not true that every patient diagnosed with ADHD needs or will benefit from behavioral treatments, psychotherapy, cognitive behavioral treatment, or accommodations in school or the workplace.

In particular, behavioral treatments may be quite helpful for some children with ADHD, particularly those with significant behavioral problems; they are less likely to be appropriate or useful for adolescents or adults with ADHD. And cognitive behavioral treatment or counseling might be beneficial for some persons with ADHD who have significant problems with self-esteem or are stuck in maladaptive patterns of social interaction, but these treatments do not alleviate the core problems of ADD syndrome that are essentially biochemical.

Marital or family therapy sessions, too, may help to identify unrecognized misunderstandings and may improve maladaptive patterns of interaction between partners or other family members, but these techniques do not, in themselves, change the chemical problems underlying ADD syndrome. Finally, accommodations such as extended time for taking examinations or a minimally distracting workplace may provide some help for students or workers with ADHD, but they are not needed by every patient with ADD syndrome and, in any case, do not alleviate the underlying problems.

In each individual case, decisions must be made to determine the specific treatment needs of the patient with ADD syndrome and, if needed, his family or household. It is also essential to consider what treatment resources are actually available, desirable, and feasible for the patient. Peter Jensen and Howard Abikoff (2000) identified seven patient characteristics useful to guide clinicians' decisions about treatments for children with ADHD:

Age and intellectual ability of the child and family

Severity and urgency of the condition itself

Patient's treatment history and effects of those treatments

Presence of comorbidity or other complicating conditions that also must be addressed as part of a comprehensive treatment plan

Family factors, including presence of psychopathology in parents or other family members

The parents' ability and willingness to apply recommended treatments

Families' wish for input and preferences about specific treatment types. (p. 638)

In addition to these patient characteristics, Jensen and Abikoff also noted that the nature of available resources to the family (for example, medical insurance, or school-based treatment resources in the community) are important factors in treatment planning. In many communities in the United States and elsewhere, too, there are even more basic resource questions such as:

Is there a psychologist or other clinician available and competent to
assess and diagnose a patient who has ADD with or without comorbid disorders?

Is a physician who understands ADHD available to examine the
patient, to prescribe appropriate medication, and to monitor responses to the medication, adjusting it as needed to optimize care?

Is appropriate medication available in the local pharmacy at a price
the patient can afford to pay?

If the patient would benefit from behavioral treatment, cognitive
behavioral treatment, or counseling, is it available for a price the
patient can pay and at a time and distance the patient can manage?

If needed resources are available locally, how long is the waiting list
to receive them?

If the patient needs accommodations in school or the workplace, are
the policies and attitudes there supportive?

Many of these patient, family, and community characteristics may
influence decisions about what treatment is appropriate, what treatment
is actually obtained and sustained, and how the treatment affects the patient and family. In addition, some other, less recognized factors may prevent a patient from even seeking assessment or treatment for ADD syndrome. I discuss these in the next chapter.

Chapter 10 Fears, Prejudices, and Realistic Hope

MYTH: ADD doesn't really cause much damage to a person's life.

FACT: Untreated or inadequately treated ADD syndrome often severely impairs learning, family life, education, work life, social interactions, and driving safety. Most of those with ADD who receive adequate treatment, however, function quite well.

Many in the general public and some professionals in medicine, psychology, and education remain skeptical about the validity of the ADHD diagnosis and its treatment. Fears and prejudices persist despite overwhelming evidence and recommendations derived from high-quality, peer-reviewed research.

In the mid-1990s, the American Medical Association (AMA) received questions about the possible overprescription of medications for ADHD; in response, they appointed a panel of medical experts to review all relevant research. To prevent bias, the panel members were experts in medical research, but not specialists in ADHD. The panel's findings, adopted by the AMA (Goldman et al. 1998), included some strong and definitive statements:

> ADHD is one of the best-researched disorders in medicine, and the overall data on its validity are far more compelling than for most mental disorders and even for many medical conditions. (p. 1105)

> ADHD . . . at any age increases the risk of behavioral and emotional problems at subsequent stages of life. It is thus a chronic

illness with persistence common into adolescence and beyond. (p. 1106)

Epidemiological studies . . . suggest that 3% to 6% of the school-
aged population may have ADHD. . . . The percentage of U.S.
youth being treated for ADHD is at . . . the lower end of the
prevalence range. (p. 1106)

Pharmacotherapy, particularly stimulants, has been extensively
studied. Medication alone generally provides significant short-
term symptomatic and academic improvement. . . . The risk-
benefit ratio of stimulant treatment in ADHD must be evaluated
and monitored on an ongoing basis in each case, but in general
is highly favorable. (p. 1106)

At about the same time, the American Academy of Child and Adolescent Psychiatry (1997) published guidelines on ADHD that included the
following:

Attention-deficit/hyperactivity disorder (ADHD) is one of the
most common psychiatric disorders of childhood and adolescence. . . . In most cases a stimulant is the first-choice medication . . . from large numbers of research studies and 60 years of
clinical experience . . . more is known about stimulant use in
children than about any other drug. (pp. 85S–92S)

Recent clinical experience and research document the continua-
tion of symptoms into adulthood. . . . Because adults are expected to function far more independently than children, and
because they have less structure and supervision, the consequences of inattention and impulsivity often have serious implications for functioning. . . . The risk of abuse and the possibility
of tolerance or drug refractoriness are greater in adults than in
children, but still are rare. (pp. 105S–106S)

The American Academy of Pediatrics (2000, 2001) published similar
reports documenting the wealth of scientific evidence that validates the

ADHD diagnosis and the effectiveness of available treatments. Despite these endorsements by respected guilds of medical professionals, media coverage still often describes ADHD as a controversial diagnosis, sometimes implying that medications used for treatment of ADHD are dangerous.

Frustrated by such media coverage, eighty-five scientists from leading universities in thirteen countries signed a statement arguing that there is no substantial scientific disagreement over whether ADHD is a real medical condition, any more than there is over whether smoking causes cancer or a virus causes HIV/AIDS. Summarizing the large body of scientific research cited, they stated:

> Leading international scientists . . . recognize the mounting evidence of neurological and genetic contributions to this disorder (ADHD). This evidence, coupled with countless studies on the harm posed by the disorder and hundreds of studies on the effectiveness of medication buttresses the need in many . . . cases for management of the disorder with . . . medication combined with educational, family and other social accommodations. . . .
>
> This is in striking contrast to the wholly unscientific views of some . . . media accounts that ADHD constitutes a fraud, that medicating those afflicted is questionable, if not reprehensible, and that any behavior problems associated with ADHD are merely the result of problems in the home, excessive viewing of TV or playing of video games, diet, lack of love and attention, or teacher/school intolerance. . . .
>
> To publish stories that ADHD is a fictitious disorder or merely a conflict between today's Huck Finns and their caregivers is tantamount to declaring the earth flat, the laws of gravity debatable, and the periodic table in chemistry as a fraud. (Barkley, Cook, et al. 2002, pp. 96–98)

In Europe and Asia some have questioned whether this disorder is specific to North America. They suggest that ADHD may be a byproduct of contemporary American culture; common in the United States, but relatively rare in most other parts of the world. To address this questioning, Steven Faraone and other international scientists (2003) reviewed the research literature to identify epidemiological studies of ADHD in a variety of cultures. They found that earlier studies reporting a much lower rate of ADHD outside the United States were based on different definitions of the disorder than those currently used. When they focused on studies that used the same *DSM-IV* criteria, this group found six studies of ADHD in children in the United States and nine comparable studies done in other countries.

These studies showed rates of 9.5 to 16 percent for ADHD in children in the United States. Studies done in cultures as diverse as Australia, Brazil, Colombia, Germany, Iceland, Sweden, and Ukraine reported rates of childhood incidence ranging from 3.7 to 19.8 percent; five of these studies identified a narrower range of 16 to 19.8 percent. The researchers concluded: "ADHD is not purely an American disorder . . . there is no convincing difference between the prevalence of this disorder in the U.S.A. and most other countries or cultures" (p. 111).

Despite this large body of scientific evidence about ADHD and its treatment, public skepticism persists. Criticism of ADHD in books, magazines, radio, and TV seems to emerge in two different forms: (1) fiercely ideological categorical attacks pursued with religious fervor, and (2) more modulated questioning of the diagnosis, its etiology, and its treatment.

Radical Attacks against ADHD

The most aggressive attacks against recognition of ADHD as a legitimate disorder have come from groups such as the Citizens Commission on Human Rights (CCHR), which advocates against using psychiatric or psychotropic medicines in any situation. This well-funded group and certain individuals associated with it have circulated allegations that ADHD is a fictitious disorder. One of their publications, "Psychiatry Betraying Families: The Hoax of ADD/ADHD and Other Learning Disabilities," argues, "These are made up disorders along with others including severe emotional disorder . . . and dyslexia. ADHD is a total, 100% fraud."

Often media releases and educational materials of the CCHR or comparable groups do not specify their affiliation with the Church of Scientology, an organization strongly opposed to *any* psychiatric diagnosis or psychiatric treatment for any disorder. A statement published in 2001 by the Church of Scientology includes the following:

> Scientology is unalterably opposed, as a matter of religious be-
> lief, to the practice of psychiatry, and espouses as a religious be-
> lief that the study of the mind and the healing of mentally
> caused ills should not be alienated from religion or condoned in
> nonreligous fields . . . mental problems are spiritual in nature.

Some individuals espousing such views have even persuaded legisla-tors in a few states to pass laws impeding access to such medications or forbidding school staff from talking with parents about ADHD. Radical advocates for this viewpoint have also organized letter-writing or media campaigns to challenge school boards or to attack the credibility of physi-cians, psychologists, or educators who advocate for scientific views of ADHD. In a few extreme cases in Europe and the United States, promi-nent professionals advocating for ADHD have been harassed and threat-ened in their offices and homes.

In 2000, plaintiffs promoting such radical views filed lawsuits in Texas, California, New Jersey, Florida, and Puerto Rico against the Amer-ican Psychiatric Association, the Novartis pharmaceutical company (man-ufacturer of Ritalin), and Children and Adults with ADHD (CHADD), an advocacy group with over twenty thousand members that has led national efforts to provide scientific information about ADHD to parents and pro-fessionals. These suits alleged a conspiracy among Novartis, CHADD, and the American Psychiatric Association to foist the ADHD diagnosis on the public in order to increase sales of medications for ADHD. All five suits were eventually withdrawn or dismissed by the courts, in some cases with prejudice because the suits were deemed frivolous.

More Moderate Criticisms about ADHD

A somewhat less ideological criticism of the ADHD diagnosis and its treatment has occurred in some media, including a variety of books like Thomas Armstrong's *The Myth of the ADD Child* (1995). Armstrong argues that although there are some children who won't behave or pay attention despite appearing normal in other ways, these problems are caused not by inherited impairments of brain function, but by a variety of societal or family problems. Armstrong referred to ADD as "a social invention," a "symptom of societal breakdown," a "response to boring classrooms," a "'bad fit' between parent and child," and "a different way of learning." He acknowledged that stimulant medication might be appropriate for some affected children, but only briefly and for specific situations.

As alternatives to medication for ADHD, Armstrong advises that parents "provide a balanced breakfast," "find out what interests your child," "enroll your child in a martial arts program," "use background music to focus and calm," "provide a variety of stimulating learning activities," "provide positive role models," and employ a variety of other strategies to give the child more attention, flexible but supportive structure, and positively toned discipline.

Most of the strategies recommended by Armstrong would be helpful for any child, including those with ADD syndrome, but in themselves they are not likely to alleviate the persisting problems of those children whose impairments are sufficient to warrant the diagnosis of ADHD.

Arguments from critics like Armstrong and others such as Lawrence Diller—who described ADD as "a catch-all condition encompassing a variety of children's behavioral problems" (Diller 1998, p. 63)—are useful because they caution against overly simplistic medical understandings of ADHD and its treatment. They remind readers of the importance of optimizing classroom environments and providing direct, consistent parental support for each child. They also warn against inadequate evaluations and inadequate monitoring of medications, as well as the assumption that every problem can be fixed with medication. Most reasonable persons would readily agree with many of their fundamental arguments.

These authors, however, seem to be working with a simplistic notion of ADHD. They characterize the disorder as unpleasant misbehavior, excessive restlessness, or intermittent distractibility. They fail to grasp the broad complexity of impairments associated with ADD syndrome, or the power of this disorder to disrupt and seriously impair the daily functioning of affected individuals and their families over months, years, and lifetimes.

ADD Syndrome Can Cause Tragic, Sustained Suffering

Throughout the United States and around the world I have spoken with many individuals who have ADD syndrome and with their family members. Repeatedly they have shown me compelling evidence that ADD syndrome can seriously impair daily functioning, disrupt ongoing development, and, in some severe cases, threaten life itself.

One especially poignant example involves Joel, a bright, lively boy whom I met a few years ago in Scotland. Joel's mother had told me about how her son had struggled from his earliest years. He was unable to control his chronic restlessness and hyperactivity, and despite his mother's persistent efforts, there was no treatment available for him. Though very bright, he had great difficulty learning and was often seriously disruptive in class. He had been repeatedly suspended from school and was finally expelled.

When I met Joel at age fifteen, he was a handsome, well-developed, appealing boy in a wheelchair. He was unable to walk and could move his arms and fingers only in contorted ways. He was unable to speak, but he could smile and was able to understand much of what was said to him. His ADHD had not been diagnosed or treated until he was twelve years old, and even then the treatment had been insufficient. Joel had continued to struggle with severe ADHD impairments that were extremely disruptive at school and at home.

At age fourteen, Joel had attempted to hang himself at home. According to a local newspaper:

> His mother said, "Since [his] earliest years he went haywire in class. He couldn't even sit down for five minutes. At the age of nine he had been suspended from school 11 times . . . Joel was an intelligent boy with an IQ of 126 (superior range) . . . he could be really affectionate and he had a wonderful sense of humor. . . . He was eventually excluded from school and it hit

him hard. . . . He felt very low, very lousy and isolated. . . . On the evening of November 14, 1999 I found Joel lying on the floor where he fell after he hanged himself. He was blue and not breathing. I thought he was dead."

Joel was eventually resuscitated, but only after parts of his brain had been permanently damaged by lack of sufficient oxygen. Since that time he has remained bound to a wheelchair, completely dependent on assistance for even the most basic tasks of eating and self-care. His mother commented to the newspaper reporter, "I think that there are a lot of children and adults out there who have taken their own lives because of this disorder [ADHD] . . . but so many times another explanation is found for a suicide and the truth stays hidden."

Another mother wrote a letter that was passed to me one morning shortly before the start of a workshop I was teaching in the Midwest. It read:

Last year my son, Jason, attended your talks on ADHD. He was very interested in what you had to say, especially about persons with ADHD who have high IQ. . . . I planned to attend your talk today, but instead we are planning Jason's memorial service for tomorrow. He committed suicide on January 28th. . . . He was 23.

Suffice it to say, Jason has had a long history of academic problems, anxiety, depression, self-esteem issues, and social isolation going all the way back to elementary school, maybe even nursery school. But because he was so bright, so likeable by adults, good-looking, and never outwardly complained . . . his conglomerate of characteristics was not labeled until last year.

Jason was attempting college for the third time. . . . I'm sure he became anxious and convinced of failure again. . . . He shot himself with a high-gauge shotgun. . . . He left a beautiful, kind and gentle letter. . . . I think he died of a broken heart, feeling he could never garner what it would take to conquer his "fatal flaws." I feel Jason's story is important for others to know. This disability, ADHD, killed him! We are devastated by his loss.

For some like Joel and Jason, the consequences of living for years with untreated or inadequately treated ADD syndrome and related problems can be devastating. In many other cases, the consequences are less dramatic, but nevertheless costly in a variety of ways.

The Many Costs of ADD Syndrome

A cute little six-year-old boy sat in my office with his parents. His big brown eyes were downcast and he looked deeply sad. I asked him, "Why are you here to talk with me today?" He kept staring down at the rug and mumbled, "Because I'm bad; I'm very, very bad." How does one assess the costs in self-esteem and diminished hope for a child who persistently sees himself in this way at the age of six? How can one anticipate the costs of living with such a view of oneself over the longer term, especially if no treatment is provided to interrupt the cycle of negative behaviors and the reactions of others?

And how does one assess the costs to an individual who receives appropriate treatment, but only late in his schooling? One high school senior came into my office for a follow-up session three months after his ADHD had been diagnosed and treated for the first time. Throughout junior high and high school this student had been chided repeatedly by his parents and teachers. They had reminded him about his very superior abilities demonstrated in standardized tests. They had confronted him about how he had been placed in classes for gifted students throughout elementary school and then removed from such classes in junior high because he was too inconsistent about studying and completing homework assignments. They had warned him that despite his strong abilities and high ambitions, he would be unable to gain admission to a good university unless he improved his grades.

It was the time in March when most colleges and universities let applicants know whether they will be admitted. The student said:

> You know, I'm grateful that my ADD has finally been diagnosed and I'm glad I have this medicine now. It helps me a lot. Every one of my teachers has commented about how now I'm doing a lot better. They noticed within a week of my starting the medi-

cine, and none of them knew I had started it. They just saw that all of a sudden I was consistent in getting my homework done and was really participating in class discussions.

What I'm not grateful for is the fact that nobody recognized and did anything about this until the middle of my last year in high school. When I was in elementary school I was always in the gifted classes. When I got to middle school and high school I got kicked out of those and put in lower-level classes because I couldn't keep up with the work and wasn't prepared enough for class.

I still hang out with those kids who were my classmates in the gifted classes back then. We all get along. We enjoy the same jokes and share the same interests. Now they're all getting admitted to top-tier universities and I'll be lucky to get into a third-rate college because my grades have been so pathetic. I'm just as smart as those friends of mine, but there is no way now that I can go back and redo the years that got me that lousy transcript! It pisses me off that I didn't have this treatment six or eight years ago! If I had, my life would have been very different and I'd have a lot more opportunities open to me today.

Even in the large number of cases where ADD syndrome impairments are not life-threatening, the consequences of not treating this syndrome can be constricting and damaging in persistent and significant ways. To go through school with untreated ADD syndrome is like trying to run a marathon carrying a knapsack of bricks. One can do it, but it is much harder to run with the bricks, and one's race time—the result of all of that hard work—will probably be much worse than the times of others who are running without the extra load.

For many, not all, with ADD syndrome the burden of frustration and discouragement begins very early and gets progressively worse. Some educators refer to the "Matthew effect" to describe how children who get a good start in learning to read tend to do increasingly well in their schooling as they grow older. In contrast, children who get a weak or late start in reading tend to get further and further behind as they go through school. The reference is biblical, from the Gospel according to Matthew, chapter 25:

> For unto everyone that hath shall be given, and he shall have
> abundance; but from him that hath not shall be taken away even
> that which he hath.

Keith Stanovich (2000) illustrated how this process can unfold in the development of vocabulary and reading skills:

> Children who are reading well and who have good vocabulary
> will read more, learn more word meanings, and hence read even
> better. Children with inadequate vocabularies—who read slowly
> and without enjoyment—read less, and as a result have slower
> development of vocabulary knowledge, which inhibits further
> growth in reading ability. (p. 184)

If this line of reasoning is extended to cover not just reading, math, and other academic skills, but also the ability to utilize executive functions throughout each stage of development, the implications are staggering. When a young child suffers from untreated ADD syndrome, that child is likely to encounter persisting difficulties with academic and social demands in many aspects of life: school, family, and social tasks and interactions. Depending on the severity of impairment and the adequacy of supports available, the child is likely to experience frustrations and delays that at best will make life more difficult, and at worst, may cause life to feel unmanageable.

It is clear that individuals with ADD syndrome often suffer considerably from their inherited impairments of executive function. It is also clear that there are safe and effective treatments available that can alleviate these impairments in 70 to 80 percent of those afflicted. So why do most individuals with ADD syndrome still not receive adequate diagnosis or treatments?

Patients, parents, and professionals throughout the United States and in twenty-five other countries have described to me barriers to effective treatment of ADD syndrome that seem persistent in every culture: (1) fears due to inadequate understanding of ADD syndrome and its treatment, (2) a lack of adequate resources for assessment and treatment,

(3) prejudice against considering genes as a major cause of ADD syndrome, and (4) prejudice against using medications to treat apparent "lack of willpower."

Fears Due to Inadequate Understanding

When a child, adolescent, or adult repeatedly fails to do what they should be able to do, most people have an explanation. In such situations many quickly assume that the person is performing poorly simply because they are lazy, stupid, stubborn, unmotivated, defiant, or some combination of these. Sometimes such assumptions are correct. Often they are not.

In every culture in every generation there probably have been substantial numbers of individuals who failed to meet performance expectations because they suffered from ADD syndrome. In most cases, their failures have probably been explained by their parents, teachers, bosses, coworkers, spouses, and friends as due to lack of motivation, lack of ability, or poor attitude. Undoubtedly many chronically failing individuals explained their shortcomings to themselves in similar ways.

Significantly, these explanations for failures are usually infused with emotion. Parents, teachers, and others feel discouragement, worry, frustration, and anger when they are repeatedly disappointed in their efforts to encourage a struggling individual to work harder, longer, and better to do what should be done.

Moreover, these mistaken assumptions are deeply entrenched in the public consciousness. Educating the public about ADHD is thus no simple matter. In explaining ADD to most people, we are trying to counter strongly held misunderstandings with more accurate, scientifically based information about the disorder and its treatment, but often people see no need for a different explanation. Many believe that they clearly understand this disorder when they truly do not.

Yet helping people develop a scientifically accurate understanding of ADD syndrome is vitally important, because common misunderstandings of ADD syndrome perpetuate the suffering of children, adolescents, and adults afflicted with this disorder. Parents and professionals who believe ADHD is an insignificant and transient problem of childhood or just a diagnostic fad are not likely to help those who are suffering find adequate assessment and treatment.

Unrealistic fears of the diagnosis and treatment are also a problem for many, and those who do not understand that ADHD is a complicated and significantly impairing problem are not likely to learn enough about the disorder to alleviate those fears. For example, many parents worry that if they provide stimulant treatment for their son or daughter with ADHD, the child might have an increased risk of drug addiction later in life. Ironically, by not seeking information about ADHD treatment, they are not likely to find out that a child who has ADHD, if untreated or inadequately treated, has *double* the risk of suffering, at some point in life, from substance abuse severe enough to warrant diagnosis. Indeed, five scientific studies involving almost a thousand children with ADHD have demonstrated that children whose ADHD is consistently treated with appropriate medications during childhood and adolescence have their elevated risk of substance abuse *reduced,* essentially to that of a child without ADHD (Wilens, Faraone, et al. 2003).

Lack of Adequate Resources for Assessment and Treatment

Not every community has adequate resources to provide assessment and treatment of ADD syndrome for children; most do not yet have any resources for treating adolescents and adults with this disorder. For most families in developing countries and for many even in the more developed countries, access to medical care is extremely limited. Many do not have access to adequately trained physicians for life-threatening medical conditions, let alone services for mental health. Even in communities where psychologists and physicians are available, patients are often put on waiting lists for many months or even years. Moreover, even when accessible, these caregivers may or may not be familiar with current understandings of ADD and its appropriate treatment.

Clinicians tend to interpret each patient's presenting complaints within the framework of diagnoses they know well. If they have been trained to recognize and treat depression and anxiety, but lack adequate training to identify and treat ADHD, clinicians are likely to interpret patients' presenting complaints about impaired short-term memory, inattention, disorganization, underachievement, and so on as signs of anxiety or depressive problems. They also are likely to provide treatments appropriate for those disorders without even considering the possibility that these may be symptoms of ADHD, with or without comorbid anxiety or depression.

Even in those communities where physicians and medications are available, such services and medications remain inaccessible to many because of cost. If family members are struggling to pay rent and to put food on the table each day, they are not likely to be able to afford visits to a doctor or medications, especially for a disorder that does not present any immediate, obvious threat to physical health or to life. Even if a family wants very much to provide appropriate treatment for a member with impairments of ADD, the costs may be prohibitive and insurance often does not cover them. Medication costs, especially for the newer, longer-acting formulations, are significant. The expense of consultations with psychologists and physicians for assessment and ongoing treatment can also be substantial. Many families simply cannot afford to begin—or to continue—treatment for ADD syndrome.

When behavioral treatments are added to medication, the costs increase substantially. Peter Jensen (2003) showed that the cost of alleviating impairments of children with ADHD to the point of "normalization" using MTA behavioral treatment alone or in combination with medication management was four times the cost of typical community care. In that study, the most cost-effective treatment for ADHD was careful medication management. (Combined behavioral and medication management treatments were somewhat more cost-effective for children with ADHD and comorbid disorders.)

Many are quick to argue that every patient with ADHD should receive all relevant treatments. Such an outlook makes sense only to those who hold unrealistic views of what professional and financial resources are actually available to most of the world's families. The unfortunate truth is that in many parts of the world at this time, only the most fortunate are likely to have access to appropriate assessment and treatments for ADD.

Prejudice against Recognizing Genes as a Major Cause

Even when resources for assessment and treatment are available and affordable, and even if individuals have been exposed to scientific information about ADD, some are reluctant to believe that problems of cognitive functioning associated with ADD are not simply the result of poor parenting or poor schooling.

Many hold persistently to a view of human nature first introduced in the sixteenth century and labeled "blank slate" by Steven Pinker (2002): that human nature is almost infinitely malleable, fully open to the shaping influences of parents, teachers, and other influences of culture, with few significant constraints. Pinker argues instead that genetic influences and other extrafamilial forces are far more powerful in shaping human nature and behavior than are family influences. He proposes three "laws" to explain influences on human behavior:

1. All human behavioral traits are heritable.
2. The effect of being raised in the same family is smaller than the effect of genes.
3. A substantial portion of the variation in complex human behavioral traits is not accounted for by the effects of genes or families.
   (p. 373)

Pinker recognizes that many studies show similarities between children and their parents. He suggests that such similarities may not result from the child learning to adopt parental behavior styles, but rather can be explained by genetic similarities between parent and child—for example, aggressive parents may have aggressive children, talkative parents may end up with talkative children, and so on. He believes that genetic factors are the most powerful shapers of a child's development and behavior, and that unique aspects of their environment contribute much of the rest.

A substantial body of research has demonstrated that genetic factors play a very large role in the etiology of ADHD. Steven Faraone and colleagues (1998) and Rosemary Tannock (1998) have summarized findings of multiple twin and adoption studies that indicate high heritability rates for ADHD and components of ADHD: from .75 to .98, with an average of about .80. By comparison, the heritability index for height is .95. At the group level, approximately 80 percent of the variance in whether an individual has ADHD can be explained by genetic factors.

The high heritability index for ADHD does not mean that these impairments are caused by a single gene. Modern genetic research thus far has identified several specific genes that contribute to ADHD, but no single gene (Thapar 2002). For this disorder, as for most others, its emergence appears to be related to small effects of multiple genes interacting rather than a large effect from one or two specific genes.

Genes are substantial risk factors for ADHD, but they do not completely explain its occurrence. Environmental factors contribute at least 20 percent to the variation in emergence of the ADD syndrome. These factors may include smoking, alcohol use, or drug use by the mother during pregnancy (Mick, Biederman, et al. 2002); complications of pregnancy, delivery, or early infancy such as toxemia or eclampsia; fetal distress; low birth weight; and difficult delivery (Sprich-Buckminster, Biederman, et al. 1993; Faraone and Biederman 1998). Psychosocial adversity such as severe marital discord, paternal criminality, and poverty have also been shown to increase vulnerability to ADHD in those genetically at risk (Biederman, Milberger, et al. 1995b; Biederman, Faraone, et al. 1996).

The main point here is that impairments of ADHD result not from a choice made by the person with ADHD nor from parental negligence. ADHD results primarily from genetic factors interacting with prenatal, perinatal, and postnatal experiences that together cause significant impairment in the brain. Given these findings, it makes little sense to blame victims of ADHD for having the disorder or to censure their parents for causing it.

The Bias against Treating a Presumed "Lack of Willpower"

Many who understand this biologically based view of ADHD remain reluctant to see medication used as the primary treatment. They tend to think of cognitive problems in ADD syndrome as a special category of impairment, very different from malfunctions of the pancreas, heart, eyes, or other bodily organs. For malfunctions of virtually every other organ system, most educated people today see prescription medication as an appropriate and often necessary treatment. Yet when the problem relates to workings of the brain, these same individuals may object to medication treatments and insist that the individual ought to fix the problems by "willpower" or some other variant of conscious effort.

Indeed, many believe that all cognitive processes can be brought under conscious control, that any individual can make changes in how he thinks, what he feels, and how he acts, if only his determination is strong enough. This is the view that Daniel Wegner (2002) has challenged as "the illusion of free will." Although he acknowledges that this illusion has adaptive functions, Wegner quotes approvingly Bernard Schlink's (1997) words,

> I don't mean to say that the thinking and reaching decisions
> have no influence on behavior. But behavior does not merely
> enact what has already been thought through and decided. It has
> its own sources. (p. 342)

Opposite to the view that willpower, or conscious effort, can control all mental processes is the view that most mental processes operate outside the realm of consciousness. As I have explained, executive functions are quick, subtle, and complex, usually operating without much input from conscious thought. Executive-function processes are not usually responsive to "willpower" on any substantial or sustained basis. But this "non-willpower" view of mental functioning is misunderstood by many and strongly opposed by some.

Resistance to the idea that much of the work of the mind is unconscious is not new. In 1917 Sigmund Freud published a short paper as a response to the strong emotional reaction many professionals and lay people had to his emphasis on the role of unconscious processes in mental life.

> You believe that you are informed of all that goes on in your
> mind if it is of any importance at all, because your conscious-
> ness gives you news of it. . . . Indeed, you go so far as to regard
> "the mind" as coextensive with "consciousness," that is, with

what is known to you, in spite of the most obvious evidence that
a great deal more is perpetually going on in your mind than can
be known to your consciousness. (p. 189)

Freud concluded that people generally felt offended by his assertions that
"the ego is not master in its own house," that persons are not in conscious
and deliberate control of all that they do. He recognized that many individuals are threatened by the idea that their thoughts and actions are
shaped by internal forces as well as external events and that these internal
forces are, in many ways, not at all under their conscious control or even
within their own awareness.

   Since Freud's time, much more has been learned about the unconscious workings of the mind. A new view of "the unconscious," quite
different from psychoanalytic formulations, is emerging in psychology
and neuroscience (see Hassin, Uleman, and Bargh 2005). But still many
persons are reluctant to believe that their conscious thought does not
reign supreme over their cognition. Even though they do not expect to
control by willpower the endocrine malfunctions of diabetes or the growth
of a cancer, they want to believe that willpower can sustain control over
malfunctioning cognitive processes that, among other important tasks,
organize and prioritize, maintain working memory, activate effort, and
regulate alertness.

   It is ironic that many who strongly resist the notion that prescription
medications may be needed to alleviate ADHD have no problem with
using everyday stimulants to aid their own cognitive functioning. Richard
Rudgley (1993) has described the longstanding and widespread use of
stimulants such as coffee, tea, cola, tobacco, and betel nut throughout the
world to improve alertness and concentration in daily life. Because one or
another of these substances is usually readily available and socially sanc-
tioned, many do not recognize that they are providing—on a more transient, erratic, and somewhat less potent basis—stimulation to cognitive
processes very similar to the actions of medications commonly prescribed
for ADHD. Use of these nonprescription agents is not seen by most as
compromising self-discipline and willpower. But in many cases they are
nevertheless prejudiced against the use of such medications to alleviate

ADD syndrome impairments that, they believe, should be corrected by force of conscious will.

This prejudice against use of medications to alleviate cognitive impairments is not merely a philosophical issue. It has very important practical implications for decisions about how persons with impaired executive functioning are to be understood and treated. If one maintains that an individual suffering from ADD syndrome can overcome these impairments simply by trying harder, then intensified instruction and reinforcement with rewards and punishments alone would seem to be sufficient intervention.

But if one understands impairments of ADD syndrome as malfunctions of cognitive processes that operate essentially outside conscious control, then intensified instruction, rewards, and punishment are not enough: medication is required. In this book I have argued that ADD syndrome results from chronic impairments in cognitive processes that, for the most part, operate outside the realm of conscious control, that are not responsive on any sustained basis to "willpower."

Realistic and Unrealistic Hope

Any discussions of hope usually emphasize that one should use willpower and determination to overcome adversity. This view often is used to challenge persons with ADD syndrome. Children, adolescents, and adults with ADD syndrome often are told that if only they will push themselves hard enough and long enough, if only they will put forth enough determined effort, then they will be able to overcome their problems with inconsistency, disorganization, working memory, emotional regulation, and so on. Such exhortations are not helpful and may be damaging. This advice is equivalent to urging a driver to step more forcefully on the accelerator to move a car with a nonfunctioning transmission.

Parents, educators, and clinicians who insist that those with ADD syndrome can overcome their impairments without medication treatment are offering unrealistic hope, which is likely ultimately to lead those who suffer from ADD syndrome to feel only more frustrated and more persistently hopeless.

Psychologists Peg Dawson and Richard Guare (2004) have contributed to the problem of unrealistic hope with their manual intended to guide educational professionals, clinicians, and parents in providing interventions for children and adolescents who demonstrate "weak executive skills." They discuss reasonably how school and home environments might be modified to support a child with these impairments. And they acknowledge the need for children to learn to carry out executive functions with progressively less adult support. But these authors refer to executive functions as though they are simply a set of skills to be learned and consciously exercised, much as one might learn how to type or to speak a foreign language. For example, they offer strategies

> to change the child's capacity for using her own executive skills. This can be done in one of two ways: 1) by motivating her to use executive skills she has but is reluctant to employ, or 2) by teaching her ways to develop or fine-tune executive skills she needs. . . . most youngsters who fail to use executive skills do so not because they don't care but because they don't yet have the executive skill. Thus, we generally recommend that parents and teachers assume this is true and begin tackling executive skill development by *teaching the desired skills.* (p. 39; italics added)

The executive functions impaired in ADD syndrome are not simply skills that need to be learned. Trying to improve the lives of persons with ADD syndrome simply by attempting to teach them "executive skills" and then "motivating them" to utilize this pedagogy is somewhat like installing improved software on a computer that lacks sufficient memory to run that software. It is comparable to providing didactic instruction in "social skills" to individuals with the "mindblindness" of autism and then expecting them to interact empathically with others. Such efforts at intervention for ADD syndrome may be well-intentioned, but they offer fundamentally unrealistic hope.

Antimedication attitudes about ADHD are not the only way to foster unrealistic hope. Some people burden patients by minimizing the suffering that often comes with ADD syndrome. They claim that this syndrome is not a disorder, but simply a different cognitive style, an approach to life that may in fact be preferable because it is not constrained much by routines and timetables. This is reminiscent of an argument made decades ago by a British psychiatrist, R. D. Laing (1997), who claimed that schizophrenia is not an illness, but simply a more creative way to experience the world. Such views ignore the reality of chronic suffering experienced by many impaired by ADD syndrome and illustrated in many examples in this book.

The issue here is not whether persons with ADD are totally helpless unless they take medication. There is good evidence that most persons with ADD have talents, abilities described by Robert Brooks and Sam Goldstein (2001) as "islands of competence," that can bring benefits to them and others whether they are taking medication or not. The hockey player discussed in Chapter 1 is one of many examples. The point here is simply that such talents often are not those needed to succeed in school or at work. Realistic hope recognizes ADD syndrome as a complex disorder that may significantly impair those affected in important ways, despite their strengths.

A third source of unrealistic hope is excessive optimism about the benefits of medication treatment. Some parents and professionals have been very impressed by dramatic and sustained improvements in ADD patients they know who have responded very well to medication treatment. They assume that anyone who takes such medication is likely to have equally transforming results. Advocates for medication treatment sometimes forget that 20 to 30 percent of those with ADD syndrome do not respond well to currently available medications. Eight out of ten are good odds—as long as one is among the eight.

When those who suffer impairments of ADD syndrome hear a promise of dramatic improvement from medication treatment and subsequently find that their symptoms do not respond well (or respond only partially) to currently available medications, they are likely to feel intense disappointment, frustration, and loss of hope. It is thus not only unrealistic, but also unfair to promise any patient that their ADD impairments will be substantially alleviated by medication or any other treatment. All one can responsibly say is that there is a substantial possibility that one or another of the available medication treatments for ADD will significantly improve that individual's ADD impairments, during periods when the medication is taken, if the kind and amount of medication are tailored to the individual.

Even when medication is optimally effective, for many with ADD syndrome medication alone is not sufficient treatment. Medication does not teach individuals skills that they have not learned. Moreover, medication treatments, when they do work, may help patients to mobilize the effort and cognitive functions required to make the changes they need to make, but success is never guaranteed. Realistic hope recognizes up front that the problems of life do not always have a fully adequate solution.

Luckily for some, suffering from ADD syndrome may ease as one gets out of school. The most difficult period for many with ADD syndrome is the time from about sixth grade through the first couple of years after high school, whether they then are in college or are engaged in another pursuit. It is during those years that individuals in most cultures are faced with the widest range of task demands with the least opportunity to escape from those tasks one finds especially difficult. If one is fortunate, it gradually becomes possible to specialize—to study or gain employment in a field where one can utilize one's strengths and avoid some areas of weakness by delegating tasks to others at work or at home. Some persons with significant ADD impairments struggle mightily throughout their schooling with poor or mediocre results but are able to achieve considerable success in, for example, business or the arts.

One factor that can help to create and sustain realistic hope in persons with ADD syndrome is ongoing emotional support provided by a parent, mentor, friend, or therapist who understands ADD syndrome and recognizes the patient's strengths. Adequate support and sufficient education about the disorder can help family members to cope with their own frustrations and may enable them to be less destructively critical and more reasonably supportive of one another.

Yet realistic hope also is tempered by the awareness that despite such interventions, untreated or inadequately treated ADD syndrome can take a great toll on one's self-esteem and on one's learning, critical capacities that may powerfully influence one's future. And timing can make a difference. Some are fortunate enough to have their ADD impairments recognized and effectively treated relatively early, before they have become too demoralized and before too many opportunities have been squandered or cut off. Others are not so fortunate. Their ADD impairments may not be recognized or treated until after the "Matthew effects" have substantially limited what might have been.

More and better research into these processes promises a clearer understanding of ADD and executive functions. Joaquin Fuster (2003) wrote that in contemporary neuroscience a new paradigm is emerging that "requires a Copernican shift in the way we construe how the cognitive code is represented and processed in the brain" (p. viii). He describes this revolution as a turn away from thinking of associative cognitive functions as residing in different locations of the brain. He argues that "cognitive functions per se have no definite cortical topography"— that perception, memory, attention, language, and intelligence all share the same common neural substrate.

Fuster emphasizes the almost seamlessly integrated operation of functions that many researchers currently think of as separate:

> Perception is part of the acquisition and retrieval of memory; memory stores information acquired by perception; language and memory depend on each other; language and logical reasoning are special forms of cognitive action; *attention serves all the other functions.* (p. 16; italics added)

Fuster's view of integrated cognitive functioning fits well with the way most persons with ADD syndrome describe their complex, interacting symptoms. It also is consistent with the view discussed in Chapter 8 that current diagnostic categories do not adequately reflect the pervasive and essential role of attention in both normal and abnormal functioning. Hopefully the years ahead will yield a clearer understanding of how these complicated workings of the human brain are related to ADD syndrome and how they add to the amazingly rich complexity of everyday human experience.

Resources

The websites listed here offer a variety of free information about attention deficit disorders. Most specialize in issues concerning children and adolescents; some focus more on adults. Many are sponsored by ADD support and advocacy organizations and provide detailed, downloadable information that has been evaluated and approved by a professional advisory board; others are less selective and may include reports that are not adequately supported by scientific research. Some list contact information for local support and advocacy groups concerned with attention deficit disorders. Many have links to related organizations, and all are nonprofit.

International Websites Based in the United States

- chadd.org offers scientifically reliable information in English and Spanish about ADD in children, adolescents, and adults. Sponsored by Children and Adults with ADHD (CHADD), the largest ADHD support and advocacy organization in the United States, it has downloadable fact sheets of science-based information for parents, educators, professionals, the media, and the general public. The site also includes contact information for two hundred local chapters of CHADD throughout the United States.

- help4adhd.org presents evidence-based information in English and Spanish about ADD in children, adolescents, and adults. This national clearing house of downloadable information and resources concerning many aspects of ADHD is funded by the U.S. government's Centers for Disease Control and Prevention and operated by CHADD. New material is added frequently, and questions directed to the site are responded to by knowledgeable health-information specialists.
- add.org is a resource in English for adults with ADD. Sponsored by Attention Deficit Disorder Association (ADDA), the world's largest organization for adults with ADHD, it provides information, resources, and networking opportunities.

International Websites Based in the United Kingdom

- info@addiss.co.uk presents information in English about ADHD across the lifespan. It serves patients, parents, teachers, and health professionals, and questions received by phone or email are answered. This site is sponsored by the National Attention Deficit Disorder Information and Support Service in the United Kingdom.
- adders.org provides a wide variety of information about ADHD in English, French, German, and Spanish. It posts websites and email addresses for support groups in forty different countries.

Websites with a National Focus

The following websites are sponsored by ADHD education and advocacy organizations in various countries. Some are much better established and provide much more reliable information than others. Many list addresses for local groups within their country. Usually the material is presented in the dominant language of the country listed.

Argentina
http://www.tdah.org.ar
Australia
ADD Association, Queensland (ADDAQ), http://www.addaq.org.au

Learning and Attentional Disorders Society (LADS),
  http://www.ladswa.com.au
Learning Difficulties Coalition NSW,
  http://www.learningdifficultiescoalition.org.au

Austria
http://www.adapt.at

Belgium
Balans, http://www.balansdigitaal.nl

Brazil
http://www.tdah.org.br/

Canada
http://www.ldac-taac.ca/

Denmark
http://www.adhd.dk

Estonia
http://www.elf.ee/

Finland
http://www.adhd-liitto.fi

France
http://hypersupers.org

Germany
Juvemus, http://www.juvemus.de
Ads, http://www.ads-ev.de
http://www.BV-AH.de

Hong Kong
http://www.snn.org.hk

Iceland
http://www.obis.is/adhd

Ireland
http://www.T.R.A.D.D.

Italy

AIFA, http://www.aifa.it

http://www.aidai.org/

Japan

http://www.e-club.jp

Mexico

http://www.deficitdeatencion.org/

The Netherlands

http://www.balansdigitaal.nl/

http://www.adhd.nl/

New Zealand

http://www.adhd.org.nz

Norway

http://www.adhd-foreningen.no

Romania

http://www.intermeding.com/speranta/

Spain

ADANA Fundación, http://www.f-adana.org

ANSHDA, http://www.anshda.org

APNADAH, http://www.tdah.org

References

Adler, L., R. C. Kessler, and T. Spencer. 2004. *Adult ADHD Self-Report Scale (ASRS v1.1)*, from www.med.nyu.edu/Psych/training/adhd.html.

Ainsworth, M. D. S., M. C. Blehar, et al. 1978. *Patterns of Attachment: A Psychological Study of the Strange Situation.* Hillsdale, N.J.: Erlbaum.

Akiskal, H. S. 1997. "Overview of Chronic Depressions and Their Clinical Management." In *Dysthymia and the Spectrum of Chronic Depressions*, ed. H. S. Akiskal and G. B. Cassano. New York: Guilford Press.

Alderman, N., P. W. Burgess, et al. 2003. "Ecological Validity of a Simplified Version of the Multiple Errands Shopping Task." *Journal of the International Neuropsychological Society* 9: 31–44.

Aman, M. G., C. Binder, et al. 2004. "Risperidone Effects in the Presence/Absence of Psychostimulant Medication in Children with ADHD, Other Disruptive Behavior Disorders, and Subaverage IQ." *Journal of Child and Adolescent Psychopharmacology* 14(2): 243–254.

American Academy of Child and Adolescent Psychiatry. 1997. "Practice Parameters for the Assessment and Treatment of Children, Adolescents, and Adults with Attention-Deficit/Hyperactivity Disorder." *Journal of the American Academy of Child and Adolescent Psychiatry* 36(10 Supplement): 85S–121S.

————. 2002. "Practice Parameter for the Use of Stimulant Medications in the Treatment of Children, Adolescents and Adults." *Journal of the American Academy of Child and Adolescent Psychiatry* 41(2 Supplement): 26S–49S.

American Academy of Pediatrics. 2000. "Clinical Practice Guideline: Diagnosis and Evaluation of the Child with Attention-Deficit/Hyperactivity Disorder." *Pediatrics* 105(5): 1158–1170.

————. 2001. "Clinical Practice Guideline: Treatment of the School-Aged Child with Attention-Deficit/Hyperactivity Disorder." *Pediatrics* 108(4): 1033–1044.

American Psychiatric Association. 1980. *Diagnostic and Statistical Manual of Mental Disorders.* Washington, D.C.: American Psychiatric Association.

————. 1994. *Diagnostic and Statistical Manual of Mental Disorders.* 4th ed. Washington, D.C.: American Psychiatric Association.

————. 2001. *Diagnostic and Statistical Manual of Mental Disorders.* 4th ed., text rev. Washington, D.C.: American Psychiatric Press.

Anastopoulos, A. D., and L. M. Gerrard. 2003. "Facilitating Understanding and Management of Attention-Deficit/Hyperactivity Disorder." In *Cognitive Therapy with Children and Adolescents,* ed. M. A. Reinecke, F. M. Dattilio, and A. Freeman. New York: Guilford Press. Pp. 19–42.

Anastopoulos, A. D., J. M. Smith, et al. 1998. "Counseling and Training Parents." In *Attention-Deficit Hyperactivity Disorder: Handbook for Diagnosis and Treatment,* ed. R. A. Barkley. New York: Guilford Press.

Anderson, C. M., A. Polcari, et al. 2002. "Effects of Methylphenidate on Functional Magnetic Resonance Relaxometry of the Cerebellar Vermis in Boys with ADHD." *American Journal of Psychiatry* 159(8): 1322–1328.

Armstrong, T. 1995. *The Myth of the ADD Child.* New York: Penguin Putnam.

Arnold, L. E. 2000. "Methylphenidate versus Amphetamine: A Comparative Review." In *Ritalin: Theory and Practice.* 2d ed., ed. L. L. Greenhill and B. B. Osman. Larchmont, N.Y.: Mary Ann Liebert. Pp. 127–137.

————. 2002. "Treatment Alternatives for Attention Deficit Hyperactivity Disorder." In *Attention Deficit Hyperactivity Disorder: State of the Science— Best Practices,* ed. P. S. Jensen and J. R. Cooper. Kingston, N.J.: Civic Research Institute. 13:1–29.

Backman, L., N. Ginovart, et al. 2000. "Age-Related Cognitive Deficits Mediated by Changes in the Striatal Dopamine System." *American Journal of Psychiatry* 157(4): 635–637.

Bargh, J. A. 2005. "Bypassing the Will: Toward Demystifying the Nonconscious Control of Social Behavior." In *The New Unconscious*, ed. R. A. Hassin, J. S. Uleman, and J. A. Bargh. New York: Oxford University Press. Pp. 37–58.

Barkley, R. A. 1993. "A New Theory of ADHD." *ADHD Report* 1(5): 1–4.

———. 1997. *ADHD and the Nature of Self-Control*. New York: Guilford Press.

———. 1998. *Attention-Deficit Hyperactivity Disorder: Handbook for Diagnosis and Treatment*. New York: Guilford Press.

———. 2000. *Taking Charge of ADHD*. New York: Guilford Press.

———. 2003. "EEG and Neurofeedback Findings in ADHD: Editorial Commentary." *ADHD Report* 11(3): 7–8.

Barkley, R. A., and J. Biederman. 1997. "Toward a Broader Definition of the Age-of-Onset Criterion for Attention-Deficit Hyperactivity Disorder." *Journal of the American Academy of Child and Adolescent Psychiatry* 36(9): 1204–1210.

Barkley, R. A., E. A. Cook, et al. 2002. "Consensus Statement on ADHD." *European Child and Adolescent Psychiatry* 11(2): 96–98.

Barkley, R. A., and K. R. Murphy. 1998. *Attention-Deficit Hyperactivity Disorder: A Clinical Workbook*. New York: Guilford Press.

Barkley, R. A., K. R. Murphy, et al. 1996. "Psychological Adjustment and Adaptive Impairments in Young Adults with ADHD." *Journal of Attention Disorders* 1(1): 41–54.

———. 2001a. "Time Perception and Reproduction in Young Adults with Attention Deficit Hyperactivity Disorder." *Neuropsychology* 15(3): 351–360.

———. 2001b. "The Inattentive Type of ADHD as a Distinct Disorder: What Remains to Be Done?" *Clinical Psychology: Science and Practice* 8(4): 489–501.

———. 2002. "Driving in Young Adults with Attention Deficit Hyperactivity Disorder: Knowledge, Performance, Adverse Outcomes and Role of Executive Functioning." *Journal of the International Neuropsychological Society* 8: 655–672.

Baron-Cohen, S. 2003. *The Essential Difference: The Truth about the Male and Female Brain.* New York: Basic Books.

Baxter, M. G., and E. A. Murray. 2002. "The Amygdala and Reward." *Nature Reviews: Neuroscience* 3: 563–573.

Bear, M. F., B. W. Connors, and M. A. Paradiso. 1996. *Neuroscience: Exploring the Brain.* Baltimore, Md.: Williams and Wilkins.

Bedard, A.-C., A. Ickowicz, et al. 2003. "Selective Inhibition in Children with Attention-Deficit Hyperactivity Disorder Off and On Stimulant Medication." *Journal of Abnormal Child Psychology* 31(3): 315–327.

Beitchman, J. H., E. B. Brownlie, et al. 1996. "Linguistic Impairment and Psychiatric Disorder: Pathways to Outcome." In *Language, Learning, and Behavior Disorders: Developmental, Biological and Clinical Perspectives,* ed. J. H. Beitchman, N. J. Cohen, M. M. Konstantareas, and R. Tannock. Cambridge, Eng.: Cambridge University Press. Pp. 493–514.

Benedetto-Nasho, E., and R. Tannock. 1999. "Math Computation, Error Patterns, and Stimulant Effects in Children with Attention Deficit Hyperactivity Disorder." *Journal of Attention Disorders* 3(3): 121–134.

Benes, F. 2001. "The Development of Prefrontal Cortex: The Maturation of Neurotransmitter Systems and Their Interactions." In *Handbook of Developmental Cognitive Neuroscience,* ed. C. A. Nelson and M. Luciana. Cambridge, Mass.: MIT Press. Pp. 79–92.

Benes, F. M., M. Turtle, et al. 1994. "Myelination of a Key Relay Zone in the Hippocampal Formation Occurs in Human Brain during Childhood, Adolescence and Adulthood." *Archives of General Psychiatry* 51: 477–484.

Berninger, V. W., and T. L. Richards. 2002. *Brain Literacy for Educators and Psychologists.* New York, Academic Press.

Biederman, J., S. V. Faraone, et al. 1993. "Patterns of Psychiatric Comorbidity, Cognition, and Psychosocial Functioning in Adults with Attention Deficit Disorder." *American Journal of Psychiatry* 150(12): 1792–1798.

———. 1995. "High Risk for Attention Deficit Hyperactivity Disorder among Children of Parents with Childhood Onset of the Disorder: A Pilot Study." *American Journal of Psychiatry* 152(3): 431–435.

———. 1999. "Clinical Correlates of ADHD in Females: Findings from a Large Group of Girls Ascertained from Pediatric and Psychiatric Referral

Sources." *Journal of the American Academy of Child and Adolescent Psychiatry* 38(8): 966–975.

———. 2004. "Gender Effects on Attention-Deficit/Hyperactivity Disorder in Adults: Revisited." *Biological Psychiatry* 55: 692–700.

Biederman, J., E. Mick, et al. 2000. "Therapeutic Dilemmas in the Pharmacotherapy of Bipolar Depression in the Young." *Journal of Child and Adolescent Psychopharmacology* 10(3): 185–192.

———. 2002. "Influence of Gender on Attention Deficit Hyperactivity Disorder in Children Referred to a Psychiatric Clinic." *American Journal of Psychiatry* 159(1): 36–42.

Biederman, J., S. Millberger, et al. 1995a. "Family-Environment Risk Factors for Attention-Deficit Hyperactivity Disorder: A Test of Rutter's Indicators of Adversity." *Archives of General Psychiatry* 52: 464–470.

———. 1995b. "Impact of Adversity on Functioning and Comorbidity in Children with Attention-Deficit Hyperactivity Disorder." *Journal of the American Academy of Child and Adolescent Psychiatry* 34(11): 1495–1503.

Biederman, J., J. A. Rosenbaum, et al. 1993. "A Three-Year Follow-up of Children with and without Behavioral Inhibition." *Journal of the American Academy of Child and Adolescent Psychiatry* 32: 814–821.

Biederman, J., and T. Spencer. 1999. "Attention-Deficit/Hyperactivity Disorder (ADHD) as a Noradrenergic Disorder." *Biological Psychiatry* 46: 1234–1242.

Biederman, J., S. Faraone, et al. 1996. "Predictors of Persistence and Remission of ADHD into Adolescence: Results from a Four-Year Prospective Follow-up Study." *Journal of the American Academy of Child and Adolescent Psychiatry* 35(3): 343–351.

Biederman, J., R. A. Thisted, et al. 1995. "Estimation of the Association between Desipramine and the Risk of Sudden Death in Five- to Fourteen-Year-Old Children." *Journal of Clinical Psychiatry* 56(3): 87–93.

Biederman, J., T. E. Wilens, et al. 1997. "Is ADHD a Risk Factor for Psychoactive Substance Abuse Disorders? Findings from a Four-Year Prospective Follow-up Study." *Journal of the American Academy of Child and Adolescent Psychiatry* 36(1): 21–29.

———. 1998. "Does Attention-Deficit Hyperactivity Disorder Impact the Developmental Course of Drug and Alcohol Abuse and Dependence?" *Biological Psychiatry* 44: 269–273.

Bird, H. R. 2002. "Diagnostic Classification, Epidemiology, and Cross-Cultural Validity of ADHD." In *Attention Deficit Hyperactivity Disorder: State of the Science—Best Practices,* ed. P. S. Jensen and J. R. Cooper. Kingston, N.J.: Civic Research Institute. 2: 1–16.

Bird, H. R., M. S. Gould, et al. 1993. "Patterns of Diagnostic Comorbidity in a Community Sample of Children Aged Nine through Sixteen Years." *Journal of the American Academy of Child and Adolescent Psychiatry* 32(2): 361–368.

Blachman, D. K., and S. P. Hinshaw. 2002. "Patterns of Friendship among Girls with and without Attention-Deficit/Hyperactivity Disorder." *Journal of Abnormal Child Psychology* 30(6): 625–640.

Blair, R. J. R. 1995. "A Cognitive Developmental Approach to Morality: Investigating the Psychopath." *Cognition* 57: 1–29.

Bowlby, J. 1978. "Attachment Theory and Its Therapeutic Implications." In *Adolescent Psychiatry: Developmental and Clinical Studies,* ed. S. Feinstein and P. L. Giovacchini. Chicago: University of Chicago. 6: 5–33.

Bradley, C. 1937. "Behavior of Children Receiving Benzedrine." *American Journal of Psychiatry* 94(11): 577–585.

Brooks, R., and S. Goldstein. 2001. *Raising Resilent Children.* Chicago: Contemporary Books.

Brown, T. E. 1996a. *Brown ADD Diagnostic Form for Adolescents.* San Antonio, Tex.: Psychological Corporation.

———. 1996b. *Brown ADD Diagnostic Form for Adults.* San Antonio, Tex.: Psychological Corporation.

———. 1996c. *Brown Attention Deficit Disorder Scales for Adolescents and Adults: Manual.* San Antonio, Tex.: Psychological Corporation.

———, ed. 2000. *Attention Deficit Disorders and Comorbidities in Children, Adolescents, and Adults.* Washington, D.C.: American Psychiatric Press.

———. 2001a. *Brown ADD Diagnostic Form for Adolescents—Revised.* San Antonio, Tex.: Psychological Corporation.

———. 2001b. *Brown ADD Diagnostic Form for Children.* San Antonio, Tex.: Psychological Corporation.

———. 2001c. *Brown Attention Deficit Disorder Scales for Children and Adolescents: Manual.* San Antonio, Tex.: Psychological Corporation.

———. 2004. "Atomoxetine and Stimulants in Combination for Treatment of ADHD: Four Case Reports." In *Journal of Child and Adolescent Psychopharmacology* 14(1): 131–138.

Burgess, P. W. 1997. "Theory and Methodology in Executive Function Research." In *Methodology of Frontal and Executive Function,* ed. P. Rabbit. East Sussex, Eng.: Psychology Press. Pp. 81–116.

Bush, G., J. A. Frazier, et al. 1999. "Anterior Cingulate Cortex Dysfunction in Attention-Deficit/Hyperactivity Disorder Revealed by fMRI and the Counting Stroop." *Biological Psychiatry* 45: 1542–1552.

Campbell, S. B. 2002. *Behavior Problems in Preschool Children: Clinical and Developmental Issues.* New York: Guilford Press.

Cantwell, D. P., and L. Baker. 1991. *Psychiatric and Developmental Disorders in Children with Communication Disorder.* Washington, D.C.: American Psychiatric Press.

Carlson, C. L., W. E. Pelham, et al. 1991. "A Divided Attention Analysis of the Effects of Methylphenidate on the Arithmetic Performance of Children with Attention-Deficit Hyperactivity Disorder." *Journal of Child Psychology and Psychiatry* 32(3): 463–471.

Carlson, G. A., M. D. Rapport, et al. 1992. "Effects of Methylphenidate and Lithium on Attention and Activity Level." *Journal of the American Academy of Child and Adolescent Psychiatry* 31: 262–270.

Castellanos, F. X. 1999. "Psychobiology of ADHD." In *Handbook of Disruptive Behavior Disorders,* ed. H. C. Quay and A. E. Hogan. New York: Kluwer Academic and Plenum. Pp. 179–198.

Castellanos, F. X., and R. Tannock. 2002. "Neuroscience of Attention-Deficit/Hyperactivity Disorder: The Search for Endophenotypes." *Nature Reviews: Neuroscience* 3: 617–628.

Chelonis, J. J., M. C. Edwards, et al. 2002. "Stimulant Medication Improves Recognition Memory in Children Diagnosed with Attention-Deficit/

Hyperactivity Disorder." *Experimental and Clinical Psychopharmacology* 10(4): 400–407.

Churchland, P. M. 1995. *The Engine of Reason, the Seat of the Soul.* Cambridge, Mass.: MIT Press.

Church of Scientology. 2001. Advance Directive, Church of Scientology Flag Service Organization.

Cohen, N. J. 1996. "Unsuspected Language Impairments in Psychiatrically Disturbed Children: Developmental Issues and Associated Conditions." In *Language, Learning, and Behavior Disorders,* ed. J. H. Beitchman, N. J. Cohen, M. M. Konstantareas, and R. Tannock. Cambridge, Eng.: Cambridge University Press. Pp. 105–127.

Cohen, N. J., M. A. Barwick, et al. 1996. "Comorbidity of Language and Social-Emotional Disorders: Comparison of Psychiatric Outpatients and Their Siblings." *Journal of Clinical Child Psychology* 25(2): 192–200.

Cohen, N. J., M. Davine, et al. 1993. "Unsuspected Language Impairment in Psychiatrically Disturbed Children: Prevalence and Language and Behavioral Characteristics." *Journal of the American Academy of Child and Adolescent Psychiatry* 32(3): 595–603.

Collett, B. R., J. L. Ohan, et al. 2003. "Ten Year Review of Rating Scales. Part 5: Scales Assessing Attention-Deficit/Hyperactivity Disorder." *Journal of the American Academy of Child and Adolescent Psychiatry* 42(9): 1015–1037.

Comings, D. E., and B. G. Comings. 1988. "Tourette's Syndrome and Attention Deficit Disorder." In *Tourette's Syndrome and Tic Disorders: Clinical Understanding and Treatment,* ed. D. J. Cohen, R. D. Bruun, and J. F. Leckman. New York: Wiley. Pp. 111–147.

Conners, C. K. 1997. *Conners' Rating Scales—Revised Manual.* North Tonawanda, N.Y.: Multi-Health Systems.

———. 2002. "Forty Years of Methylphenidate Treatment in Attention-Deficit/Hyperactivity Disorder." *Journal of Attention Disorders* 6(Supplement 1): S17–S30.

Conners, C. K., D. Erhardt, et al. 1999. *Conners' Adult ADHD Rating Scales.* North Tonawanda, N.Y.: Multi-Health Systems.

Craik, F. I. M., M. Byrd, et al. 1987. "Patterns of Memory Loss in Three Elderly Samples." *Psychology and Aging* 2: 79–86.

Csikszentmihalyi, M., and R. Larson. 1984. *Being Adolescent: Conflict and Growth in the Teenage Years.* New York: Basic Books.

Csikszentmihalyi, M., and B. Schneider. 2000. *Becoming Adult: How Teenagers Prepare for the World of Work.* New York: Basic Books.

Cunningham, C. E. 1998. "A Large-Group Community-Based, Family Systems Approach to Parent Training." In *Attention-Deficit Hyperactivity Disorder: Handbook for Diagnosis and Treatment,* ed. R. A. Barkley. New York: Guilford Press.

Damasio, A. R. 1994. *Descartes' Error: Emotion, Reason, and the Human Brain.* New York: G.P. Putnam's Sons.

———. 1999. *The Feeling of What Happens.* New York: Harcourt Brace.

———. 2003. *Looking for Spinoza: Joy, Sorrow, and the Feeling Brain.* New York: Harcourt.

Dawson, P., and R. Guare. 2004. *Executive Skills in Children and Adolescents: A Practical Guide to Assessment and Intervention.* New York: Guilford Press.

de Fockert, J. W., G. Rees, et al. 2001. "The Role of Working Memory in Visual Selective Attention." *Science* 291(2): 1803–1805.

Denckla, M. B. 1996. "A Theory and Model of Executive Function." In *Attention, Memory, and Executive Function,* ed. G. R. Lyon and N. A. Krasnegor. Baltimore, Md.: Paul H. Brookes. Pp. 263–278.

———. 2000. "Learning Disabilities and Attention Deficit Hyperactivity Disorder in Adults: Overlap with Executive Dysfunction." In *Attention-Deficit Disorders and Comorbidities in Children, Adolescents, and Adults,* ed. T. E. Brown. Washington, D.C.: American Psychiatric Press. Pp. 297–318.

Dendy, C. A. Z. 1995. *Teenagers with ADD: A Parents' Guide.* Bethesda, Md.: Woodbine House.

———. 2000. *Teaching Teens with ADD and ADHD.* Bethesda, Md.: Woodbine House.

Diamond, A., and C. Taylor. 1996. "Development of an Aspect of Executive Control: Development of the Abilities to Remember What I Said and to 'Do As I Say, Not as I Do.'" *Developmental Psychobiology* 29(4): 315–334.

Diller, L. H. 1998. *Running on Ritalin: A Physician Reflects on Children, Society, and Performance in a Pill.* New York: Bantam Books.

Disney, E. R., I. J. Elkins, M. McGue, and W. G. Iacono. 1999. "Effects of

ADHD, Conduct Disorder, and Gender on Substance Use and Abuse in Adolescence." *American Journal of Psychiatry* 156(10): 1515–1521.

Douglas, V. I. 1999. "Cognitive Control Processes in Attention-Deficit/Hyperactivity Disorder." In *Handbook of Disruptive Behavior Disorders,* ed. H. C. Quay and A. E. Hogan. New York: Kluwer Academic and Plenum. Pp. 105–138.

Doyle, A. E., J. Biederman, et al. 2000. "Diagnostic Efficiency of Neuropsychological Test Scores for Discriminating Boys with and without Attention-Deficit/Hyperactivity Disorder." *Journal of Consulting and Clinical Psychology* 68(3): 477–488.

DuPaul, G., K. McGoey, et al. 2001. "Preschool Children with Attention-Deficit/Hyperactivity Disorder: Impairments in Behavioral, Social, and School Functioning." *Journal of the American Academy of Child and Adolescent Psychiatry* 40(5): 508–515.

DuPaul, G. J., and T. J. Power. 2000. "Educational Interventions for Students with Attention-Deficit Disorders." In *Attention Deficit Disorders and Comorbidities in Children, Adolescents, and Adults,* ed. T. E. Brown. Washington, D.C.: American Psychiatric Press. Pp. 607–635.

DuPaul, G. J., and G. Stoner. 2003. *ADHD in the Schools: Assessment and Intervention Strategies.* New York, Guilford Press.

Durston, S., N. T. Tottenham, K. M. Thomas, M. C. Davidson, I.-M. Eigsti, Y. Yang, et al. 2003. "Differential Patterns of Striatal Activation in Young Children with and without ADHD." *Biological Psychiatry* 53: 871–878.

Edelman, G. M. 1992. *Bright Air, Brilliant Fire: On the Matter of the Mind.* New York, Basic Books.

Edelman, G. M., and G. Tononi. 2000. *A Universe of Consciousness: How Matter Becomes Imagination.* New York: Basic Books.

Erhardt D., and S.P. Hinshaw. 1994. "Initial Sociometric Impressions of Attention-Deficit Hyperactivity Disorder and Comparison Boys: Predictions from Social Behaviors and from Nonbehavioral Variables." *Journal of Consulting and Clinical Psychology* 62(4): 833–842.

Erikson, E. H. 1960. *Childhood and Society.* New York: W.W. Norton.

———. 1968. *Identity: Youth and Crisis.* New York: W.W. Norton.

Ernst, M., A. S. Kimes, et al. 2003. "Neural Substrates of Decision Making in Adults with Attention Deficit Hyperactivity Disorder." *American Journal of Psychiatry* 160(6): 1061–1070.

Ernst, M., A. J. Zametkin, et al. 1999. "High Midbrain DOPA Accumulation in Children with Attention Deficit Hyperactivity Disorder." *American Journal of Psychiatry* 156(8): 1209–1215.

Eslinger, P. J. 1996. "Conceptualizing, Describing, and Measuring Components of Executive Function." In *Attention, Memory, and Executive Function,* ed. G. R. Lyon and N. A. Krasnegor. Baltimore, Md.: Paul H. Brookes. Pp. 367–395.

Everett, C. A., and S. V. Everett. 1999. *Family Therapy for ADHD: Treating Children, Adolescents and Adults.* New York: Guilford Press.

Fabiani, M., and E. Wee. 2001. "Age-Related Changes in Working Memory and Frontal Lobe Function: A Review." In *Handbook of Developmental Cognitive Neuroscience,* ed. C. A. Nelson and M. Luciana. Cambridge, Mass.: MIT Press. Pp. 473–488.

Faraone, S. V., and J. Biederman. 1998. "Neurobiology of Attention-Deficit Hyperactivity Disorder." *Biological Psychiatry* 44: 951–958.

Faraone, S. V., J. Biederman, et al. 1996. "Cognitive Functioning, Learning Disability, and School Failure in Attention Deficit Hyperactivity Disorder: A Family Study Perspective." In *Language, Learning and Behavior Disorders,* ed. J. H. Beitchman, N. J. Cohen, M. M. Konstantareas, and R. Tannock. Cambridge, Eng.: Cambridge University Press. Pp. 247–271.

Faraone, S. V., J. Sergeant, et al. 2003. "Worldwide Prevalence of ADHD: Is It an American Condition?" *World Psychiatry* 2(2): 104–113.

Faraone, S., T. J. Spencer, et al. 2004. "Meta-Analysis of the Efficacy of Methylphenidate for Treating Adult Attention-Deficit Hyperactivity Disorder." *Journal of Clinical Psychopharmacology* 24(1): 24–29.

Feldman, R. S., J. S. Meyer, and L. F. Quenzer. 1997. *Principles of Neuropsychopharmacology.* Sunderland, Mass.: Sinauer Associates.

Fitzsimons, G. M., and J. A. Bargh. 2004. "Automatic Self-Regulation." In *Handbook of Self-Regulation: Research, Theory and Applications,* ed. R. F. Baumeister and K. D. Vohs. New York: Guilford Press. Pp. 151–170.

Fox, N. A., et al. 2001. "The Biology of Temperament: An Integrative Approach." In *Handbook of Developmental Cognitive Neuroscience,* ed. C. A. Nelson and M. Luciana. Cambridge, Mass.: MIT Press. Pp. 631–645.

Frazier, J. A., J. Biederman, et al. 2001. "Should the Diagnosis of Attention-Deficit/Hyperactivity Disorder Be Considered in Children with Pervasive Developmental Disorder?" *Journal of Attention Disorders* 4(4): 204–211.

Freud, S. 1917. "One of the Difficulties of Psychoanalysis." In *Sigmund Freud: Character and Culture,* ed. P. Rieff. New York: Collier.

Fuster, J. M. 2003. *Cortex and Mind: Unifying Cognition.* New York: Oxford University Press.

Gagnon, J. H., and W. Simon. 1973. *Sexual Conduct: The Social Sources of Human Sexuality.* Chicago: Aldine.

Gammon, G. D., and T. E. Brown. 1993. "Fluoxetine and Methylphenidate in Combination for Treatment of Attention Deficit Disorder and Comorbid Depressive Disorder." *Journal of Child and Adolescent Psychopharmacology* 3(1): 1–10.

Geary, D. C. 1994. *Children's Mathematical Development: Research and Practical Applications.* Washington, D.C.: American Psychological Association.

Geller, B., J. L. Craney, et al. 2003. "Phenomenology and Longitudinal Course of Children with a Prepubertal and Early Adolescent Bipolar Disorder Phenotype." In *Bipolar Disorder in Childhood and Early Adolescence,* ed. B. Geller and M. P. DelBello. New York: Guilford Press. Pp. 25–50.

Geller, B., B. Zimmerman, et al. 2002a. "DSM-IV Mania Symptoms in a Prepubertal and Early Adolescent Bipolar Disorder Phenotype Compared to Attention-Deficit Hyperactive and Normal Controls." *Journal of Child and Adolescent Psychopharmacology* 12(1): 11–25.

———. 2002b. "Phenomenology of Prepubertal and Early Adolescent Bipolar Disorder: Examples of Elated Mood, Grandiose Behaviors, Decreased Need for Sleep, Racing Thoughts and Hypersexuality." *Journal of Child and Adolescent Psychopharmacology* 12(1): 3–9.

Geller, D. A., J. Biederman, et al. 1996. "Comorbidity of Juvenile Obsessive-Compulsive Disorder with Disruptive Behavior Disorders." *Journal of the American Academy of Child and Adolescent Psychiatry* 35(12): 1637–1646.

———. 2002. "Attention-Deficit/Hyperactivity Disorder in Children and Adolescents with Obsessive-Compulsive Disorder: Fact or Artifact?" *Journal of the American Academy of Child and Adolescent Psychiatry* 41(1): 52–58.

Gerring, J. P., K. D. Brady, et al. 1998. "Premorbid Evidence of ADHD and

Development of Secondary ADHD after Closed Head Injury." *Journal of the American Academy of Child and Adolescent Psychiatry* 37(6): 647–654.

Giedd, J. N., J. Blumenthal, et al. 1999. "Brain Development during Childhood and Adolescence: A Longitudinal MRI Study." *Nature Neuroscience* 2(10): 861–863.

Giedd, J. N., J. W. Snell, et al. 1996. "Quantitative Magnetic Resonance Imaging of Human Brain Development: Ages 4–18." *Cerebral Cortex* 6:551–560.

Goldberg, E. 2001. *The Executive Brain: Frontal Lobes and the Civilized Mind.* New York: Oxford University Press.

Goldman, L. S., M. Genel, et al. 1998. "Diagnosis and Treatment of Attention-Deficit/Hyperactivity Disorder in Children and Adolescents." *Journal of the American Medical Association* 279(14): 1100–1107.

Goldman-Rakic, P. 1987. "Circuitry of the Primate Prefrontal Cortex and the Regulation of Behavior by Representational Memory." In *Handbook of Physiology: The Nervous System. Vols. 1 and 2: Higher Functions of the Brain,* ed. F. Plum. Bethesda, Md.: American Physiological Society. (sec. 5): 373–417.

Gottwald, B., Z. Mihajlovic, et al. 2003. "Does the Cerbellum Contribute to Specific Aspects of Attention?" *Neuropsychologia* 41: 1452–1460.

Greenberger, E., and L. Steinberg. 1986. *When Teenagers Work: Psychological and Social Costs of Adolescent Employment.* New York: Basic Books.

Greene, R. W. 1998. *The Explosive Child.* New York: HarperCollins.

Greene, R. W., J. Biederman, et al. 2002. "Psychiatric Comorbidity, Family Dysfunction, and Social Impairment in Referred Youth with Oppositional Defiant Disorder." *American Journal of Psychiatry* 159(7): 1214–1224.

Greenhill, L. 2004. "Outcome Results from NIMH, Multi-Site Preschool ADHD Treatment Study." Symposium presented at the Fifty-first Annual Meeting of the American Academy of Child and Adolescent Psychiatry, Washington, D.C.

Greenhill, L., J. M. Halperin, and H. Abikoff. 1999. "Stimulant Medications." *Journal of the American Academy of Child and Adolescent Psychiatry* 38(5): 503–512.

Hassin, R. A., J. S. Uleman, and J. A. Bargh, eds. 2005. *The New Unconscious.* New York: Oxford University Press.

Hazell P. L., and J. E. Stuart. 2003. "A Randomized Controlled Trial of Clonidine Added to Psychostimulant Medication for Hyperactive and Aggressive
Children." *Journal of the American Academy of Child and Adolescent Psychiatry*
42(8): 886–894.

Hervey, A. S., J. N. Epstein, et al. 2004. "Neuropsychology of Adults with
Attention Deficit Hyperactivity Disorder: A Meta-Analytic View." *Neuropsychology* 18(3): 485–503.

Hinshaw, S. P. 2002a. "Is ADHD an Impairing Condition in Childhood and
Adolescence?" In *Attention Deficit Hyperactivity Disorder: State of the Sci-
ence—Best Practices,* ed. P. S. Jensen and J. R. Cooper. Kingston, N.J.:
Civic Research Institute. 5:1–21.

———. 2002b. "Preadolescent Girls with Attention-Deficit/Hyperactivity
Disorder. I: Background Characteristics, Comorbidity, Cognitive and Social Functioning and Parenting Practices." *Journal of Consulting and Clinical Psychology* 70(5): 1086–1098.

Hinshaw, S. P., and C. A. Anderson. 1996. "Conduct and Oppositional
Defiant Disorders." In *Child Psychopathology,* ed. E. J. Mash and R. A.
Barkley. New York: Guilford Press. Pp. 113–149.

Hinshaw, S. P., E. T. Carte, et al. 2002. "Preadolescent Girls with Attention-
Deificit/Hyperactivity Disorder. II: Neuropsychological Performance in
Relation to Subtypes and Individual Classification." *Journal of Consulting
and Clinical Psychology* 70(5): 1099–1111.

Horner, B. R., and K. E. Scheibe. 1997. "Prevalence and Implications of
Attention-Deficit Hyperactivity Disorder among Adolescents in Treat-
ment for Substance Abuse." *Journal of the American Academy of Child and
Adolescent Psychiatry* 36(1): 30–36.

Jackson, S. W. 1992. "The Listening Healer in the History of Psychological
Healing." *American Journal of Psychiatry* 149(12): 1623–1632.

James, W. 1890. *Principles of Psychology.* New York: Dover.

Jensen, P. S. 2003. "Cost Effectiveness of Treatment Options for Attention-
Deficit/Hyperactivity Disorder." Paper given at the Fiftieth Anniversary
Meeting of the American Academy of Child and Adolescent Psychiatry,
Miami, Fla.

Jensen, P. S., and H. Abikoff. 2000. "Tailoring Treatments for Individuals with Attention-Deficit/Hyperactivity Disorder: Clinical and Research Perspectives." In *Attention Deficit Disorders and Comorbidities in Children, Adolescents, and Adults,* ed. T. E. Brown. Washington, D.C.: American Psychiatric Press. Pp. 637–652.

Johnson, S. H., and J. M. Rybash. 1993. "A Cognitive Neuroscience Perspective on Age-Related Slowing: Developmental Changes in the Functional Architecture." In *Adult Information Processing: Limits on Loss,* ed. J. Cerella, J. Rybash, W. Hoyer, and M. L. Commons. San Diego: Academic Press. Pp. 143–173.

Kagan, J. 1994. *Galen's Prophecy: Temperament in Human Nature.* New York, Basic Books.

Kagan, J., and N. Snidman. 2004. *The Long Shadow of Temperament.* Cambridge, Mass.: Harvard University Press.

Katz, L. J., G. Goldstein, et al. 2001. *Learning Disabilities in Older Adolescents and Adults: Clinical Utility of the Neuropsychological Perspective.* New York: Kluwer Academic and Plenum.

Kendell, R., and A. Jablensky. 2003. "Distinguishing between the Validity and Utility of Psychiatric Diagnoses." *American Journal of Psychiatry* 160: 4–12.

Kessler, R. C. 2004. "Prevalence of Adult ADHD in the United States: Results from the National Comorbidity Study Replication (NCS-R)." Paper presented at the 157th American Psychiatric Association Annual Meeting, New York.

Kessler, R. C., K. A. McGonagle, et al. 1994. "Lifetime and Twelve-Month Prevalence of DSM-III-R Psychiatric Disorders in the United States." *Archives of General Psychiatry* 51: 8–19.

Kosslyn, S. M., and O. Koenig. 1995. *Wet Mind: The New Cognitive Neuroscience.* New York: Free Press.

Krusch, D. A., R. Klorman, et al. 1996. "Methylphenidate Slows Reactions of Children with Attention Deficit Disorder during and after an Error." *Journal of Abnormal Child Psychology* 24(5): 633–650.

Lahey, B. B., W. E. Pelham, et al. 1998. "Validity of DSM-IV Attention-Deficit/Hyperactivity Disorder for Younger Children." *Journal of the American Academy of Child and Adolescent Psychiatry* 37(7): 695–702.

Laing, R. D. 1997. *Politics of Experience*. New York, Ballantine.

Latham, P. S., and P. H. Latham. 1996. *Documentation and the Law: For Professionals Concerned with ADD/LD*. Washington, D.C.: JKL Publications.

———. 1999. *Higher Education Services for Students with LD or ADHD*. Washington, D.C.: JKL Communications.

———. 2005. *Learning Disabilities/ADD and the Law: 2005 Case Update*. Washington, D.C.: JKL Communications.

Lawrence, V., S. Houghton, et al. 2002. "ADHD Outside the Laboratory: Boys' Executive Function Performance on Tasks in Videogame Play and on a Visit to the Zoo." *Journal of Abnormal Child Psychology* 30(5) : 447–462.

LeDoux, J. 1996. *The Emotional Brain*. New York: Simon and Schuster.

———. 2002. *Synaptic Self: How Our Brains Become Who We Are*. New York: Penguin Putnam.

Leiner, H. C., A. L. Leiner, and R. S. Dow. 1989. "Reappraising the Cerebellum: What Does the Hindbrain Contribute to the Forebrain?" *Behavioral Neuroscience* 103(5): 998–1008.

Levine, M. 2003. *The Myth of Laziness*. New York: Simon and Schuster.

Levinson, D. J., C. N. Darrow, et al. 1978. *Seasons of a Man's Life*. New York: Alfred A. Knopf.

Levinson, D. J., and J. D. Levinson. 1996. *Seasons of a Woman's Life*. New York: Alfred A. Knopf.

Levy, F. 2004. "Synaptic Gating and ADHD: A Biological Theory of Comorbidity of ADHD and Anxiety." In *Neuropsychopharmacology* 29(9): 1589–1596.

Loo, S. K. 2003. "EEG and Neurofeedback Findings in ADHD." *ADHD Report* 11(3): 1–9.

Luciana, M. 2001. "Dopamine-Opiate Modulations of Reward-Seeking Behavior: Implications for the Functional Assessment of Prefrontal Development." In *Handbook of Developmental Cognitive Neuroscience*, ed. C. A. Nelson and M. Luciana. Cambridge, Mass.: MIT Press. Pp. 647–662.

MacCoon, D. G., J. F. Wallace, and J. P. Newman. 2004. "Self-Regulation: Context-Appropriate Balanced Attention." In *Handbook of Self-Regulation: Research, Theory, and Applications*, ed. R. F. Baumeister and K. D. Vohs. New York: Guilford Press. Pp. 422–444.

Marrocco, R. T., and M. C. Davidson. 1998. "Neurochemistry of Attention." In *The Attentive Brain,* ed. R. Parasuraman. Cambridge, Mass.: MIT Press. Pp. 35–50.

Max, J. E., S. Arndt, et al. 1998. "Attention-Deficit Hyperactivity Disorder Symptomatology after Traumatic Brain Injury: A Prospective Study." *Journal of the American Academy of Child and Adolescent Psychiatry* 37(8): 841–847.

Mayberg, H. S., M. Liotti, et al. 1999. "Reciprocal Limbic-Cortical Function and Negative Mood: Converging PET Findings in Depression and Normal Sadness." *American Journal of Psychiatry* 156(5): 675–682.

Mayes, S. D., S. L. Calhoun, et al. 2000. "Learning Disabilities and ADHD: Overlapping Spectrum Disorders." *Journal of Learning Disabilities* 33(5): 417–424.

McDermott, S. P. 2000. "Cognitive Therapy for Adults with Attention-Deficit/Hyperactivity Disorder." In *Attention Deficit Disorders and Comorbidities in Children, Adolescents, and Adults,* ed. T. E. Brown. Washington, D.C.: American Psychiatric Press. Pp. 569–606.

McEwen, B. S. 1991. "Non-Genomic and Genomic Effects of Steroids on Neural Activity." *Trends in Pharmacological Science* 12:141–147.

Melnick, S. M., and S. P. Hinshaw. 1996. "What They Want and What They Get: The Social Goals of Boys with ADHD and Comparison Boys." *Journal of Abnormal Child Psychology* 24(2): 169–185.

Mennin, D., J. Biederman, et al. 2000. "Towards Defining a Meaningful Anxiety Phenotype for Research in ADHD Children." *Journal of Attention Disorders* 3(4): 192–199.

Merry, S., and L. K. Andrews. 1994. "Psychiatric Status of Sexually Abused Children Twelve Months after Disclosure of Abuse." *Journal of the American Academy of Child and Adolescent Psychiatry* 33:939–944.

Mick, E., J. Biederman, et al. 2002. "Case-Control Study of Attention-Deficit/Hyperactivity Disorder and Maternal Smoking, Alcohol Use, and Drug Use during Pregnancy." *Journal of the American Academy of Child and Adolescent Psychiatry* 41(4): 378–385.

———. 2005. "Revisiting the Diagnostic Utility of Irritability in Pediatric Bipolar Disorder. *Biological Psychiatry* (in press).

Milham, M. M., K. I. Erickson, et al. 2002. "Attentional Control in the Aging

Brain: Insights from an fMRI study of the Stroop Task." *Brain and Cognition* 49(3): 277–296.

Milich, R., C. Carlson, et al. 1991. "Effects of Methylphenidate on the Persistence of ADHD Boys Following Failure Experiences." *Journal of Abnormal Child Psychology* 19(5): 519–536.

Millstein, R. B., T. E. Wilens, et al. 1997. "Presenting ADHD Symptoms and Subtypes in Clinically Referred Adults with AHHD." *Journal of Attention Disorders* 2(3): 159–166.

Minde, K., L. Eakin, et al. 2003. "Psychosocial Functioning of Children and Spouses of Adults with ADHD." *Journal of Child Psychology and Psychiatry* 44(4): 637–646.

Miyake, A., and P. Shah, eds. 1999. *Models of Working Memory: Mechanisms of Active Maintenance and Executive Control.* New York: Cambridge University Press.

Mota, V. L., and R. J. Schachar. 2000. "Reformulating Attention-Deficit/ Hyperactivity Disorder According to Signal Detection Theory." *Journal of the American Academy of Child and Adolescent Psychiatry* 39(9): 1144–1151.

MTA Cooperative Group. 1999. "A Fourteen-Month Randomized Clinical Trial of Treatment Strategies for Attention-Deficit/Hyperactivity Disorder." *Archives of General Psychiatry* 56:1073–1086.

Murphy, K., and R. A. Barkley. 1996. "Prevalence of DSM-IV Symptoms of ADHD in Adult Licensed Drivers: Implications for Clinical Diagnosis." *Journal of Attention Disorders* 1(3): 147–162.

Murphy, P., and R. Schachar. 2000. "Use of Self-Ratings in the Assessment of Symptoms of Attention Deficit Hyperactivity Disorder in Adults." *American Journal of Psychiatry* 157(7): 1156–1159.

Nada-Raja, S., J. D. Langley, et al. 1997. "Inattentive and Hyperactive Behaviors and Driving Offenses in Adolescence." *Journal of American Academy of Child and Adolescent Psychiatry* 36(4): 515–522.

Nestler, E. J., and R. C. Malenka. 2004. "The Addicted Brain." *Scientific American* 290: 50–57.

O'Doherty, J., M. L. Kringlebach, E. T. Rolls, J. Hornak, and C. Andrews. 2001. "Abstract Rewards and Punishment Representations in the Human Orbitofrontal Cortex." *Nature* 4(1): 95–102.

Ornstein, R. 1997. *The Right Mind: Making Sense of the Hemispheres.* New York: Harcourt Brace.

Ortiz, J., and A. Raine. 2004. "Heart Rate Level and Antisocial Behavior in Children and Adolescents: A Meta-Analysis." *Journal of the American Academy of Child and Adolescent Psychiatry* 43(2): 154–162.

Parasuraman, R., J. S. Warm, et al. 1998. "Brain Systems of Vigilance." In *The Attentive Brain,* ed. R. Parasuraman. Cambridge, Mass.: MIT Press. Pp. 221–256.

Park, D. C., and T. Hedden. 2001. "Working Memory and Aging." In *Perspectives on Human Memory and Cognitive Aging: Essays in Honor of Fergus Craik,* ed. M. Naveh-Benjamin, M. Moscovitch, and H. L. Roediger III. New York: Psychology Press. Pp. 148–160.

Pelham, W. E., and D. A. Waschbusch. 1999. "Behavioral Intervention in Attention-Deficit/Hyperactivity Disorder." In *Handbook of Disruptive Behavior Disorders,* ed. H. C. Quay and A. E. Hogan. New York: Kluwer Academic and Plenum. Pp. 255–278.

Pennington, B. P. 2002. *Development of Psychopathology: Nature and Nurture.* New York: Guilford Press.

Phelan, T. W. 2003. *1-2-3 Magic: Effective Discipline for Children 2–12.* 3d ed. Glen Ellyn, Ill.: Child Management.

Phelps, E. A. 2005. "The Interaction of Emotion and Cognition: The Relation between the Human Amygdala and Cognitive Awareness." In *The New Unconscious,* ed. R. A. Hassin, J. S. Uleman, and J. A. Bargh. New York: Oxford University Press. Pp. 61–76.

Phillips, M. L., W. C. Drevets, et al. 2003a. "Neurobiology of Emotion Perception I: The Neural Basis of Normal Emotion Perception." *Biological Psychiatry* 54: 504–514.

———. 2003b. "Neurobiology of Emotion Perception II: Implications for Major Psychiatric Disorders." *Biological Psychiatry* 54: 515–528.

Pinker, S. 2002. *The Blank Slate: The Modern Denial of Human Nature.* New York: Viking Penguin.

Pochon, J. B., R. Levy, et al. 2002. "The Neural System That Bridges Reward and Cognition in Humans: An fMRI study." *Proceedings of the National Academy of Sciences* 99(8): 5669–5674.

Posner, M. I., and M. E. Raichle. 1994. *Images of Mind*. New York: Scientific American Library.

Prince, J. B., T. E. Wilens, et al. 1996. "Clonidine for Sleep Disturbances Associated with Attention-Deficit Hyperactivity Disorder: A Systematic Chart Review of Sixty-two Cases." *Journal of the American Academy of Child and Adolescent Psychiatry* 35(5): 599–605.

Purvis, K. L., and R. Tannock. 1997. "Language Abilities in Children with Attention Deficit Hyperactivity Disorder, Reading Disabilities, and Normal Controls." *Journal of Abnormal Child Psychology* 25(2): 133–144.

Quinlan, D. M., and T. E. Brown. 2003. "Assessment of Short-Term Verbal Memory Impairments in Adolescents and Adults with ADHD." *Journal of Attention Disorders* 6(4): 143–152.

Rabbitt, P. 1997. "Methodologies and Models in the Study of Executive Function." In *Methodology of Frontal and Executive Function*, ed. P. Rabbitt. East Sussex, Eng.: Psychology Press Publishers. Pp. 1–38.

Rabiner, D., J. D. Coie, et al. 2000. "Early Attention Problems and Children's Reading Achievement: A Longitudinal Investigation." *Journal of the American Academy of Child and Adolescent Psychiatry* 39(7): 859–867.

Ramachandran, V. S., and S. Blakeslee. 1998. *Phantoms in the Brain*. New York: William Morrow.

Ramsay, J. R., and A. L. Rostain. 2003. "A Cognitive Therapy Approach for Adult Attention Deficit Disorder." *Journal of Cognitive Psychotherapy* 17(4): 319–334.

Rapport, M. D., and C. B. Denney. 2000. "Attention Deficit Hyperactivity Disorder and Methylphenidate: Assessment and Prediction of Clinical Response." In *Ritalin: Theory and Practice*. 2d ed., ed. L. L. Greenhill and B. B. Osman. Larchmont, N.Y.: Mary Ann Liebert. Pp. 45–83.

Ratey, J., M. S. Greenberg, et al. 1992. "Unrecognized Attention-Deficit Hyperactivity Disorder in Adults Presenting for Outpatient Psychotherapy." *Journal of Child and Adolescent Psychopharmacology* 2(4): 267–275.

Rief, S. F. 2005. *How to Reach and Teach Children with ADD/ADHD*. San Francisco: Jossey-Bass.

Robin, A. L. 1998. *ADHD in Adolescents: Diagnosis and Treatment*. New York: Guilford Press.

Rourke, B. P., and K. D. Tsatsanis. 2000. "Nonverbal Learning Disabilities and Asperger Syndrome." In *Asperger Syndrome*, ed. A. Klin, F. R. Volkmar, and S. S. Sparrow. New York: Guilford Press. Pp. 231–253.

Rowland, A. S., D. M. Umbach, et al. 2001. "Studying the Epidemiology of Attention-Deficit Hyperactivity Disorder: Screening Method and Pilot Results." *Canadian Journal of Psychiatry* 46: 931–940.

Rudgley, R. 1993. *The Alchemy of Culture: Intoxicants in Society.* London: British Museum Press.

Safer, D. J., J. M. Zito, and S. dosReis. 2003. "Concomitant Psychotropic Medication for Youths." *American Journal of Psychiatry* 160(3): 438–449.

Safer, J. 2002. *The Normal One: Life with a Difficult or Damaged Sibling.* New York: Free Press.

Salthouse, T. A. 1991. *Theoretical Perspectives on Cognitive Aging.* Hillsdale, N.J.: Lawrence Erlbaum.

Sampaio, R. C., and C. L. Truwit. 2001. "Myelination in the Developing Human Brain." In *Handbook of Developmental Cognitive Neuroscience*, ed. C. A. Nelson and M. Luciana. Cambridge, Mass.: MIT Press. Pp. 35–44.

Scahill, L., M. Schwab-Stone, et al. 1999. "Psychosocial and Clinical Correlates of ADHD in a Community Sample of School-Age Children." *Journal of the American Academy of Child and Adolescent Psychiatry* 39(8): 976–984.

Schacter, D. L. 1996. *Searching for Memory: The Brain, the Mind, and the Past.* New York: Basic Books.

Scheffer, R. E., R. A. Kowatch, et al. 2005. "Randomized, Placebo-Controlled Trial of Mixed Amphetamine Salts for Symptoms of Comorbid ADHD in Pediatric Bipolar Disorder after Mood Stabilization with Divalproex Sodium." *American Journal of Psychiatry* 162 (1): 58–64.

Schlink, B. 1997. *The Reader*, trans. C. B. Janeway. New York: Pantheon.

Schmidt, L. A., N. A. Fox, et al. 1999. "Behavioral and Psychophysiological Correlates of Self-Presentation in Temperamentally Shy Children." *Developmental Psychobiology* 35: 119–135.

Sergeant, J. A., H. Guerts, et al. 2002. "How Specific Is a Deficit of Executive Functioning for Attention-Deficit/Hyperactivity Disorder?" *Behavioural Brain Research* 130: 3–28.

Shallice, T., and P. Burgess. 1991. "Deficits in Strategy Application Following Frontal Lobe Damage in Man." *Brain* 114: 727–741.

Shaywitz, S. E. 2003. *Overcoming Dyslexia.* New York: Alfred A. Knopf.

Shaywitz, S. E., B. A. Shaywitz, et al. 1999. "Effects of Estrogen on Brain Activation Patterns in Postmenopausal Women during Working Memory Tasks." *Journal of the American Medical Association* 281(13): 1197–1202.

———. 2002. "Disruption of Posterior Brain Systems for Reading in Children with Developmental Dyslexia." *Biological Psychiatry* 52: 101–110.

Sherwin, B. B. 1998. "Estrogen and Cognitive Functioning in Women." *Society for Experimental Biology and Medicine* 217: 17–22.

Siegel, D. J. 1999. *The Developing Mind: How Relationships and the Brain Interact to Shape Who We Are.* New York: Guilford Press.

Smalley, S. L., J. J. McGough, et al. 2000. "Familial Clustering of Symptoms and Disruptive Behaviors in Multiplex Families with Attention-Deficit/Hyperactivity Disorder." *Journal of the American Academy of Child and Adolescent Psychiatry* 39(9): 1135–1143.

Snyder, J. M. 2001. *AD/HD and Driving: A Guide for Parents of Teens With AD/HD.* Whitefish, Mont.: Whitefish Consultants.

Solanto, M. V., A. F. T. Arnsten, et al. 2001. "Neuroscience of Stimulant Drug Action in ADHD." In *Stimulant Drugs and ADHD: Basic and Clinical Neuroscience,* ed. M. V. Solanto, A. F. T. Arnsten, and F. X. Castellanos. New York: Oxford University Press. Pp. 355–379.

Solanto, M. V., E. H. Wender, et al. 1997. "Effects of Methylphenidate and Behavioral Contingencies on Sustained Attention in Attention-Deficit Hyperactivity Disorder: A Test of the Reward Dysfunction Hypothesis." *Journal of Child and Adolescent Psychopharmacology* 7(2): 123–136.

Sonuga-Barke, E. J. S., L. Dalen, et al. 2003. "Do Executive Deficits and Delay Aversion Make Independent Contributions to Preschool Attention-Deficit/Hyperactivity Disorder Symptoms?" *Journal of the American Academy of Child and Adolescent Psychiatry* 42(11): 1335–1342.

Sonuga-Barke, E. J. S., D. Daley, et al. 2002. "Does Maternal ADHD Reduce the Effectiveness of Parent Training for Preschool Children's ADHD?" *Journal of the American Academy of Child and Adolescent Psychiatry* 41(6): 696–702.

Spencer, T., J. Biederman, et al. 1996a. "Growth Deficits in ADHD Children Revisited: Evidence for Disorder-Associated Growth Delays?" *Journal of the American Academy of Child and Adolescent Psychiatry* 35(11): 1460–1469.

———. 1996b. "Pharmacotherapy of Attention-Deficit Hyperactivity Disorder across the Life Cycle." *Journal of the American Academy of Child and Adolescent Psychiatry* 35(4): 409–432.

———. 1998. "Disentangling the Overlap between Tourette's Disorder and ADHD." *Journal of Child Psychology and Psychiatry* 39(7): 1037–1044.

Spencer, T., and L. Greenhill. 2003. "OROS Methylphenidate Treatment for Adolescent Attention-Deficit/Hyperactivity Disorder." Paper presented at the American Academy of Child and Adolescent Psychiatry, Miami, Fla.

Spencer, T., T. E. Wilens, et al. 2000. "Attention-Deficit/Hyperactivity Disorder with Mood Disorders." In *Attention-Deficit Disorders and Comorbidities in Children, Adolescents, and Adults,* ed. T. E. Brown. Washington, D.C.: American Psychiatric Press. Pp. 79–124.

Sprich-Buckminster, S., J. Biederman, et al. 1993. "Are Perinatal Complications Relevant to the Manifestation of ADD? Issues of Comorbidity and Familiality." *Journal of the American Academy of Child and Adolescent Psychiatry* 32(5): 1032–1037.

Stanovich, K. E. 2000. *Progress in Understanding Reading: Scientific Foundations and New Frontiers.* New York: Guilford Press.

Strauch, B. 2003. *The Primal Teen: What the New Discoveries about the Teenage Brain Tell Us about Our Kids.* New York: Doubleday.

Stuss, D. T., and M. Binns. 2001. "Aging: Not An Escarpment, But Many Different Slopes." In *Perspectives on Human Memory and Cognitive Aging: Essays in Honor of Fergus Craik,* ed. M. Naveh-Benjamin, M. Moscovitch, and H. L. Roediger III. New York: Psychology Press. Pp. 334–347.

Swanson, H. L., and L. Sáez. 2003. "Memory Difficulties in Children and Adults with Learning Disabilities." In *Handbook of Learning Disabilities,* ed. H. L. Swanson, K. R. Harris, and S. Graham. New York: Guilford Press. Pp. 182–198.

Swanson, J. M., H. C. Kraemer, et al. 2001. "Clinical Relevance of the Primary Findings of the MTA: Success Rates Based on Severity of ADHD and ODD Symptoms at the End of Treatment." *Journal of the American Academy of Child and Adolescent Psychiatry* 40(2): 168–179.

Tannock, R. 1998. "Attention Deficit Hyperactivity Disorder: Advances in Cognitive, Neurobiological, and Genetic Research." *Journal of Child Psychology and Psychiatry* 39(1): 65–99.

———. 2000. "Attention-Deficit/Hyperactivity Disorder with Anxiety Disorders." In *Attention Deficit Disorders and Comorbidities in Children, Adolescents, and Adults,* ed. T. E. Brown. Washington, D.C.: American Psychiatric Press. Pp. 125–170.

Tannock, R., and T. E. Brown. 2000. "Attention Deficit Disorders with Learning Disorders in Children and Adolescents." In *Attention-Deficit Disorders and Comorbidities in Children, Adolescents, and Adults,* ed. T. E. Brown. Washington, D.C.: American Psychiatric Press. Pp. 231–295.

Tannock, R., and R. Schachar. 1996. "Executive Dysfunction as an Underlying Mechanism of Behavior and Language Problems in Attention Deficit Hyperactivity Disorder." In *Language, Learning, and Behavior Disorders,* ed. J. H. Beitchman, N. J. Cohen, M. M. Konstantareas, and R. Tannock. New York: Cambridge University Press. Pp. 128–155.

Thapar, A. 2002. "Attention Deficit Hyperactivity Disorder: New Genetic Findings, New Directions." In *Behavioral Genetics in the Postgenomic Era,* ed. R. Plomin, J. C. Defries, I. W. Craig, and P. McGuffin. Washington, D.C.: American Psychological Association. Pp. 445–462.

Thompson, P. M., J. N. Giedd, et al. 2000. "Growth Patterns in the Developing Brain Detected by Using Continuum Mechanical Tensor Maps." *Nature* 404: 190–193.

Tourette's Syndrome Study Group. 2002. "Treatment of ADHD in Children with Tics: A Randomized Controlled Trial." *Neurology* 58: 527–536.

Voeller, K. K. S. 2001. "Attention-Deficit/Hyperactivity Disorder as a Frontal-Subcortical Disorder." In *Frontal-Subcortical Circuits in Psychiatric and Neurological Disorders,* ed. D. G. Lichter and J. L. Cummings. New York: Guilford Press. Pp. 334–371.

Vohs, K. D., and R. F. Baumeister. 2004. "Understanding Self-Regulation." In *Handbook of Self-Regulation: Research, Theory, and Applications,* ed. R. F. Baumeister and K. D. Vohs. New York: Guilford Press.

Volkmar, F. R., and A. Klin. 2000. "Diagnostic Issues in Asperger Syndrome." In *Asperger Syndrome,* ed. A. Klin, F. R. Volkmar and S. S. Sparrow. New York: Guilford Press. Pp. 25–71.

Volkow, N. D., J. S. Fowler, et al. 2002. "Mechanism of Action of Methylphenidate: Insights from PET Imaging Studies." *Journal of Attention Disorders* 6(supplement 1): S31–S43.

Volkow, N. D., J. Logan, et al. 2000. "Association between Age-Related Decline in Brain Dopamine Activity and Impairment in Frontal and Cingulate Metabolism." *American Journal of Psychiatry* 157(1): 75–80.

Volkow, N. D., and J. M. Swanson. 2003. "Variables That Affect the Clinical Use and Abuse of Methylphenidate in the Treatment of ADHD." *American Journal of Psychiatry* 160(11): 1909–1918.

Volkow, N. D., G.-J. Wang, et al. 1997. "Effects of Methylphenidate on Regional Brain Glucose Metabolism in Humans: Relationship to Dopamine D_2 Receptors." *American Journal of Psychiatry* 154(1): 50–55.

———. 1999. "Prediction of Reinforcing Responses to Psychostimulants in Humans by Brain Dopamine D_2 Receptor Levels." *American Journal of Psychiatry* 156(9): 1440–1444.

———. 2004. "Evidence That Methylphenidate Enhances the Saliency of a Mathematical Task by Increasing Dopamine in the Human Brain." *American Journal of Psychiatry* 161(7): 1173–1180.

Wechsler, D. 1991. *Wechsler Intelligence Scale for Children.* 3d ed. San Antonio, Tex.: Psychological Corporation.

———. 1997a. *Wechsler Adult Intelligence Scale: Third Edition Administration and Scoring Manual.* San Antonio, Tex.: Psychological Corporation.

———. 1997b. *Wechsler Memory Scale.* 3d ed. San Antonio, Tex.: Psychological Corporation.

———. 2003. *Wechsler Intelligence Scale for Children.* 4th ed. San Antonio, Tex.: Psychological Corporation.

Wegner, D. M. 2002. *The Illusion of Conscious Will.* Cambridge, Mass.: MIT Press.

Weinberg, W. A., and R. A. Brumback. 1990. "Primary Disorder of Vigilance: A Novel Explanation of Inattentiveness, Daydreaming, Boredom, Restlessness, and Sleepiness." *Journal of Pediatrics* 116: 720–725.

Wender, P. 1987. *Hyperactive Child, Adolescent, and Adult: Attention Deficit Disorder through the Lifespan.* New York: Oxford University Press.

———. 1995. *Attention-Deficit Hyperactivity Disorder in Adults.* New York: Oxford University Press.

West, R., K. J. Murphy, et al. 2002. "Lapses of Intention and Performance Variability Reveal Age-Related Increases in Fluctuations of Executive Control." *Brain and Cognition* 49(3): 402–419.

Wilens, T. E., J. Biederman, et al. 1998. "Does ADHD Affect the Course of Substance Abuse? Findings from a Sample of Adults with and without ADHD." *American Journal of Addictions* 7: 156–163.

———. 2002. "Attention Deficit/Hyperactivity Disorder across the Lifespan." *Annual Review of Medicine* 53: 113–131.

Wilens, T. E., S. V. Faraone, et al. 2003. "Does Stimulant Therapy of Attention-Deficit/Hyperactivitiy Disorder Beget Later Substance Abuse? A Meta-analytic Review of the Literature." *Pediatrics* 111(1): 179–185.

Wilens, T. E., T. J. Spencer, et al. 2000. "ADHD and Psychoactive Substance Abuse Disorders." In *Attention Deficit Disorders and Comorbidities in Children, Adolescents, and Adults,* ed. T. E. Brown. Washington, D.C.: American Psychiatric Press.

Winnicott, D. W. 1965. *The Family and Individual Development.* London: Tavistock Publications.

Wise, R. A. 1989. "The Brain and Reward." In *The Neuropharmacological Basis of Reward,* ed. J. M. Liebman and S. J. Cooper. Oxford, Eng.: Clarendon. Pp. 377–424.

Wise, R. A., and P. P. Rompre. 1989. "Brain Dopamine and Reward." *Annual Review of Psychology* 40:191–225.

Wozniak, J. R., J. Biederman, et al. 1995. "Mania-Like Symptoms Suggestive of Childhood-Onset Bipolar Disorder in Clinically Referred Children." *Journal of the American Academy of Child and Adolescent Psychiatry* 34(7): 867–876.

Zametkin, A. J., T. E. Nordahl, et al. 1990. "Cerebral Glucose Metabolism in Adults with Hyperactivity of Childhood Onset." *New England Journal of Medicine* 323(20): 1361–1366.

Index